CONTESTED CELLS

GLOBAL PERSPECTIVES ON THE STEM CELL DEBATE

CONTESTED CELLS

GLOBAL PERSPECTIVES ON THE STEM CELL DEBATE

editors
Benjamin J Capps
Alastair V Campbell
National University of Singapore

ICP
Imperial College Press

Published by

Imperial College Press
57 Shelton Street
Covent Garden
London WC2H 9HE

Distributed by

World Scientific Publishing Co. Pte. Ltd.
5 Toh Tuck Link, Singapore 596224
USA office: 27 Warren Street, Suite 401-402, Hackensack, NJ 07601
UK office: 57 Shelton Street, Covent Garden, London WC2H 9HE

British Library Cataloguing-in-Publication Data
A catalogue record for this book is available from the British Library.

CONTESTED CELLS
Global Perspectives on the Stem Cell Debate

ISBN-13 978-1-84816-437-6
ISBN-10 1-84816-437-8

Typeset by Stallion Press
Email: enquiries@stallionpress.com

Printed in Singapore by Mainland Press Pte Ltd

CONTENTS

Abstracts xiii

Foreword (by Thomas H. Murray) xxix

Contested Cells: Global Perspectives on the Stem Cell Debate — A Critical Introduction **1**

Benjamin Capps and Alastair V. Campbell

Introduction: The Source of Controversy 1
Part One — Contested Cells: Understanding the Ethical Controversy 4
Part Two — Global Perspectives 29
Closing Remarks 52

Part One Contested Cells: Understanding the Ethical Controversy **55**

(a) The Problems of Regulation **55**

1. A Case Study of Experimental Stem Cell Therapy and the Risks of Over-Regulation 57

Anthony Hollander

2. Stem Cell Technology: From Research Regulation to Clinical Applications 63

Donald Chalmers

Introduction 63
The Derivation of Stem Cells and the Current Science 65
Regulation of Stem Cell Research 72
Towards the Clinical Use of Stem Cell Technology 82
Conclusions 92
Acknowledgements 93

3. Legal Imperialism in the Regulation of Stem Cell Research and Therapy: The Problem of Extraterritorial Jurisdiction 95

Daniela Cutas and Christian Munthe

Introduction 95
The Vision of Global Regulation of ES Cell Research 98
Research and Researchers 101
Clinicians 106
Patients 109
Concluding Discussion 116
Postscript 119

4. Governing Cloning: United Nations' Debates and the Institutional Context of Standards 121

W. Calvin Ho

Cloning and the United Nations 124
Stem Cells, Cloning and the Bioethics Committee of Singapore 132
Domestic and Institutional Responses in the UK 135
Some Observations 146
Conclusion 152

(b) The Enduring Ethical Debate **155**

5. Sociological Reflections on Ethics, Embryonic Stem Cells and Translational Research 157

Claire Williams and Steven Wainwright

Sociology and Bioethics 157
Empirical Ethics: Embryonic Stem Cells and Translational Research 159
Translational Research, Hybrid Embryos and Experimental Neuroscience 172
Towards Multidisciplinary Translational Ethics? 184
Acknowledgements 188

6. Rhetoric, Power and Legitimacy in Public Discourse: A Critical Analysis of the Public Debate Surrounding the Review of Embryo Research and Cloning Legislation in Australia in 2005 189

Tamra Lysaght and Ian Kerridge

Introduction 189
Contested Notions of Science 193
Rhetoric, Power and Legitimacy 195
Conclusion 201

7. New Developments in Stem Cell Science: iPS Cells and the Challenge to Consent 207

Jonathan Mackenney and Benjamin Capps

Introduction 207
The Perpetuation of a Great Mistake: Immortals in Research 210
Reappraising Consent: Where's the Harm in iPS Cell Science? 221
Conclusion 239
Acknowledgements 240

8. 'Reasonable Suffering': The Application of Stem Cell Technologies to Non-Human Animals 241

James Yeates

Introduction 241
The Contexts 243
The Legal Status Quo 248
Unfairness 256
A Proposed Solution: Rawls and Fairness 258
Application to SCTs in the Veterinary Context 271
Application to Applied Stem Cell Research in Laboratory Context 275

9. Ontological Status of Human–Non-Human Embryonic Chimeras 279

Josef Kuře

Introduction: From the Mythological Chimera, to the Chimera in Biomedical Research 279
Chimerism and Semantics: Problems With Terminology and Definitions 293
Human–Non-Human Embryonic Chimeras: Demarcation of the Semantic Scope 303
Chimera Ontological Status 317
Conclusions 318

10. Religion, Civic Virtue and the Stem Cell Debate 321

Teoh Chin Leong

Introduction 321
Setting the Context: Substantive and Procedural Ethics 322
The Cultivation of an Ethic of Citizenship 324
Three Principles of Civic Virtue 325
An Institutional Ethics of Citizenship 333
Five Objections 334

Procedural Virtues in Public Ethical Discourse 339
Religion and the Cultivation of Exploratory Openness 341
Civic Virtue and the Stem Cell Debate 344
Conclusion 356
Acknowledgements 356

Part Two Global Perspectives **357**

11. Rejuvenated Federalism: State-Based Stem Cell Research Policy 359

Geoffrey Lomax

Introduction 359
Sovereign Action and Social Controversy 361
Social Controversy and Administrative Legitimacy 362
Procedural Frameworks and Legitimacy 363
Developing Normative Ethical Standards for Research 364
State-State Interactions in Policy Development 366
Stem Cell Science and Federalism 368
Critiques of a State-Based Approach 371
Plurality and Levels of Engagement 371
The Emergence of Federal Stem Cell Policy 373
The Pathway Towards Clinical Application 374
Conclusion 375

12. Hybrid Embryos — Ethics, Law and Rhetoric in the United Kingdom's Stem Cell Policy 377

Natasha Hammond-Browning and Søren Holm

Hybrids and the HFEA 379
Debate 382
Derivation of Stem Cells from Hybrid Embryos 387
The Future of Hybrids in Clinical Medicine 391
Conclusion 393

13. Stem Cell Research and Its Clinical Application in China: Interactions Between Science, Ethics and Society 395

Renzong Qiu and Xiaomei Zhai

Introduction 395
Stem Cell Research in China's Social Environment 396
Stem Cell Research and Chinese Culture 398
Awareness of Patients' and Human Subjects' Rights 404
Regulatory Gaps and Challenges 409
Clinical Application of Stem Cell Products: The Concerns of Under Regulation 416
Conclusion: Hope for Future Regulation 418
List of Chinese Laws and Regulations 419

14. Neither a 'Person' Nor a 'Thing': The Controversy Concerning the Moral and Legal Status of Human Embryos in Japan 421

Satoshi Kodama and Akira Akabayashi

Introduction: Neither a 'Person' Nor a 'Thing' 421
The Bioethics Committee of the Council for Science and Technology 422
Committee Discussions Regarding the Regulation of Human Cloning 425
Human Embryo Research 430
Life Sciences and Bioethics: Checks *or* Balances? 434
Conclusion 437
Acknowledgements 439

15. A Tale of Two Countries: Czech and Slovak Stem Cell Biopolicies 441

Peter Sýkora

Introduction 441
Historical and Cultural Context 443

Legislation 444
Searching for Reasons 457
Conclusion 475
Acknowledgements 477

Index 479

ABSTRACTS

1. A CASE STUDY OF EXPERIMENTAL STEM CELL THERAPY AND THE RISKS OF OVER-REGULATION

Professor Anthony Hollander
Department of Cellular and Molecular Medicine
School of Medical Sciences
University of Bristol
United Kingdom

Anthony Hollander considers the objectives of effective regulation. He presents a case study in which a group of scientists, of which Hollander was a member, successfully transplanted a human trachea into a patient grown from mesenchymal stem cells. Professor Hollander's chapter sets out the challenges that the researchers faced in respect to meeting the burden of regulatory requirements. The problem of over-regulation, he argues, sometimes means that opportunities — or even lives — are lost. This is not to say that research should be deregulated; but unnecessary delay and over cautiousness may hamper innovative research. He discussed the special permissions granted by the UK and Spanish regulatory authorities, concluding that regulators skilled in ethical review should appreciate that sometimes specified risks are worth taking.

2. STEM CELL TECHNOLOGY: FROM RESEARCH REGULATION TO CLINICAL APPLICATIONS

Professor Donald Chalmers
Faculty of Law
University of Tasmania
Australia

Since the cloning of Dolly the sheep in 1996, and the isolation and culture of human embryonic stem cells in 1998, there has been widespread international coverage, substantial research effort and considerable investments in stem cell science and technology. This is due to the prospect of using stem cells for finding cures for novel disease targets, and for developing therapies for previously untreatable cell, tissue and organ damage. Stem cells are also a valuable tool for basic scientific research on embryogenesis, normal growth and disease development. This chapter examines the current stage of experimentation in stem cell technology; the regulatory frameworks established for the derivation of stem cells, particularly human embryonic stem cells; and the protections and procedures for the applications of stem cells generally in clinical practice.

Additionally, the chapter provides an analysis and assessment of whether the *International Society for Stem Cell Research Guidelines* represent an acceptable, best-practice model for the future development of international policies and national regulation of stem cell research as it translates to clinical applications. The chapter concludes that the ISCCR *Guidelines* are an important contribution to the future development of responsible stem cell applications and therapies. These *Guidelines* provide a foundation of core principles for the transitional phase from research to clinical trials and for the integrated harmonisation of international approaches to the translation of stem cell research to clinical applications. The *Guidelines* should be used as compliance standards in any assessments of clinical applications of stem cell technology.

3. LEGAL IMPERIALISM IN THE REGULATION OF STEM CELL RESEARCH AND THERAPY: THE PROBLEM OF EXTRATERRITORIAL JURISDICTION

Daniela Cutas, Ph.D.
Department of Philosophy, Linguistics and Theory of Science
University of Gothenburg
Sweden

Professor Christian Munthe
Department of Philosophy, Linguistics and Theory of Science
University of Gothenburg
Sweden

Countries worldwide have very different national regulations on human embryonic stem (ES) cell research, informed by a range of ethical values. Some countries find reason to extend the applicability of their regulations on such research to its citizens when they visit other countries. Extraterritorial jurisdiction has recently been identified as a potential challenge towards global regulation of ES cell research. This chapter explores the implications and impact of extraterritorial jurisdiction and global regulation of ES cell research on researchers, clinicians and national health systems, and how this may affect patients. The authors argue that it would make ethical sense for ES cell restrictive countries to extend its regulations on ES cell research beyond its borders, because, if these countries really consider embryo destruction to be objectionable on the basis on the status of the embryo, then they ought to count it morally on par with murder (and thus have a moral imperative to protect embryos from the actions of its own citizens). However, doing so could lead to a legal situation that would result in substantial harm to central values in areas besides research, such as health care, the job market, basic freedom of movement, and strategic international finance and politics. Thus, it seems that restrictive extraterritorial jurisdiction in respect to ES cell research would be deeply problematic, given that the ethical permissibility of ES cell research is characterised by deep and wide disagreement.

4. GOVERNING CLONING: UNITED NATIONS' DEBATES AND THE INSTITUTIONAL CONTEXT OF STANDARDS

W. Calvin Ho
Secretariat of the Bioethics Advisory Committee
Singapore

To what extent are ethical standards dependent on institutions? Is it possible to speak of such standards without reference to particular institutions and their developmental history? How do different institutions come to share certain standards but not others?

In this chapter, Ho argues that the initiative by the United Nations to create a legally binding standard to govern cloning technology failed to recognise the range of variation in the moral and cognitive orientations of different nations. The major impediment for a binding Declaration was the impossibility within the international forum to distinguish between therapeutic and reproductive cloning. Vague concepts, such as 'dignity', were a hindrance to effectual consensus, because it was not a sufficiently generic 'immutable mobile' that could be easily transplanted from one socio-political setting to another.

In contrast, social and political conditions operating within the more limited context of a nation appeared to have been more effective in managing not only the variety of orientations, but also the imagined possibilities that cloning entailed. Two different approaches to standards creation by Singapore's Bioethics Advisory Committee and the UK's Human Fertilisation and Embryology Authority are considered. Legitimisation, in both cases, appeared as a kind of 'social contract': In exchange for permitting limited therapeutic cloning the state would assure its strict regulation (and prohibition of reproductive cloning) subject to the very highest standards of public accountability.

5. SOCIOLOGICAL REFLECTIONS ON ETHICS, EMBRYONIC STEM CELLS AND TRANSLATIONAL RESEARCH

Professor Clare Williams
School of Social Science and Public Policy
King's College London
University of London
United Kingdom

Professor Steven Wainwright
School of Social Science and Public Policy
King's College London
University of London
United Kingdom

This chapter offers some sociological reflections on bioethics, embryonic stem cells and translational research. The authors argue that ethical reasoning is traditionally presented in a disembodied way within philosophical bioethics. Wainwright and Williams' sociological research examines the views of laboratory scientists and transplant clinicians in two areas: first, the ethics of biomedical science research using human embryonic stem cells; and second, the ethics of translational research (the shift from lab to clinic). The chapter outlines some of the ways in which these two strands of empirical research add to the small number of sociological studies which explore the ways in which ethical dilemmas and reasoning occur in the clinical setting, and to an even smaller body of work exploring scientists' views on the ethical issues relating to their research. In the second part of the chapter, some of the ethical issues raised in two related key areas are discussed: the creation of hybrid embryos; and experimental neuroscience. These two areas are used to explore the potential for multidisciplinary research on translational ethics. The chapter concludes with some broader reflections on the interrelationships between philosophy and sociology for future research on stem cells, translational research, and bioethics.

6. RHETORIC, POWER AND LEGITIMACY IN PUBLIC DISCOURSE: A CRITICAL ANALYSIS OF THE PUBLIC DEBATE SURROUNDING THE REVIEW OF EMBRYO RESEARCH AND CLONING LEGISLATION IN AUSTRALIA IN 2005

Tamra Lysaght, Ph.D.
Centre for Biomedical Ethics
National University of Singapore
Singapore

Associate Professor Ian Kerridge
Centre for Values, Ethics and Law in Medicine
The University of Sydney
Australia

In December 2006, the Australian Parliament passed an amendment bill to liberalise federal legislation governing stem cell research in Australia. The public debate that surrounded the eventual passage of this legislation turned, as it had in other countries, on the moral status of the embryo (and contested over whether embryos could be deliberately created or destroyed for research), on the one hand, and the potential medical and scientific benefit to be gained from stem cell research, on the other.

This chapter draws on qualitative research conducted on the Australian stem cell policy episode between 2005 and 2006, and which examined how science and scientific knowledge was deployed in the claims participants in these debates used to support their arguments. This analysis demonstrated that science was often used for rhetorical purposes and to establish moral, epistemic and political authority. The authors suggest that it may be possible to achieve clarity about the issues at stake by understanding how science is deployed rhetorically in situations where science is contested and moral positions are irreconcilable. Lysaght and Kerridge conclude with some predictions about the future direction of public discourse surrounding stem cell research as the debates shift in response to new scientific developments.

7. NEW DEVELOPMENTS IN STEM CELL SCIENCE: iPS CELLS AND THE CHALLENGE TO CONSENT

Dr. Jonathan Mackenney
Visiting Fellow, Centre for Biomedical Ethics
National University of Singapore
Singapore

Benjamin Capps Ph.D.
Centre for Biomedical Ethics
National University of Singapore
Singapore

The successful reprogramming of somatic cells to become induced pluripotent stem (iPS) cells have led some to claim that iPS cell research advances an ethically preferable approach compared to human embryonic stem cell research. However, iPS cell research is not without its ethical challenges. Indeed, the tremendous promise of iPS cells research could lead to an appetite for rapid progress and increased pressure for human tissue to derive iPS cells, thereby expanding the practice of appropriating tissue from patients without informed consent. Such a practice is not without precedence and is typically justified by an expedient utilitarian reasoning.

This chapter argues that tissue should not be appropriated without explicit consent, as patients have proprietary interest in controlling the way their body parts or cells are used. Radin's interpretation of property as empowering agents to control the external world grounds such an interest. Thus, unauthorised appropriation of tissue jeopardises the patient's interests by misappropriating control. One implication of Radin's view is that patients retain privacy interest even if after severing their proprietary interest through valid consent. Nevertheless, this chapter also argues that the right may be justifiably curtailed if the donor's interest in the tissue ceases to exist and the researcher has the authoritative interest instead. This can happen when an iPS cell line is developed by modifying the tissue such that the original (unaltered) tissue no longer exists.

8. 'REASONABLE SUFFERING': THE APPLICATION OF STEM CELL TECHNOLOGIES TO NON-HUMAN ANIMALS

James Yeates
Department of Clinical Veterinary Science and Centre for Ethics in Medicine
University of Bristol
United Kingdom

Stem cell technologies are applied to non-human animals in two contexts: animals are used in the laboratory context in the development and testing of stem cell therapies intended for human therapeutic applications, and in the veterinary context as recipients of stem cell technologies for therapeutic purposes. The regulation of the laboratory and veterinary contexts in the UK legislature is intended to limit suffering of animals to what is reasonable, where reasonableness is considered as based on balances between costs and benefits. Such a compromise allows unfair suffering for at least some animals, for the benefit of others, human or non-human. In order to address this issue, it is necessary to look outside the concepts of reasonableness in the cost-benefit model.

The political philosophy of John Rawls's writings on fairness are applied to these contexts as an alternative view on reasonableness. There are good reasons why consideration of non-human suffering could be included in Rawls's heuristic process, so that distributive decisions could include non-human animal interests. It is argued in this chapter that the application of one Rawlsian principle — the Difference Principle — would mandate that each and every animal should be spared a life not worth living. This principle is applied to the use of animals in development and testing of stem cell therapies and veterinary use of stem cell technologies.

9. ONTOLOGICAL STATUS OF HUMAN–NON-HUMAN EMBRYONIC CHIMERAS

A/Prof Josef Kuře
University Centre for Bioethics and Department of Medical Ethics
Masaryk University
Czech Republic

This chapter concerns the premise that clarification of ontological status of an entity is a necessary element for any ethical considerations. In this respect, this chapter is about the current search for the ontological status of human–non-human chimeras; and specifically focuses on the embryonic level of human-animal mixtures. Clarification of the status has become a central issue in the stem cell debate; and in particular, with respect to the creation of animal-human mixtures in embryonic research. A central problem in these debates is that no one definition is suitable for all kinds of mixtures (for example, 'chimeras' as distinct from 'hybrids'). A spectrum of these various possible animal-human combinations or mixtures is presented with respect to the cultural and historical context of chimerism. The term chimera has different meaning and connotations in various languages; there are difficulties in finding an appropriate equivalent for the term 'chimera' in the Asian and African languages. An overview of approaches that attempt to make sense of the ontological status of these human-animal combinations is provided, covering both preformistic and epigenetic positions, and their diverse supporting theories. Based on these theories and the proposed matrix as a framework for the ontological status of human-animal embryonic chimeras, the chapter attempts to provide a critical analysis to the fundamental question: What is a human-animal embryonic chimera?

10. RELIGION, CIVIC VIRTUE AND THE STEM CELL DEBATE

Teoh Chin Leong
Centre for Biomedical Ethics
National University of Singapore
Singapore

In order to provide citizens the conditions for flourishing in a liberal pluralistic democracy, values such as freedom and equality must be respected. Due to the fact of pluralism, an 'ethics of citizenship' that includes the cultivation of civic virtues must also exist so as to meet the flourishing goals of reducing resentment, alienation and divisiveness, and increasing cooperation, harmony and respect. These goals remain in focus when debating public policies. This chapter argues for the instilling of an overlapping consensus on a set of normative standards in the form of procedural civic virtues that ought to apply when engaging in public debates on policies over complex areas of morality. It also argues that religious considerations need not be occluded from these debates as long as the considerations are forwarded without contravening the procedural virtues. The chapter considers how the procedural virtues can delineate civically admissible approaches of ethical deliberation on public policies and rule out inadmissible forms of deliberation, in the context of the permissibility of human embryonic stem cell research. In particular, it considers whether two instances of public speech may be considered civically virtuous: one religiously-based, the other, secular. The chapter concludes that there is a need to go beyond terms of fair-process or substantive argumentation in considering ethical legitimacy, through the cultivation and application of procedural civic virtue in public discourse.

11. REJUVENATED FEDERALISM: STATE-BASED STEM CELL RESEARCH POLICY

Dr. Geoffrey Lomax
California Institute for Regenerative Medicine
San Francisco, CA
Co-chair Interstate Alliance on Stem Cell Research
United States of America

From 2001 to 2008 federally sponsored stem cell science in the United States was subjected to restrictive policies. This restrictive federal context served as a catalyst for state jurisdictions to develop flexible policies designed to accommodate the advancement of stem cell science. The emergence of state research programmes has resulted in a unique developmental trajectory for stem cell science in the United States. Experience with state research programme-development suggests this trajectory incorporates three general phases: (1) programme initiation, (2) development and implementation, and (3) creation of support networks. These phases may be viewed as elements of a common procedural framework incorporating principals of constitutional democracy, participatory governance, proceduralism, and network theory. This framework may be further explicated by considering the development of normative ethical standards for state-based research programmes.

This chapter will describe the development of ethical norms with particular attention given to the procedural mechanisms and support networks that have enabled state research programmes to develop in a transparent and compatible manner. While the emphasis is on the development of ethical standards, the framework is equally applicable to a range of policy issues related to stem cell research programming.

The stem cell experience in the United States is unique given that the biomedical research enterprise has historically been dominated by federal policy. The 'organic' emergence of state-based programmes is illustrative of a 'bottom up' approach, where state and federal policy interact resulting in a hybrid framework. This framework may provide useful insights for addressing social and ethical concerns in relation to the clinical application of stem cell science and biomedicine generally within a pluralistic setting.

12. HYBRID EMBRYOS — ETHICS, LAW AND RHETORIC IN THE UNITED KINGDOM'S STEM CELL POLICY

Natasha Hammond-Browning
Cardiff Law School
Cardiff University
United Kingdom

Professor Søren Holm
Centre for Social Ethics and Policy
School of Law
University of Manchester
United Kingdom

In 2008, there was significant interest in the creation of animal-human 'cybrid' embryos for human embryonic stem cell research, as it had the potential to solve the problem of procuring human oocytes for research. However, recent developments in creating induced pluripotent stem (iPS) cells have been used by some to suggest that interest in funding research involving cybrid embryos will wane. This chapter considers the UK's policy developments on research involving animal-human embryo research (principally, inserting human nuclear DNA into an enucleated animal oocyte). In the account of the debate, the chapter focuses on the various attempts to control and alter the debate by renaming the entities that are contemplated. In the light of developments concerning iPS cells, it also discusses some common challenges in bringing iPS and hybrid cells towards clinical use. Holm and Hammond-Browning reason that the usefulness of research involving hybrid embryos may be significantly limited due to the advent of iPS cells. However, it is still too early to say whether hybrid embryo research is obsolete: such research could contribute to the perfection of methods or the discovery of alternative methods of stem cell derivation.

13. STEM CELL RESEARCH AND ITS CLINICAL APPLICATION IN CHINA: INTERACTIONS BETWEEN SCIENCE, ETHICS AND SOCIETY

Professor Renzong Qiu
Program in Bioethics
Chinese Academy of Social Sciences
People's Republic of China

Professor Xiaomei Zhai
Centre for Bioethics
Chinese Academy of Medical Sciences and
Peking Union Medical College
People's Republic of China

Science and technology is held in high regard among the Chinese population; and since publication of the *Nature* paper on the first cloned sheep, Dolly, in 1997, there has been an ongoing debate about cloning and stem cell research. Subsequent to the publication, an unprecedented meeting of scientists, physicians, bioethicists and lawyers was held in China to discuss the ethical, legal and social issues that such developments in biotechnology raised. The meeting reached a consensus on the need for regulation and the setting up of a national ethics committee. This chapter examines China's engagement with bioethics through a discussion of the development of biotechnology within its social environment. It sheds light on the cultural and legal factors influencing the cloning and stem cell debate. Such factors include the strong support for science and technology, firmly rooted Confucian beliefs and pre-existing legal and regulatory factors that favoured stem cell research. Another relevant factor is the growth of bioethics in China which has led to bioethicists playing a more active role in the debates. These debates led to the promulgation of the *Ethical Guiding Principles for Research on Human Embryonic Stem Cells (2003)*. The chapter also draws attention to some regulatory gaps of the *Ethical Guiding Principles*, and emerging ethical and governance challenges engendered by issues arising from advancement of science and technology. It concludes with a call for further regulations to fill the gaps and meet the emerging challenges adequately.

14. NEITHER A 'PERSON' NOR A 'THING': THE CONTROVERSY CONCERNING THE MORAL AND LEGAL STATUS OF HUMAN EMBRYOS IN JAPAN

Assistant Professor Satoshi Kodama
Department of Biomedical Ethics, Graduate School of Medicine
University of Tokyo
Japan

Professor Akira Akabayashi
Department of Biomedical Ethics, Graduate School of Medicine
University of Tokyo
Japan

Since the birth of Dolly the sheep in 1997, several developments have shaped human embryo research in Japan. These developments include the establishment of the *Bioethics Committee* under the *Council for Science and Technology Policy*; the release of the two reports: 'Regarding the Production of Human Individuals Through Cloning', and 'Regarding Human Embryo Research Focusing Primarily on Human Embryonic Stem Cells'; and the enactment of 'The Law Concerning Regulation Relating to Human Cloning Techniques and Other Similar Techniques'. This chapter summarises and examines these developments with focus on the discussions of the *Bioethics Committee.* It also examines the conflicts that took place between advocates and sceptics of human embryo research.

The chapter concludes that although several issues surfaced during the discussions, the *Bioethics Committee* managed to reach a compromise in a distinctly 'Japanese way'. By describing human embryos as the 'sprout of human life', the *Committee* found an eclectic solution, in part imported from other Western jurisdictions, which allowed regulated embryo research to proceed.

15. A TALE OF TWO COUNTRIES: CZECH AND SLOVAK STEM CELL BIOPOLICIES

Associate Professor Peter Sýkora
Centre for Bioethics and Philosophy Department
University of Saints Cyril and Methodius
Slovak Republic

Despite sharing centuries of the same laws, cultural history, and tradition, and existing as a common state — Czechoslovakia, until a recent breakup in 1993 — the Czech Republic and Slovak Republic have developed opposite biopolicies regarding research on human embryos and human embryonic stem cells. In the Slovak Republic, any research which would involve destroying human embryos is prosecuted by the Penal Code (2005) with a sanction of up to 15 years in prison. In contrast, the Czech Republic passed the Embryonic Stem Cell Research Act in 2006 allowing procurement of embryonic stem cells from supernumerary embryos. At first glance it may seem that the differences in biopolicies could be attributed to religious differences: where the Czech Republic tends towards an atheistic biopolicy, and has no ideological objections to human embryo research, the Slovak Republic has a regulatory position informed by Catholic ethics.

This chapter provides a comparison of key political and historical developments in the Czech Republic and Slovak Republic regulatory policies, and demonstrates that the differences in biopolicies may actually be the result of other factors, such as the status of science in society and the amount of public debate on human embryo research. Instead of religious differences, it is reasoned that the probable key factor is the impact national research lobbies had on the preparation of each countries' biopolicies.

FOREWORD

Stem cell research, along with cloning, only recently emerged as major research fronts, and they have just as quickly gone global. What makes them especially interesting for those concerned with the ethics, law, and regulation of medicine and science has been the remarkable diversity of responses among nations. Understanding the causes and nature of that diversity, and the challenges it poses to international cooperation, is the ambitious task set by the editors and authors of *Contested Cells: Global Perspectives on the Stem Cell Debate — A Critical Introduction.* To a remarkably commendable extent, they are successful.

This book offers a healthy mix of perspectives and content: from science, ethics, political philosophy, law, and sociology; with fine-grained, nuanced analyses of responses in different countries from Asia, Oceania, Europe and North America; it offers sophisticated and original insights into moral disagreements, cultural framings, and civic virtue. Readers will find their understanding of fundamental concepts such as dignity and respect in the context of international bioethical discourse becoming deeper and more complex.

I invite and encourage you to engage with the authors of this volume, some of whom may not yet be well known outside their regions — but should and soon will be. You can be assured of time well spent in the company of serious, thoughtful, and creative scholars who care deeply about their subject matter, and about the world in which we live, a world just beginning to come to terms with the clinical implications of stem cell research, and the challenges of living and working in a global community.

Thomas H. Murray, Ph.D.
The Hastings Center
Garrison, NY, USA

CONTESTED CELLS: GLOBAL PERSPECTIVES ON THE STEM CELL DEBATE — A CRITICAL INTRODUCTION

Benjamin Capps and Alastair V. Campbell

INTRODUCTION: THE SOURCE OF CONTROVERSY

This book is entitled 'Contested Cells'. We might have prefixed this with *essentially*, because many of the concepts seen as fundamental to the debate — for example, 'dignity', as used in reference to the human embryo — resist analytic and philosophical scrutiny, perhaps even to the degree that they have become meaningless in sensible debate; such protean usage may be nothing more than a pretext for equivocation. The result, for some, has been for the debate to become a political debacle. And furthermore, these disputes 'cannot be settled by appeal to empirical evidence, linguistic usage, or the canons of logic alone'.[1] In the stem cell debates, disagreement is the rule, rather than the exception.

The potential for the clinical application of stem cells to revolutionise medicine — especially in the field of regenerative medicine — is generally not challenged. But an enduring issue concerns the morally acceptable sources of human stem cells — whether pluripotent or multipotent. The derivation of human pluripotent embryonic stem cells requires the destruction of nascent human life; and this technique has been followed by the creation of animal-human mixtures, or 'cybrids', which according

[1] J. Gray. On the Contestability of Social and Political Concepts. *Political Theory* 1977; 5(3): 331–348.

to some commentators, inevitably entails the illegitimate crossing of fundamental species boundaries.[2] These developments have raised wider concerns about our failure to respect the 'dignity' of human life, and the danger of an inexorable slide to reproductive cloning.

Another aspect of the debate is the contention that there is not even a need to do these experiments, because there are alternatives in the form of somatic stem cells. But this claim ought to be tempered by the current scientific uncertainty. For example, the question of whether induced pluripotent stem cells (iPS cells) are functionally equivalent to the 'gold standard' embryonic stem cells, remains to be answered.[3] This means that communication of the science should be moderated to avoid ambitious claims, misinforming stakeholders, or manufacturing uncertainty (and the subsequent insistence on the legitimacy of precautionality has the tendency to encourage the prohibition of controversial science).

However, we should not forget that the stem cell debate is not only about embryo research; and, indeed, closing off this contentious path merely forces researchers down others. For example, some point to the inducement that must accompany the procurement of oocytes for research from women[4]; or the consequences of rampant technological advance, resulting, for example, in the commodification of stem cell lines. Stem cells economics may fuel an industry of irrepressible commercialisation, and this potentially threatens the integrity of transactions between scientists and donors.[5]

Another key ethical issue, considered in number of the following contributions, is the clinical translation of stem cell research ahead of reliable

---

[2] See: Kure, this volume.

[3] A recent paper suggests that there are molecular differences between iPS cells and embryonic stem cells. It is unknown whether the differences in gene expression are biologically significant; M. Chin *et al.* Induced Pluripotent Stem Cells and Embryonic Stem Cells are Distinguished by Gene Expression Signatures. *Cell Stem Cell* 2009; 5: 111–123.

[4] See: B. Capps and A.V. Campbell. Why (only some) Compensation for Oocyte Donation for Research Makes Ethical Sense. *Journal of International Biotechnology Law* 2007; 4: 89–102.

[5] See: Mackenney & Capps, this volume.

clinical evidence.[6] While often charging high costs for such treatment (thus revealing that they are not intended to be seen as clinical trials), practitioners (often part of global networks, and not always limited to regulatory havens, as one might expect) are reluctant to make available data for review and scrutiny, relying instead on patchy reports and hearsay. This risks patients' well-being by exposing them to potentially unsafe therapies, and is almost certainly exploitative of their sometimes desperate plight.[7] Some countries are becoming acutely aware of these concerns, and are implementing new rules which are designed to curtail a growing business in unproven treatments. The availability of stem cells as lifestyle treatments may not be as much of a concern to the vulnerable or unwell; but it does risk a catastrophic error or unforeseen side-effect which becomes a setback for the reputation of validated science.[8]

In Part One of this volume, the reader will find a valuable collection of theoretical papers, which, when taken together, illustrate the connections — as well as the disparities — between different ideas of stem cell legitimacy. It is noticeable, for example, that many countries have been keen to advocate that there is an 'ethically right' way to conduct stem cell science. While this has taken countries in the direction of a number of regulatory paths, it also shows that few welcome a regulatory vacuum. The complexity of the regulatory responses also highlights that frameworks have been sophisticated enough to accommodate issues beyond the

---

[6] International Society for Stem Cell Research. 2008. *ISSCR Guidelines for the Clinical Translation of Stem Cells.* 3 Dec.

[7] A recent report describes a patient who developed glioneuronal neoplasms after undergoing repeated transplants of 'fetal neural stem cells' in Russia starting in 2001. The article, by an Israeli team who removed the tumours, reports that the growths originated from donor cells derived from two or more tissue sources. See: N. Amariglio *et al.* Donor-Derived Brain Tumor Following Neural Stem Cell Transplantation in an Ataxia Telangiectasia Patient. *PLoS Medicine* 2009; 6(2): e29.

[8] New anti-aging 'stem cell' products available in the EU do not contain stem cells, or even parts of stem cells, because under European law, it is illegal for cosmetics sold to contain human tissue or human-tissue extracts. If they did, they would have to meet strict regulatory criteria as medicinal products, not cosmetics. While these products are mostly harmless, the marketing of these products is accused of being misleading (although most, on closer examination, claim to only 'harness' stem cell 'potential'.)

question of the status of the embryo. Within these regulatory responses, there is evidence that, even if new or foreseeable threats to 'dignity' or liberty remain conceptually befuddling in how exactly they are 'threats', there is a willingness to tackle regulatory issues as a matter of political accountability. These national developments require careful consideration in the global context.

The national perspectives, to be found in Part Two of this volume, recognise that unregulated practices threaten the wellbeing of donors and recipients alike. The challenge for international bodies, such as the United Nations, is to create for an environment which is supportive of regulative cooperation with respect to these specific groups, whilst striving to avoid issues seemingly destined for inevitable conflict. This, in turn, will require nations to submit to covenants which protect the interests of donors in non-embryonic areas of stem cell science, while allowing recipients of therapies to benefit from safe and proven technologies.

We now consider in more detail how these broad ethical and regulatory issues play out in the contributions to this volume.

PART ONE

CONTESTED CELLS: UNDERSTANDING THE ETHICAL CONTROVERSY

a) The Problems of Regulation

Stem cell science is just one aspect of a widespread technological transformation involving, among others, neuroscience, nanotechnology and reproductive medicine. This kind of progress drives technocratic solutions that permeate into all aspects of life, whether they are welcome or not. These technologies are a challenge to traditional regulatory frameworks found in many technologically-advanced countries. As Roger Brownsword explains: the changes that we are witnessing are 'highly significant for the future of law and the way that we regulate social life'; and this sea change makes regulation an unwieldy concept.[9] Time and again, our laws,

[9] R. Brownsword. 2008. *Rights, Regulation, and the Technological Revolution.* Oxford NY. Oxford University Press. 6–7 and 130.

condemned as archaic, and often hard pressed to keep up, become wholly inadequate.

The first part of the collection begins with a case study, written by Anthony Hollander, which confronts the objectives of effective regulation. The case concerns a group of scientists, of which Hollander was a member, who successfully transplanted a human trachea grown from mesenchymal stem cells into a patient.[10] Professor Hollander's chapter sets out the challenge for the researchers; he writes:

> '...therapies will never reach clinical trial or commercial exploitation because the burden of meeting regulatory requirements is so heavy that resources will not be available. Patients may continue to suffer and some may die because a new treatment could not be exploited' [61].[11]

Hollander clearly brings into focus the problem of overregulation; of the fastidious and protracted assessment of risk, and which sometimes means that opportunities — or even lives — are lost. Society's response to controversy inevitably swings to conservative-minded principles. This is not to say that research should be deregulated; but unnecessary delay and over cautiousness may hamper innovative research. Hollander writes: 'As a scientist I have been trained to pay attention to every detail, make no assumptions, test every theory to the limit of technical capability and even then to be aware that my hypotheses may be wrong' [58]. But, the urgency of the situation in this case meant that normal regulatory measures would have to be circumvented — not because of a maverick irresponsibility and disregard for time-wasting measures — but because 'we might, just might, make a real difference to this lady's life and surely it was worth trying' [59]. Hollander and his colleagues decided to 'plunge headlong into helping those who are suffering' [62]; and through numerous special permissions granted by the UK and Spanish regulatory

---

[10] The transplantation is reported in: P. Macchiarini *et al.* Clinical Transplantation of a Tissue-Engineered Airway. *Lancet* 2008; 372: 2023–2030.

[11] Where a quote appears in the text followed by a page reference enclosed by square brackets, it should attributed to the proximate named author(s), and the page to his or her contribution in this volume.

authorities, were able to transplant the new organ successfully. Hollander's plea, therefore, is not to deregulate, but to ensure that regulators are skilled in ethical review; and that they appreciate that sometimes, specified risks are worth taking. This may require, given the circumstances, the bending of procedural oversight. It does not suggest the breaking of ethical norms, or the justification for reckless abandon. Sometimes, it takes a certain risk-taking vision to make the significant steps in medicine: if taking these risks are worth it when the patient benefits, the patient only suffers when progress is blocked.

The problem, as Hollander acknowledges, is that while evaluators have no choice but to work within the regulatory framework that has been established in law, the challenge is to appraise translational research effectively. His observations, from the view of a scientist, imply that sometimes the bar for research approval is set too high with respect to proving the benefits; furthermore, the bureaucratic hurdles can be complicated and time consuming. However, throughout this book, the plight of patients being misled and harmed through exposure to treatments which lack scientific validity is highlighted. These cases appear principally to be a phenomenon of 'regulatory havens' which harbour unscrupulous clinicians. The difference between these jurisdictions and regulated countries is stark. Within a provisionally effective ethical regulatory framework, no patient is exposed to experiments that are not valid in principle. Nor are they forced, coerced or tricked into taking part. But there are concerns when loopholes, a lack of interest, or economic motivations, permit scientists and doctors to bypass normal scientific and ethical oversight.

Hollander and his colleagues did not operate in an ethical vacuum, and in fact were more than honest in their attempts to expedite the process. Throughout, the patient was well informed and a willing participant, albeit in an experimental procedure. (This, in itself, is not uncommon in medical innovation.) It is possible, therefore, that the kinds of risks that Hollander talks about can only plausibly happen where there are *strong* regulatory frameworks and a *willingness* to monitor research. In this context, an ethical bar is set, either through national, regional or international measures. Sometimes getting over it may be perceived as requiring an unreasonable or unattainable absence of risk. But, scientists and doctors within regulated environments operate within a culture of responsibility to patients and their peers (a high calling indeed), and the requirement for proper scientific validation. Risks, therefore, can be taken only within a framework of evaluation and oversight (because one can only know the extent of these risks after impartial due consideration). All research involves a degree of risk; and the challenge for those that are responsible for approving research is to weigh it appropriately: what this amounts to changes from case to case, and patient to patient. This balancing requires skill, and while many countries create an environment to promote adept ethical review, others have failed to ensure levels of proficiency and accountability.

International Regulation

The regulatory challenge means different things to different countries. The essay by Donald Chalmers helpfully describes some of the most important developments in this respect. The 'embryo question' continues to resist straightforward solutions (compromise, not surprisingly, is still elusive), and it is now part and parcel of the regulation of the wider reproductive enterprise, that includes human cloning, fertility medicine, genetic selection (PGD), and chimera and hybrid research. Chalmers notes that there are predominantly three kinds of control to be found: *strict regulation*, *licensing schemes*, and *guidelines regulation schemes*. All of these characterise a default 'restrictive tilt': that countries favour either *regulated* permission (the tilt is against prohibition) or prohibition (*vice-versa*) of embryo research. The corresponding laws tend to be complex in their coverage of a myriad of activities and techniques, and as a result, legislative interpretation has become intricate, and sometimes, bewildering in its ambitions. If countries bring the stem cell controversy under a *permissive* regulatory umbrella, a list of permissible activities will be drawn up; also stipulating what activities will continue to be categorically prohibited. A *prohibitive* tilt will ban the derivation of cells within national borders. In these countries, the laws are often straightforward in stipulating that embryo research is not permitted, thus implicitly prohibiting other related technologies. Sometimes they remain naive to the problems of tying up loose regulatory ends — for example, addressing the migration of patients to more permissive states; and by embracing progressive change to a degree, one wonders as to the legitimacy of the policy (for example, policies seem contradictory in their moral consistency in banning embryo research while promoting their ambitions for the import of embryonic cells from other jurisdictions).

The default of this 'tilt' depends on each country; and in closer examination, it is evident that there are a number of cultural and historical factors that determine this. There is a good deal more to know about each country's regulatory mix — there are few laws which evince a blanket prohibition or open permission — and instead an enquirer will find a patchwork of measures. One has to do some leg work to find out the terms on which research is permitted or prohibited, and then translated into the clinics (an area which is critically underdeveloped in most regulatory schemes, suggesting that most are confident, but perhaps unduly so, in current clinical regulations to adapt to stem cell science).

Chalmers concludes that the *International Society for Stem Cell Research (ISSCR) Guidelines for the Conduct of Human Embryonic Stem Cell Research (December 21st, 2006)* are a central contribution to the future development of responsible stem cell applications and therapies as stem cell research moves gradually into the clinic. The problem with any international guidance, however, is that it requires countries to assimilate common norms; a point taken up by Daniela Cutas and Christian Munthe in the next chapter. They argue that effective global or multinational regulation of stem cell research will imply some degree of imperialism; that is, to achieve effective international regulation, involved parties will have to be willing to accommodate (either permissive or prohibitive) regulations within their own laws. They explore this phenomenon in the context of extraterritorial jurisdiction and embryo research.

The authors note that extraterritorial jurisdiction is acknowledged in the ISSCR Guidelines as 'Responsibility for Conduct' of researchers.[12] However, because researchers will be expected to work between jurisdictions, the Guidelines instruct them to 'assume the responsibility for compliance with local statutes and adherence to guidelines'.[13] It is also likely that the translocation of clinicians and patients to other jurisdictions

[12] ISSCR, *op. cit.* note 6, para. 5.1.

[13] Ibid: para. 5.2.

will expose them to diverse, and sometimes bewildering, laws. As some have argued, the solution to impending accidental transgressions, and to facilitate cooperation, is to harmonise international regulation under a universal set of rules; but this is suggestive of a common ethical framework underlying those laws, as well. Cutas & Munthe argue that 'the prospect of a globally harmonised regulatory framework [is] considerably more vulnerable to the existence of very restrictive views' [97]. And they note further: any moral reasons for the '*consistent* legal application of the *moral* view underlying the restrictive legislations would imply that the ES cell research is, as a matter of fact, a case of genocide' (emphasis in original) [105]. This does not mean that we can easily discount ideas of a prohibitive nature:

> 'Since logic dictates that, on the basis of such a [prohibitive] moral evaluation, ES cell research amounts to genocide, ES cell research would look like a classic example of the sort of act where ...extraterritorial jurisdiction is often seen as acceptable within international law' [97].

But they further argue that it 'becomes a deeply problematic feature [of extraterritorial jurisdiction] in cases where deep and wide disagreement exists as to whether or not certain activities belong to one of these types' [98]. Cutas & Munthe are right to say, that, given the evidence, restrictive measures would require an unjustifiable transgression into the sovereignty of liberal pro-embryo research countries. Moreover, a restrictive position would 'risk setting in motion a chain of events that would jeopardize international financial and political stability on a scale considerably larger than merely the ES cell area and, possibly, with vast effects in terms of life and health' [118]. They conclude that the restrictive use of extraterritorial jurisdiction potentially 'clouds the vision of a global substantial regulation of ES cell research and rather inspires international conflict' [116].

The concerns that Cutas & Munthe raise are similar to those which were expressed by the European governments that objected to the proposed ethical stance of the European Union's *Tissues Directive*.[14] In the

---

[14] *Directive 2004/23/EC of the European Parliament and of the Council of 31 March 2004 on setting standards of quality and safety for the donation, procurement, testing, processing, preservation, storage and distribution of human tissues and cells* (Final Act OJ L 102 7.4.2004 48).

early drafting of the Directive, the *Liese Report* attempted to guide the ethical debate towards a harmonised conservative position, and therefore restrict embryo research that was being conducted, legally, elsewhere.[15] The restrictive tone of the Report was eventually dropped; and the final position taken echoes the view of the *European Group on Ethics and New Technologies* (EGE) that 'It is not only legally difficult to seek harmonisation of national laws at Community level, but, because of lack of consensus, it would be inappropriate to impose one exclusive moral code'.[16] The result was a set of minimal standards stipulated by the *Tissues Directive*, but which reflected inherent regulatory pluralism by remaining neutral about controversial research, stating:

> 'This Directive should not interfere with decisions made by Member States concerning the use or non-use of any specific type of human cells... including embryonic stem cells. If ...any particular use of such cells is authorised in a Member State, this Directive will require the application of all provisions necessary to protect public health...'.[17]

And furthermore, it was stated that the 'Directive shall not prevent a Member State from maintaining or introducing more stringent protective measures [which] include the prohibition or restriction of imports of human tissues or cells.'[18] Thus, the Directive set out rules which were easily transferable to established national legislatures, focussing on safety and consent issues predominantly, but which would also act as a guide for new states joining the Union.

The problem becomes more acute when countries collectively become global in their ambitions, such as those of the United Nations (UN).

[15] See: B. Capps. 2005. The Human Embryo, Stem Cell Research, and the European Union. In *Crossing Borders. Cultural, Religious, and Political Differences Concerning Stem Cell Research: A Global Approach.* W. Bender, C. Hauskeller & A. Manzei, eds. Münster: Agenda Verlag: 435–467.

[16] The European Group on Ethics in Science and New Technologies. *1998 Ethical Aspects of Research Involving the Use of Human Embryo in the Context of the 5th Framework Programme.* No. 12, 23rd November. Strasbourg. European Commission. p. 10, para 2.4.

[17] *supra.* note 14, recital 12.

[18] Ibid. Article 4(2).

Calvin Ho's contribution to this volume considers the UN's 2005 *Human Cloning Declaration* to have been largely a failure as a gesture of moral or legal authority.[19] He notes that, during the UN cloning debate, the view that there was no real distinction between therapeutic cloning and reproductive cloning, since both involved the use of a common technological process: 'proved attractive to many countries (especially those with a predominantly large Catholic population) without having first arrived at a national position on the subject' [125]. A number of compromise approaches were proposed which were 'not greeted with much enthusiasm' [125]. The impasse remained, despite the observation that reproductive cloning represented an 'imminent threat and prompt response on the part of the international community would be politically expedient' [126]. Ho suggests a number of economic, socio-political and ethical arguments that may have been behind the prolonged wrangling. Noting also that the problem for large, diverse fora, such as the UN, is that there is a substantial group of member states which are largely disinterested in the technology (the remoteness of the issues of human cloning in many developing countries where far more urgent medical and health concerns need to be prioritised); thus weakening the pro-therapeutic and anti-cloning coalitions alike.

Ho remarks, however, that the Declaration did have the effect of motivating countries to get their domestic laws in order. Ho points to the fact that the 'absence of a sufficiently generic "immutable mobile" or "boundary object" that could be easily transplanted from one sociopolitical setting' [123] was a root impediment to progress in the UN:

> 'The notion of human dignity was itself too vague to inspire action, and also too ambiguous to enable consensus to be forged across a community with varied, and in some respects conflicting interests and concerns' [123].

For Ho, however, this ought not to be considered as necessarily fatal for cooperative international law. His analysis locates shared ethical premises

---

[19] A/Res/59/280 (23 Mar 2005).

in the separate adjudication work on cloning of the Bioethics Advisory Committee (Singapore) and the Human Fertilisation and Embryology Authority (UK). Both tended to use the ideas of 'tolerance, compromise and regulation' [153] as valid responses to questions about effective societal coherence (what has been called the 'Warnock Strategy', after the UK philosopher, Mary Warnock)[20]; and Ho argues that, although their approaches were somewhat different (holistic and incremental respectively), this points to the existence of the 'immutable mobile'. The question both bodies asked was: How would it be possible to legitimise a permissive tilt — if this seems as rightly being ethical — given the wide disagreement in society (and that a proportion of the population was known to object to embryo research)? Legitimisation, in both cases, appeared as a kind of 'social contract': 'in exchange for permitting a limited amount of embryo research the state would assure its strict regulation subject to the very highest standards of public accountability'.[21]

Would such an approach have been applicable to the UN Declaration? Was there a way to countenance both the willingness to ban reproductive cloning, and, to allow those countries that wanted to permit therapeutic cloning to do so within a robust national legal framework? If they could have, instead of concluding the Fifty-Ninth General Assembly with the rather toothless *Declaration on Cloning*, a potentially powerful tool to stop reproductive cloning may have resulted, all the while assuring the global public that therapeutic cloning, where legal, would be subject to the very highest standards of public accountability.

Given the failures of international law, what, then, could be the point of regulatory harmonisation? One should note, for instance, that a number of states had already enacted bans on reproductive cloning by the time the UN's Declaration had been ratified; and that most countries that were obdurate in rejecting the outright international ban had set high standards of oversight for therapeutic cloning. Moreover, the inevitable

[20] S. Franklin & C. Roberts. 2006. *Born and Made: An Ethnography of Pre-implantation Genetic Diagnosis*. Princeton, NJ: Princeton University Press: 197–198; Cf. Department of Health & Social Security. 1984 (reprinted 1988). *Report of the Committee of Inquiry into Human Fertilisation and Embryology*. London: Her Majesty's Stationary Office.

[21] Franklin & Roberts, ibid, p. 197.

consequence it would seem, as pointed out by Cutas & Munthe in the previous chapter, is an impasse when international law instruments are used in ways to compromise sovereign interest. We may, however, postulate at least three reasons for the specific calls for regulation in this field of research: 1) It gets important issues onto the agendas of states yet to address them. Granted that some states have more immediate concerns, the international forum serves to redirect attention and awareness, and may provide a future environment constructive for collaborative action in this respect. 2) It provides the means for states to try again to gain legal ground on issues they feel strongly about. For example, there are a number of European states which may have considered the permissive tilt of the EU as an abject moral failure; international condemnation may have (although it was unlikely) reversed this trend, or at least resolved ambiguities (where EU law remained silent) in favour of prohibition. 3) Anyone who thought that prohibiting reproductive cloning would face few obstacles, ought to have noted the considerable obstacles that the European Union and Council of Europe had to overcome when creating laws in medicine and science. But, what was forthcoming in these European fora were minimal standards of research, and these have been seen as instrumental in protecting the rights of donors and recipients, and guiding acceding states towards an agreed level of regulation (which in some states was altogether absent at the time of accession).

In the final analysis, the 'embryo question' — obliging a jumble of political, religious, and scientific answers, and dispersing into many aspects of technology that force us to look at what it means to be 'human' — faces considerable hurdles when transposed onto the global setting. Ho finds some hope, in that countries have 'developed in ways that have meaning within their local context, and it is also within this context that the political and socio-cultural impetus and resources in resolving conflicts over meaning are found' [152]. It is these local solutions that are thematic in Part Two of this volume.

b) The Enduring Ethical Debate in Translational Research

The six papers in this section of the volume turn away from the specific problems of regulation to the particular challenges of translational research. Put in rather general terms: while regulators continue to struggle with several fundamental ideas concerning, principally, the status of the embryo, clinical translation will require a nuanced appreciation of the potential developments in stem cell science.

Clare Williams and Steven P. Wainwright begin this section with an empirical investigation of the ways in which ethical dilemmas and reasoning occur in the translational research and clinical setting. They recapitulate some of their recent work in empirical ethics: exemplar of the specific approach of 'sociology *in* bioethics'. This method 'explores the links between bioethics, medicine, science and society and aims to ground more abstract philosophical ethical debates in empirical case studies which explore and describe the embodied ethics of "real actors" in particular social worlds' [157]. Williams & Wainwright are critical of the 'disembodiment' of bioethics by one-sided philosophical debates [163]; their point is that this kind of approach to ethics has tended to dominate technology debates. Enquiring of the opinions of various actors in the stem cell debate — in this case, scientists — can show that significant ethical details may be obscured by policies focused on legitimacy alone. The narrow set of explanations used — perhaps, in the final analysis, only assuring to a few like-minded of an established and worthy doctrine — fail to account for the interest of those actually involved.

These philosophical based arguments, Williams & Wainwright maintain, bring to the fore 'ethical issues that encompass issues such as: the use and destruction of embryos; informed consent; commercialisation and the commodification of bodies; the "threat" of reproductive cloning; animal rights and species integrity; [and] resource allocation' [168]. But they argue that this prevailing way of doing bioethics — a 'view from nowhere' [168] — misses the point; and they present their own data — asking scientists how they see themselves as ethical, as well as expert, actors, by drawing the boundaries of ethical scientific activity — to bear out this out. They attest that scientists, although bound by the formal legal and ethical framework, are reflective and prepared 'to venture into ethical argumentation and thereby enter the foothills of normative as opposed to merely conventional ethics' [167]. This fact leads their challenges to 'normative bioethics', and is supported by 'Our scientists' refusal to create embryos for research, even though this is legal in the UK and is something that is promoted by many bioethicists' [167]. An important supposition of their work is that:

> 'scientists must nevertheless demonstrate their commitment to "ethics" as the audiences of science include various public and regulatory constituencies who, in one way or another, lend the whole bio-scientific enterprise legitimacy' [159].

Their work does indeed shed a different light on the stem cell debate. Returning to Hollander's chapter in this volume, for example, we can immediately locate the 'ethical reflection and rectitude' [167] that Williams & Wainwright found in their studies. The rules of 'ethical' research may be deep rooted in a long history of normative debate, but in the urgent context described by Hollander, they may have become merely hindrances — indeed, the rigid imposition of these rules might well have cost Claudia Castillo her life. Williams & Wainwright's 'descriptive empirical ethics' is important in that it uncovers the inevitable loopholes and weaknesses of regulatory structures by asking of those who spend every day working within them.

Williams & Wainwright's paper is a reflection upon the 'dysfunctional marriage' between sociologists and philosophers. Much like the authors, we do not see that the social science and philosophical approaches ought to be mutually exclusive: the task, Williams & Wainwright declare, is to appreciate how they both are tasks fundamental to bioethics practice. Their position is that the former approach embodies a philosophically dominated bioethics field. But, this is also suggestive of (but does not go as far as) the 'Anti-theory' movement, which advocates that we can do without normative ethics altogether, and that our moral guides ought to be a kind of Humean reflection; that is, ethical solutions ought to be about empirically informed knowledge of sentiment and custom, rather than principles formed from intellectual reason.[22] Stuart Toddington comes to

---

[22] Cf. A. Baier. 1989. Doing Without Moral Theory. In *Anti-Theory in Ethics and Moral Conservatism.* S. Clarke & E. Simpson, eds. Albany, NY: State of New York University Press: 29–48.

the philosophers' defence in this respect: the central problems of the methodology of social science require for their resolution the resources of an objective moral theory:

> 'a "fact" is not *given*, it is the *product* of a framework of assumptions comprising an explanatory or interpretative scheme. This has undermined the notion of "empirical proof"; quite obviously, the "proof" is a product of non-empirical assumptions which themselves stand in need of justification'.[23]

Scientists' and clinicians' views about regulatory structures do not necessarily point to their inefficacy or otherwise; they are observations informed by individuals who have a stake in the permissions and restrictions of law. The law tells them what they may or may not do, restricting their freedom of action, and thereby curbing maverick, and sometimes, insidious inclinations. But, the goals, factual circumstances, and context of a particular regulatory regime may be very different from the aspirations of a particular scientist or clinician. Indeed, those that find the rule of law too restrictive will relocate to areas which are more conducive to what they want to do; or even move to regulatory havens, should their ambitions go further than any existing regulatory system. The risk of empirical ethics is to overplay cultural values and sub-cultural sensitivities as determinants of public-orientated regulatory regimes, thus leading to a disciplinary (and relativistic) understanding of legal jurisprudence. Law, thereby, becomes a pragmatic judgement of embodied actors, and only tells us about their own (the regulatee's) depiction of means to ends. But, if a regulatory regime is to avoid the thin ethics that the introduction of pragmatic solutions often leads to,[24] a prior requirement of any empirical

---

[23] S. Toddington. 1993. *Rationality, Social Action and Moral Judgment.* Edinburgh: Edinburgh University Press: x. (Italics in original).

[24] Cf. An approach that Robertson appears to support, when he argues (in respect to the creation of inter-species forms): 'when doing so serves important human needs... [as] the question of breaching species barriers is... less a matter of principle than a question of pragmatics and context'. J. Robertson. A Response to 'Crossing Species Boundaries' by Jason Scott Robert and Francoise Baylis. *American Journal of Bioethics* 2003; 3: W64–W65.

approach is for scientific facts to be delivered as neutral statements, thereby stripping them of moral underpinnings. It is worthwhile to find out what moral values different actors attach to their own statements of fact (the 'realities of situation'); and understanding these values and principles is fundamental to our sociological awareness of events. But it is only by understanding the values themselves, out in the open and in their objective entirety as expressions of *moral* theories, that we can appreciate our complex social structures and then formulate ethical solutions.

Tamra Lysaght and Ian Kerridge likewise use an 'empirical ethics' approach to analyze the Australian stem cell policy, which developed in the years 2005 and 2006. Using their own qualitative data, they examine how science was deployed in the claims of participants: observing that the policymaking debate in Australia was typified by the preferential deployment of claims with sound scientific support. The authors claim: 'Science has a special place in these and other policy contexts because it is posited as the most reliable and value-neutral source of truth and knowledge' [202]. They noted that the authority figures, such as scientists, involved in the policy process were more likely to control the shape and direction of scientific research. Scientists, therefore, were able to obscure other ideas by making them unsuitable for serious consideration by policy makers (we could imagine that their targets would be those based in religion or culture). And by having the ear of politicians, for example, they could undercut intellectual debate by making other views nothing more than anecdotal; and thus, it would seem, would have the final, and determinant, say in stem cell policies. The authors conclude:

> 'The preferential use of science claims in the Australian debate surrounding stem cell research meant that the status attached to scientific knowledge was greater than other ways of knowing and that the personal narratives and stories of those most likely to be affected by the outcomes of the policy episode were marginalised' [202].

How concerned should we be that the 'rhetorical power of science claims' [202] is entrenched in the legitimation process? Legitimation signifies a broad range of public interests i.e. that there are good reasons to choose one policy over another; this, as Lysaght & Kerridge point out: 'is because the moral positions upon which the stem cell dispute is fought are fundamentally incommensurable' [203]. Thus, the *legitimacy* of regulatory purposes and practices become secondary, because they are a difficult set of more narrow justifying reasons. Societies who fail to acknowledge the importance of science *within* a framework of public understanding (in terms of what they understand and how it is perceived, and ultimately, accepted), risk the growth of public scepticism and cynicism in the integrity of science-based policy decisions, and moreover, the marginalisation of science expertise.[25] Any professed gap between 'the public' and science may be exploited by opportunisms and expediency; thus the principal driving force to *use* science and technology is a political agendum, rather than a justification of whether a technology, in terms of legitimacy, ought to be permitted or not.

Noticing this, the authors remind us 'that science is not value-neutral and does not occur in a political vacuum' [205]. Scientists themselves will have a certain idea of legitimacy which drives their research; they might advocate policies which promote interventions that promise to assist medical research, and in due course, to deliver therapies for major human disease. However, scientists' views also appeal to a specific moral reason and this brings us back to our commentary on Williams & Wainwright's chapter, where we argued that scientists, just as much as any other agent, are under the same obligations to 'persuade' the public as to the legitimacy of their position. That is, whether an adequate ethical justification is available to them to promote their opinions.

Researchers have a central role in ensuring that stem cell science stays within the bounds that are set up by the regulatory regime in which each one of them works; so to speak, the activities of researchers are to be legal, if not necessarily 'ethical', as long as their endeavours meet the immediate jurisdiction's criteria. Researchers' transgressions can have resonating effects on public opinion; witness, for example, the Hwang scandal. Hwang, however, did not only contravene South Korea's laws,

[25] See: Lysaght & Kerridge, this volume; see also: L.J. Virelli III. *'Political' Science: Peer Reviewers as Agents of Administrative Legitimacy*. SSRN 2008. Revised (and published) as: 'Training the Elephant in the Room: Scientific Peer Review and Administrative Legitimacy'; last revised March 24, 2009; *Administrative Law Review* Fall 2009. Available at: http://papers.ssrn.com/sol3/papers.cfm?abstract_id=1259801 [Accessed 08 Sep 2009].

but also long standing, universal standards of ethics. Hwang, from his luminary status, was able to coerce junior colleagues to donate oocytes; and if we learn anything from this affair, it is that society must be watchful of other exploitative practices driven by the 'business of science'. In their contribution, Jonathan Mackenney and Benjamin Capps consider the micro-event of procuring cells for stem cell work, focusing in particular on the future of research on induced Pluripotent Stem cells (iPS cells). There have been claims that iPS cells are an 'ethically clean' alternative to contentious embryo research and cloning technologies currently used. To create these immortal cell lines, the raw material needed is procured by a simple biopsy, for which consent can easily be given. What instead has happened, however, is a culture of routinely procuring cells for research without asking the patient; this is easily done by hiding the intention to appropriate cells within the medical procedure. The justification for this is the trumping of consent requirements by the 'good of science'. But this typically utilitarian grounded vindication exploits the intimate access to the body that is generated by an ongoing physician-patient relationship. The authors argue that this research practice ought not to endorse, nor be intentionally conflated with, medical goals: if patients are not told about the research aims, or are led to believe wrongly that excised tissue is for medically indicated procedures only, then they cannot be said to have consented to its use in research (regardless of the research's propinquity to the medical procedure). Moreover, without authorisation (in any form), additional biopsies or collection of abandoned tissue entail an unacceptable level of deceit or misinformation.

The authors' argument stems not only from the non-consensual insult to the body, but also from privacy rights that endure in excised cells; and by virtue of these latter rights (rather than any proprietary rights) an interest continues in the fate of the cells, despite the transfer (consented to or not) of property. This privacy interest can be removed by first asking the patient for access to the cells, and secondly, authorising the endeavours of researchers in creating, and therefore owning, an immortal cell line. They do not argue for stringent informed consent, because, given the dynamic field of stem cell science, to give general information is not to deny the donor the facts, but truly due to the uncertainty of research aims and future technology. But, rather than duping patients about the fate of cells taken during unrelated medical procedures, which is sure to foster distrust in researchers, an acquiescence to consent norms may develop enthusiasm on the part of the donor to willingly, rather than unwittingly, take part in research. By looking at the consent procedures of UK biobank, which are designed to develop an ongoing relationship with participants, Mackenney & Capps propose that a similar partnership ought to be created between the research community and the public, which not only benefits, but also contributes to, scientific endeavour. Such a partnership may be particularly important given the physical and psychological status of patients who donate not for personal gain, but who want to contribute to the endeavour of treating those with similar illness.

James Yeates' chapter sets out to address the omission of nonhuman animals from the discussion of the ethics pertaining to stem cell therapies. He notes that, while the advent of stem cell technologies has been against a backdrop of concern about the use of increasing numbers of nonhuman animals in the laboratory context, there has been relatively less said about animal welfare. Yeates, in this respect, asks whether it is acceptable to 'inflict' suffering on nonhuman animals in the testing and development of clinical stem-cell therapies [242]. This chapter focuses on the *interests of the animals themselves*. By using a novel deployment of John Rawls' approach in Justice as Fairness, Yeates argues that life has instrumental value for animals (leaving open the question of whether their life might additionally have intrinsic value to them). He states:

> 'Life is instrumentally valuable for an animal because it permits it to have "positive" ends: enjoyable, eudaimonic states... Thus life is valuable to an animal if it affords sufficient positive value to outweigh any negative value: this is a life worth living. The desirability of a state of positive welfare is categorically valuable and this affords an instrumental value to life' [242].

The application of this Rawlsian framework reveals that a number of veterinary relationships established by UK and EU law can be considered unfair to the animal itself; they contribute to a 'Life Not Worth Living' (LNWL). As Yeates remarks, Rawls did not overtly extend Justice as Fairness to the veterinary context (but neither did he include sick humans in his distributive theory, instead hypothesising the idealised participation of healthy individuals in the Original Position). This, Yeates argues, opens up the Original Position beyond its strictly epistemic conditions; and this way into Rawls' theory allows the moral consideration of the severity and duration of suffering of animals. This is a level of welfare that we ought to avoid inflicting upon sentient animals, and should their lives fall below this, there is a moral duty to end such an existence. Instead, what society should aim for is providing 'Lives *Worth* Living' (LWL) for animals. Thus, the principles of justice as fairness would prescribe that all animals should have a guaranteed minimum opportunity, regardless of context and species, to ensure intra-contextual and intra-specific fairness. These rules potentially permeate into all aspects of animal welfare (pet ownership, husbandry and animal research). And specifically:

> 'Stem cell therapies cannot be legitimately used to provide further companionship for an animal's owner, increase performance of sports animals or increase productivity of farmed animals, if that requires the animal having a LNWL. Animals with diseases should be euthanased if the treatment cannot avoid their having a LNWL. ...The main fear with novel therapies is that they are implemented by clinicians enthusiastic about the novelty and progress, rather than about the interests of the animal itself' [274].

Such a framework can be extended to animal research, thus limiting the human 'benefits' that come at a cost to animal interests. Yeates' framework adds further philosophical strength to Russell & Burch's 3Rs — Replacement, Reduction and Refinement.[26] And while stem cell science raises the prospect of ever more animals being employed in research and therapy; it may, conversely, foster opportunities to decrease the unfair suffering of animals by using *in vitro* grown human organs and tissues as an alternative.

However, the application of Justice as Fairness, Yeates readily admits, risks foregoing significant benefits to humans: 'under Justice as Fairness

[26] W. Russell & R. Burch. 1959. *The Principle of Humane Experimental Technique.* London: Menthuen.

the benefits to other subjects would not legitimise keeping any subjects with a LNWL, any more than any other system which lowered the maximum for the benefit of any better-advantaged citizens' [276]. He does add the following caveat: 'If subjects are considered as individuals extended in stages through a lifetime, then short periods of LNWL might be balanced by periods of LWL. This would effectively be a refinement, but one focusing not on lessening pain but on increasing positive experiences as counterbalance' [276].

Yeates' chapter takes a different path from those more common arguments which see the conflict between human beings and animals as irreconcilable until we acknowledge that non-human beings have a place in our moral framework. This latter view has drawn attention to the inconsistency of denying a moral role to biological characteristics such as race or sex, while at the same time attributing a moral role to another biological characteristic such as species. These arguments tend towards a concept of a 'person', who is self-aware or sentient, and therefore brings some non-human animals into the moral community, while sometimes excluding human beings at the fringes of life.[27] The evident complexity of social structures, however, undermines simplistic 'balancing of interests' arguments (of the kind presented in modern Millian ideas), and fails to acknowledge that decisions made by thinking beings presuppose the circumstances of their own bonds and relationships to non-sentient human beings. That is not to say that human and non-human moral entitlements cannot be relationally similar, but this requires a deeper understanding of the conditions of agency and our responsibilities to other non-agents.[28] The corollary, of course, is that there is something special about human beings — their 'dignity' perhaps — and this reserves the moral sphere for only human beings, including those which are non-sentient (a point that Yeates touches upon in his concluding remarks: 'An embryo, without basic neural structures cannot suffer, and therefore *ceteris paribus* cannot have a life worth living' [276].) Yeates, in this respect, successfully

[27] Cf. P. Singer. 1975. *Animal Liberation: A New Ethics for our Treatment of Animals*. New York: New York Review/Random House.

[28] D. Beyleveld and R. Brownsword. 2001. *Human Dignity in Bioethics and Biolaw*. Oxford NY: Oxford University Press.

disassociates the 'animal debate' from the embryo question, and draws much needed attention to the improvement of animal welfare.

Returning to the Embryo Question

The 'embryo question' asks: what is it about a being that makes it worthy of moral status? The implications of this question are the background of Joseph Kure's chapter, in which he analyses the notions of human-animal biological mixtures. His chapter is a thought-provoking search for the ontological status of these beings, and specifically a clarification of what we are really talking about when we call a thing a 'chimera' or 'hybrid' (what has been called an 'admixed embryo' in UK law, to differentiate from 'true chimeras' — the fertilisation of a human egg with animal sperm or *vice versa*). His focus is on the research interest in these entities, writing that 'repeating the humanzee experiment is not a project that many researchers want to try, or one that would get support from an ethical review board given its questionable scientific merits and the moral concerns' [289].

The interest in creating human-nonhuman mixtures has been driven by the lack of human oocytes for research; the immediate solution, so some scientists claim, is to use those from animals. The controversy of such a move is well captured in Kure's essay. He traces the origin of the chimeric being back to antiquity, and notes the awe that these beings held in various cultural and historical contexts. Even modern science struggles with the intangible status of such beings: 'it is difficult to apply our classification and categories for novel beings or "in-between" species, that do not occur in nature, and which do not fall under the (well) defined categories used in biology' [306]. The apparent breakdown of the distinction between human and inhuman, human and animal, has been a familiar topic in the media. In the horror genre, for example, the beings are a feature of disgust, but also curiosity, possessing a 'half-hypnotic fascination'.[29] But the animals portrayed with human characteristics, such as speech and recognisable

[29] As an exemplar of the characterization of 'monstrous hybridity' from H.P. Lovecraft's 'The Shadow Over Innsmoth', first published in 1936, by Everett, PA: Visionary Publishing Co. Chapter IV. Available online at: http://www.hplovecraft.com/writings/fiction/texts/soi.asp. [Accessed 08 Sep 2009].

human facial expressions, are often creations that we welcome as friendly companions; and even the 'good guys' when pitted against the environmental excesses of human ascendancy. But if these beings are not 'human', then what are they? Inevitably, this uncertainly is played upon to create a format for their oft expected 'anti-human' character; or to surprise us when a non-human displays, unexpectedly, human virtues. However, while the distinction between the living and breathing human-animal creatures found in text and celluloid are far removed from the cellular entities imagined in stem cell science, the tendency is to incite deep-seated ideas of repagination. As one commentator stated:

> 'There is a lot of innate wisdom in the "yuck" factor, or repugnance as it is also known. My Question is: what will they actually create? It is simplistic or deliberately deceptive to say that they are simply making stem cells. In order to obtain stem cells they surely have to go through the blastocyst stage; they have to create a "something" from which to derive the new cells. What is this something? It must be human to be of any use to researchers'.[30]

We can split this objection into two parts: objection to transferring human genetic material into the nonhuman; and creating human-animal beings to then be destroyed in stem cell research.

The principal goal of stem cell scientists at present is to transfer the genetic coding of human beings into enucleated animal oocytes to create 'cybrids' (through interspecies somatic nuclear transfer).[31] The aim here is not the creation of postnatal beings, but to develop stem cells genetically related to the donor they were cloned from; this has been called 'therapeutic cloning' because of the possibility of deriving matched cells

[30] J. Quintavalle, quoted in: I. Sample. 2006. Stem Cell Experts Seek Rabbit-Human Embryo. *The Guardian*. Friday 13 Jan.

[31] They would carry mitochondria of both human and animal origin. The first report of such an entity was reported in: Y. Chen *et al.* Embryonic Stem Cells Generated by Nuclear Transfer of Human Somatic Nuclei into Rabbit Oocytes. *Cell Research* 2003; 13: 251–263; also see: S. Minger. Interspecies SCNT-derived Human Embryos — A New Way Forward for Regenerative Medicine. *Regenerative Medicine* 2007; 2: 103–106.

for treatment. One justification is to address the current paucity of oocytes available for use in human embryonic research, and meet the inevitable demand that clinical transition will create. Scientists are also attempting to create modified embryos and cells which mimic the genetic defects found in humans.[32]

The recombinant procedures scientists employ to move DNA from one cell to another are adapted from processes found in nature, and which have been used in research and therapy for some time. Genetically modified bacteria are used to produce human insulin to treat diabetes, and clotting factors to treat haemophilia (these are 'cellular hybrids', because daughter cells will have identical human-bacterial genomes).[33] Pig heart valves have already been introduced into humans. But on a much larger scale, the future may see human organs developing inside animals, forming a chimeric being with two distinct cell populations: the human organs within the animal vessel.

While these experiments do present certain risks, for example, the chance that animal viral vectors may be encouraged to cross over into human infection,[34] conceding the repugnance of such experiments is more problematic. The ethical question is whether a human genome, or parts thereof, relocated into an animal cell really does warrant the aforementioned response? Genetic modification has always tended to incite a degree of trepidation: witness, for example, the rejection of GMO crops.[35] The response continues to be indicative of the permeation of the precautionary principle (and scientific scepticism) into regulatory policy. But for some, it is too easily appropriated by those who have their own moral or

---

32 For example: P. Catalina *et al.* Genetics Stability of Human Embryonic Stem Cells: A First-Step Towards the Development of Potential hESC-Based Systems for Modeling Childhood Leukemia. *Leukemia Research* 2009; 33: 980–990.

33 G. Walsh. Therapeutic Insulins and their Large-Scale Manufacture. *Applied Microbiology and Biotechnology* 2005; 67: 151–159; S. Pipe. Recombinant Clotting Factors. *Journal of Thrombosis and Haemostasis* 2008; 99: 840–850.

34 National Health and Medical Research Council. 2005. *Statement on Animal-to-Human Transplantation (Xenotransplantation) Research.* 10 March/Final report and advice to the National Health and Medical Research Council; Sep 2004.

35 L. Levidow. Precautionary Uncertainty: Regulating GM Crops in Europe. S*ocial Studies of Science* 2001; 31: 842–874.

political agenda in relation to objectionable biotechnology.[36] However, while precaution may in some circumstances unjustifiably restrain the free hand of scientists, it also allows policy makers to avoid foreseen (or merely hypothesised) threats and irreversible damage — a factor often overlooked by those overly optimistic about science.[37]

The second objection reflects the still deep-rooted controversy concerning the status of the human embryo. For some, this technology means creating ever more of human lives from an unlimited supply of animal oocytes, and this compounds the unacceptable destruction and commodification of human life. There has been little headway in resolving this issue; with religious doctrine and philosophical ideas of potentially and proportionality, being pitted against utilitarian-type arguments grounded in sentience, and human rights arguments derived from the concept of agency.

However, there is also a concern that these human-animal beings — cloned and genetically modified — will possess, in some way, human attributes. In this respect, *The UK Academy of Medical Sciences* stated:

> 'If the concept of "human dignity" has content, it is because there are factors of form, function or behaviour that confer such dignity or command respect. Either hybrid creatures would also possess these factors or they would not. If they do possess these factors, they would also have a specific type of dignity analogous or identical to human dignity that other creatures lack; if not, they would not'.[38]

We can surmise that the *Academy* is suggesting that human-animal mixtures would fall into either the animal or human category — not both.

---

[36] H. Somsen. 2008. Cloning Trojan Horses: Precautionary Regulation of Reproductive Technologies. In *Regulating Technologies: Legal Futures, Regulatory Frames and Technological Fixes.* R. Brownsword and K. Yeung, eds. Oxford: Hart Publishing: 221–242.

[37] Cf. S. Holm & T. Takala. High Hopes and Automatic Escalators: A Critique of Some New Arguments in Bioethics. *Journal of Medical Ethics* 2007; 33: 1–4.

[38] Academy of Medical Sciences. 2007. *Inter-Species Embryos: A Report by the Academy of Medical Sciences.* Jun. London: Academy of Medical Sciences: 29.

And if it made it into the latter, then the being would have the status of any other human being and any rights that follow. Arguments for fundamental human rights can be categorised into two broad camps: the 'dignity' view, and the 'agent' view. The former, which is prominently voiced, so it is argued, in many international conventions, stresses that human beings, by being virtue of being *human*, have rights. But, on this view, it would seem that no non-human being could ever have rights. While this claim raises the familiar charge of 'speciesism', we are left also with the perplexing question of how much 'human' is *human* enough.

The agent view narrows the focus of rights to the capacities of a being that is capable of self-regarding law; that is, a capacity for rational constraint of their conduct. When this normal capacity dips, then rights are withheld proportionally. On this view, rights are claims made by those who can, and not claims made on behalf of those who cannot.[39] While this view leaves us with the troubling question of what we can do to non-rights holders, it does mean that we have to take the potential agent status of human-nonhuman animals seriously. But, we do not know yet whether a mouse with a brain containing human neurones is a cause for concern in this respect: will it be able to think 'human'? So far, we have made few strides in affording rights to any non-human animals, which nevertheless show characteristically significant capacities of agency. And this does represent a far reaching ethical question: whether societies are comfortable with a potential widening of the circle of rights holders? If these anomalous beings are seen as 'persons', then are we willing to welcome then into our current framework of human rights? We suspect that the inherent difficulties in granting *human* rights to all human beings, the failure to recognise the fundamental interests of *all* human agents throughout the world, and the continued exclusion of all other beings from this moral framework, makes this unlikely. Since it is doubtful that we will be able to settle on how much 'humanness' makes a being a 'person', such beings, if ever created, are likely to become objects of experimentation and imprisoned in the laboratories from whence they came.

---

[39] D. Beyleveld. 2000. The Moral Status of the Human Embryo and Foetus. In *The Ethics of Human Procreation*. H. Haker & D. Beyleveld, eds. Aldershot: Ashgate: 59–85.

Teoh Chin Leong's chapter examines the role that religion can play in public discourse. He approaches the task from the ground up, using the ideas of Robert Audi about the cultivation of an ethics of citizenship: a substantive *and* procedural framework for reducing resentment, alienation and divisiveness, and increasing cooperation, harmony and respect.[40] Teoh argues that Audi's theory is a plausible account of how religion ought to be incorporated into public policy debates. Teoh's chapter is a convincing account of the development of what he sees as a false dilemma driving a wedge between substantive ethics and proceduralism (we pick up on proceduralism again, below). He sees as more important to human flourishing, given a 'presumption of undecidability' that contributes to the separation of religion and secular beliefs,[41] an idea of *virtue-based process legitimacy*: 'In a procedural account of ethical citizenship, it is the principles, values, virtues, attitudes and dispositions that accompany civic engagement that are important... these traits or virtues ...help to (procedurally) guide and facilitate fruitful dialogue amongst discoursing parties in an open, civil and respectful manner'.[42] This, Teoh claims, ought to facilitate cooperation between religious institutions and the drive for political order and public policy; however, he laments the absence of such virtues in 'newspapers, public talks, letters to the forum, on the internet or in public and interest group debates' [341]. In criticising two examples from the stem cell debates, one rooted in religious doctrine, the other from a 'pro-embryo research' commentary, Teoh argues that the '*spirit* of public debate and inquiry' [355] are lost to dogmatic (both religious and secular) beliefs. Instead of such biased discussions, Audi's three principles of *secular rationale*, *secular motivation* and *theo-ethical equilibrium*, ought to be the staring point for a 'civically-conscious discourse ...[and should] promote our flourishing goals whilst ensuring the moral legitimacy of ethical debate and public policy' [356].

[40] R. Audi. 2000. *Religious Commitment and Secular Reason*. Cambridge, UK; New York: Cambridge University Press.

[41] R. Ashcroft. Fair Process and the Redundancy of Bioethics: A Polemic. *Public Health Ethics* 2008; 1: 3–9: 3.

[42] Teoh, this volume [340–341].

Teoh's chapter concludes Part One of this volume; his observations on the virtues and the procedures of policy making, ideally set up the following chapters on global perspectives in stem cell research. Although the subsequent papers, representing various national approaches to the stem cell issue, are focussed on the grand design of regulating this controversial issue(s), it is worth while considering the characters, whether good or bad, that contribute to policy decisions: politicians, civil servants, and experts representing religion, culture or science; and how their dispositions and roles are integrated with ideas of public good or interest. Policies become 'ethical' or objectionable not only on the basis of their procedural validity, but also on the logic of substantive justifications, and the skills of those who make them. The public's confidence in these decisions depends, in part, on the conviction that they are made by virtuous players, and based on good reasons. And, whether one argues that the fact of plurality requires mechanistic frameworks to guide our public ethics, or bemoans the presumption of undecidability which discourages the real 'bioethics' task of finding normative resolution, communities will continually collide with contested issues that require some kind of ethical solution. Therefore, they will need people willing and capable to meet this calling. In the following Part Two, the reader will find examples of the ethical 'solutions' used by different countries in the stem cell debate.

PART TWO

GLOBAL PERSPECTIVES

The five papers found in Part Two of the volume represent unique perspectives on regulatory developments in seven countries active in stem cell research, and one where this kind of science is less developed (for reasons that will become apparent). In stem cell science, there are four distinct regulatory categories depending on the origin of stem cells: 1) somatic stem cells (either donated, or from 'waste' and 'discarded' tissue); 2) foetal stem cells from abortuses; 3) cord blood cells; and 4) embryonic stem cells. In this latter category would also be included the further controversies of chimera-derived stem cells, and those created through therapeutic cloning. Very little is said in the proceeding chapters about the *regulation* of first kind of stem cells; and with very few exceptions, the clinical transition 'from bench to bedside' has attracted relatively little regulatory notice. This is because although iPS cells feature as a newly conceived cell type, their regulation has tended to fall in line with existing measures to regulate cells and tissues.[43] This is not without its controversies, as discussed by Mackenney & Capps in this volume, and referred to earlier in this introduction.

Foetal Stem Cell Regulation

With respect to the second category of cells, regulation has appeared to remain fairly static. Although the potential isolation of foetal stem cells has originated a good deal of controversy, the regulation of such research has tended to be conceptually fixed to the kind of rules first promulgated by the *Polkinghorne Report* in the UK.[44] The Report was principally about deflating any possible influence that imminent foetal research may have on the decision to terminate a pregnancy. The consent of the pregnant woman was central, and the ethical debate concerned who should ask, and at what point — before or after the termination — it would it be acceptable to do so. At the time, the Report came under criticism, principally on its implication that commodification of unborn life was permissible, and because of the inexorable ethical inter-relational concerns of foetal use and abortion.[45] More recently, the Polkinghorne guidelines have been questioned as appearing disconnected from modern medical science. For example, in 'excluding clinical investigators from the clinical care of women undergoing pregnancy termination the [Polkinghorne] guidelines codified distrust of clinicians who undertake research'.[46] This situation is potentiality inhibiting progress in modern foetal medicine, because it suggests that obstetricians cannot be associated with foetal research; and, some argue, that the requirement for separation is unnecessarily hampering the collection of stem cells at the

[43] See, for example, the EU's Tissues Directive, *op. cit.* note 14.

[44] J. Polkinghorne. 1989. *Review of the Guidance on Research Use of Foetuses and Foetal Material*. HMSO: London.

[45] J. Keown. The Polkinghorne Report on Fetal Research: Nice Recommendations, Shame About the Reasoning. *Journal of Medical Ethics* 1993; 19:114–120.

[46] J. Kent & N. Pfeffer. Editorial: Regulating the Collection and Use of Fetal Stem Cells. *British Medical Journal* 2006; 332: 866–867.

time of termination — there are, it is claimed, ethical ways to connect this process.

Cord Blood Regulation

The use of cord blood-derived stem cells[47] has been thought by some to avoid the ethical constraints found in other sources, because it utilises an otherwise routinely discarded 'waste product' of maternity hospitals. For some time, cord blood has successfully been used for treatment of a number of childhood diseases.[48] This kind of allogenic, non-directed donation grew into a tradition of public, rather than private, banking of cord blood. However, because of progress in isolating and expanding its stem cell content, cord blood has become of increasing 'bio-value' as an autologous resource. Thus, the growing industry in private banking of cord blood has become a notable 'health insurance policy' for children worldwide. The UK's *Royal College of Obstetricians and Gynaecologists* summarised the current situation:

> 'There is substantial speculation about the use of cord blood non-HSC in treatment of a variety of acute and chronic conditions but there is increasing evidence of the use of fetal-derived stem cells in the treatment of neurological disease[49] and a number of preclinical studies in animal models, which suggest an improvement in cardiac function following infusion of umbilical cord stem cells for acute myocardial infarction.[50] There has also been a report of the infusion of cord blood

---

[47] C. McGuckin *et al.* Production of Stem Cells with Embryonic Characteristics from Human Umbilical Cord Blood. *Cell Proliferation* 2005; 38: 245–255.

[48] E. Gluckman. Hematopoietic Stem-Cell Transplants Using Umbilical-Cord Blood. *New England Journal of Medicine* 2001; 344: 1860–1861.

[49] S. Dunnett & A. Rosser. Cell Therapy in Huntington's Disease. *Neurotherapeutics* 2004; 1: 394–405.

[50] B. Kim *et al.* Cell Transplantation Improves Ventricular Function after a Myocardial Infarction: A Preclinical Study of Human Unrestricted Somatic Stem Cells in a Porcine Model. *Circulation* 2005; 112 (9 Suppl): 196–204; J. Leor *et al.* Human Umbilical Cord Blood Cells: A New Alternative for Myocardial Repair? *Cytotherapy* 2005; 7: 251–257; H.E. Broxmeyer. Biology of Cord Blood Cells and Future Prospects for Enhanced Clinical Benefit. *Cytotherapy* 2005; 7: 209–218.

> stem cells in a patient with longstanding spinal injury.[51] Commercial cord blood banks are citing such preliminary research as further potential uses in their literature. In addition, websites are now offering cell therapy using cord blood cells ahead of formal clinical trials'.[52]

However, the *Royal College*, along with other groups, have repeatedly voiced their reservations about the emergent trend of unregulated private banking.[53] The principal concerns are twofold. Firstly, there are concerns that the practice of collection — driven by extraneous economic interests — places the health of the neonate secondary to obtaining cord blood of sufficient volume and quality. It is also important to note that should external contracts be established for collection, this risks dividing the duties of the attending physicians, because it is not clear what their role is in the agreement between the mother and the collection/storage bank (which may be based in another jurisdiction).[54] Secondly, while it may well be prudent to store cord blood for future use, the *clinical* prospects of this future are not evident. There are no treatments currently available beyond those developed in the late 1980s; and there are no reputable scientific reports to support the imagined clinical targets of regenerative medicine. At present, banks can only

[51] K.S. Kang *et al.* A 37-Year-Old Spinal Cord-Injured Female Patient, Transplanted of Multipotent Stem Cells from Human UC Blood, with Improved Sensory Perception and Mobility, Both Functionally and Morphologically: A Case Study. *Cytotherapy* 2005; 7: 368–373.

[52] Royal College of Obstetricians and Gynaecologists. 2006. *Umbilical Cord Banking. Scientific Advisory Committee. Opinion Paper 2* (revised Jun 2002).

[53] The *European Group on Ethics in Science and New Technologies* therefore advised that: 'The legitimacy of commercial cord blood banks for autologous use should be questioned as they sell a service, which has presently, no real use regarding therapeutic options. Thus they promise more than they can deliver. The activities of such banks raise serious ethical criticisms'. European Commission. 2004. *Ethical Aspects of Umbilical Cord Blood Banking. No. 19.* 16 Mar. Strasbourg: European Commission: 20.

[54] Where hospitals believe that they will be able to provide this service safely to those who demand it, we suggest that they should make it clear to prospective parents that this agreement will be conditional upon the clinical and logistical demands on the service locally at the time.

offer the facilities for storage, because the technology for treatment does not exist beyond clinical trials; and therefore, the chances of cord blood being used for treatment remains as remote for most patients.

Thus, one might point to the fact that the *promise* of technology shapes how people prospectively (on their own terms) need it. The result is optimism and hope that drives a credulous population to expend resources to bank cord blood, but has the consequence that blood units are locked away from public use (and life-saving allogenic use). Moreover, if one looks to the future of cord blood banking, the focus on 'for-profit' banking, rather than developing public programmes, creates a culture of 'private insurance' to benefit those who can pay. The complaint is therefore one of justice; and some argue that regulatory oversight is necessary for this burgeoning industry.[55]

Embryonic Stem Cell Regulation: Political Tension and the Law

The fourth regulatory category has come under most ethical scrutiny. As was evident in the first part of this volume, many of the current questions come back to the controversies of embryo research; the concerns about cloning or creating chimeras, the commodification of human life, and debate about fundamental principles such as dignity. With the USA becoming the first country to approve human embryonic stem cell trials in humans, the urgency of sound regulatory oversight is pressing;[56] and this has taken many countries beyond embryo questions, to those of comprehensive regulatory coverage of translational aspects of stem cell science.

---

[55] R. Steinbrook. The Cord-Blood-Bank Controversies. *The New England Journal of Medicine* 2004; 351: 2255–2257.

[56] The trial is currently on hold because of the risk of rogue cells that may trigger tumours. Geron Corporation had been given Food and Drug Administration approval for Phase I trails of a cryopreserved formulation of human embryonic stem cell-derived oligodendrocytes. The new cell-based drug, GRNOPC1, will be primarily assessed for safety by injecting it into patients with functionally complete spinal cord injury. The drug has been shown to enhance re-myelination in rats. For full coverage, see: http://www.geron.com/GRNOPC1Clearance/ [Accessed 08 Sep 2009].

Geoffrey Lomax's contribution raises the tension within national law in a particular context: the separation of state and federal law in the USA. During his first term in office, Ex-President Bush was vocal in his opposition to embryo research. In his 2001 address, he described: 'Like a snowflake, each of these embryos is unique, with the unique genetic potential of an individual human being',[57] and from then established the restrictive federal policy to limit funding to 60 existing cells lines 'where the life-and-death decision has already been made'.[58] But, given the autonomous legislatures of individual states, this also set up, as Lomax remarks, an '"extraordinary tapestry", in which scientific and political threads are delicately intertwined'. Lomax's enlightening critique focuses on the distribution of authority between federal and state governments. He argues that to meet the administrative challenges encountered by sovereign states in stem cell research programs, procedural mechanisms:

> '...combined with the formation of inter-jurisdictional networks within the sphere of publically funded stem cell science programming, has served to enhance legitimacy and advance effective governance' [360].

This leads to the intriguing question as to whether such a model for responsible governance of controversies involving science and technology *through state action*, constitutes a '*rejuvenated federalism*' [360]?

Lomax's contribution invites us to look more closely at the curious phenomena which may focus regulations towards a particular objective. He describes how the procedural turn strongly influenced the *California Stem Cell Institute's* policies (more on this later). It was one of many states to initiate stem cell programmes at the time, given the prospect of adapting to federal policies in respect to their own legal peculiarities. However, many states recognised the technical challenges posed by policy interaction and the potential for border issues, leading to the formation of the *Interstate Alliance on Stem Cell Research*. The result was, perhaps remarkably, given

---

[57] President George W. Bush's Address on Stem Cell Research. *CNN*. 9 Aug 2001. Available at: http://edition.cnn.com/2001/ALLPOLITICS/08/09/bush.transcript/index.html [Accessed 08 Sep 2009].
[58] Ibid.

the controversial issues at stake, cooperation between participating states; and concurrently, the alignment of state regulations with various (but not all) federal standards, such as those referring to patents. The embryo question, not surprisingly, was not one of the issues to become part of the regulatory consensus. We can take regulation to mean the 'sustained and focussed attempt to alter the behaviour of others according to standards or goals with the intention of producing a broadly identified outcome or outcomes'.[59] In this frame, state and international cooperation is seen as shifting many different outlooks to focus in the same regulatory direction. In the USA, states responded to a restrictive federal policy. This created a patchwork of stem cell policies, and led to a characteristic decentralising of regulation. The only alternative for permissive states was to keep out of federal legitimation; but in doing so, rather ironically, that ultimately led to a welcome, cooperative research environment. Lomax argues that the states' willingness to engage in a coordinated stem cell policy forum may have been instrumental in an enlightened federal policy; albeit that George W. Bush's personal beliefs were, until now, a barrier to continued debate at this level. But, far from damaging the regulatory focus, the alignment of regulatory frameworks reflected 'the ongoing desire to ensure broad health and economic benefit from stem cell research' [370]. It was notable, according to Lomax, that states became 'laboratories for democracy' [369], were attentive to local 'justice-related concerns' [369], and were a 'source of policy innovation' [369]. In the global debates, where there are broadly similar border issues, the driving force for international harmonisation is a *lack of regulation*. But, the basic idea of an 'enlightened federal approach' is one that ought not to be lost in the international debates. We can take note, for example, that the EU (for example, see the comments we made on the *Tissues Directive*, above) has seen an increasing grouping of member states' policies; and, arguably, this ought to be the focus in further international initiatives.

The introduction of the *Food and Drug Administration's* Guidelines for Human Stem Cell Research was the most recent development in

---

[59] J. Black. 2005. What is Regulatory Innovation? In *Regulatory Innovation: A Comparative Analysis*. J. Black, M. Lodge & M. Thatcher, eds. Cheltenham: Edwards Elgar: Chap. 1: 11.

the USA, after President Barack Obama's executive order to remove Bush's previous policy. The similarity of these guidelines to many states' laws arguably showed the remarkable consistency within the USA with respect to the broader issues of stem cell science. According to Obama, these guidelines should address concerns of 'responsibility, scientific worth, and legality', suggesting that it was no longer the embryo question — for Obama at least — which was central to the American debate.[60] The *Dickey-Wicker Amendment* as part of the 2009 *Omnibus Appropriations Act*,[61] however, introduced exclusions into the guidelines: principally, the prohibition on federal funding to derive embryonic stem cells. It remains to be seen whether the *Stem Cell Enhancement Act* 2009, or some other legislative action, will lead to more permissive federal regulations (the guidelines are a step in this direction).[62] In this respect, Lomax concludes that the FDA has 'initiated efforts to promote communication and exchange between the agency and its stakeholders with the goal of facilitating development of safe and effective therapeutic products [374].'

The Procedural Fix

Lomax's paper brings into focus the mechanics of the (Californian) procedural approach. The idea of procedural justice (a theory within politics) is often distinguished from those of substantive justice (the 'business' of ethics). The procedural idea can be narrowed to the processes of politics itself,[63] or to a wider objective that also integrates comprehensive moralities.[64] Procedural ethics is referred to by Jasanoff as 'regulatory science': the use of techniques, processes and artefacts that

[60] M. Majumder & C. Cohen. Future Directions for Oversight of Stem Cell Research in the United States: An Update. *Kennedy Institute of Ethics Journal* 2009; 19: 195–200.

[61] Public Law 111–8, Division F, Title V, sec. 509.

[62] The 2005 introduction of the Act (H.R.810) was vetoed by Bush in July of that year.

[63] Cf. S. Hampshire. 1989. *Innocence and Experience.* London. Penguin Books.

[64] Cf. J. Rawls. 2005. *Political Liberalism.* Columbia University Press: 2nd Revised Edition.

further the task of policy development. This involves validation (employing, for instance, expert advice, and peer and scientific review) and 'persuasive efforts to protect the public against risks, emanating from scientific institutions and their products'.[65] The system described by Lomax is one built upon the constitutional charge granted to public officers to set policy, issue regulations, and adjudicate decisions that carry the force of law (or are transposed into law by governmental approval). Importantly, what legitimises the authority of bodies, like the *Californian Stem Cell Institute,* according to Lomax, is that officers are subject to a principled set of ground rules that must guide them as public policy agents.

Most national solutions to legitimate policies on the stem cell issue have tended towards some kind of 'procedural fix': (we only mention the key points due to space) they implement rules of transparent discussion, removing coercion and manipulation, so that policymakers are able to filter valid and justifiable paths for regulation and operative policies; or at least find those options which are suitable for political consumption. No one substantive solution ought to take precedent from the outset (otherwise making the process rather opaque, and perhaps disingenuous); but instead, the framework employs a set of principles which focus all efforts towards a legitimate and conciliatory policy outcome. The framework expects that agents freely enter the debate, and that each recognises what they must do if they reasonably expect their view to be considered; moreover, they cannot back out of the agreement if they don't get their way.[66] The proceduralist's claim is that the ethical validity of the framework ought to be readily conceded, and that outcomes, even when they are objectionable to ones' own views, are 'acceptable' because of the justness of the process. For advocates of the procedural fix, it has been necessary to consider not only how jurisdictions can optimise regulatory procedures, but also to understand the proper normative content that validates them.

---

[65] S. Jasanoff. 2005. *Designs on Nature: Science and Democracy in Europe and the United States.* Princeton, NJ: Princeton University Press: 230.

[66] Cf. D. Gauthier. 1986. *Moral by Agreement.* Oxford NY: Oxford University Press.

Roger Brownsword, perhaps with a hint of disparagement, concluded that a procedural strategy to overcome a 'legitimacy crisis' is dependent upon each protagonist judging that the:

> 'constituency's ethical commitments are better served by an adjustment of position and by reaching accommodation with one another rather than by unreflectively standing one's ground'.[67]

This is a claim that many have been unwilling to let proceduralism get away with. The principal objections are that the focus on process integrity is flawed; and proceduralism cannot meet the 'ethical' standards it virtuously broadcasts, because the outcomes are 'right' answers only in the sense that they meet a broad range of public interests. It therefore fails to impart *legitimation* to the claims of regulatory action.

With respect to the first objection, the critical enquirer questions the relative effectiveness of the procedures themselves; and is largely suspicious of the circumstances of ideal deliberation.[68] Detractors will point to the unavoidable imbalances in all conditions of discourse because of their particular sensitivity to political influence. This is because the course of action chosen is designed to achieve a set of predetermined (political) goals, and often to sustain the trajectory of the current regulatory tilt. Practitioners of the procedural art can adapt and combine leading ideas to get the 'best' results; but, as Frank Michelman argues, often the process remains legitimate only as long as certain outcomes are vouchsafed or excluded as a concluding possibility.[69] To be sure, getting the procedures right is no easy task, and ensuring political transparency is a constant challenge. But, it is not inevitable that a well thought-out procedural system is bound to

[67] Brownsword, *op. cit.* note 9, p. 130.

[68] In this regard, T. McCarthy, in A Theory of Communicative Competence (*Philosophy and Social Science* 1973; 3: 135–156) considers that Habermas' criteria necessary for the 'Ideal speech situation' is practically unattainable. See: J. Habermas. 1970. Towards a Theory of Communicative Competence. In *Recent Sociology No. 2*. H. Dreitzel, ed. New York: Macmillan: 114–148.

[69] F. Michelman. Constitutional Legitimation for Political Acts. *Modern Law Review* 2003; 65: 1–15.

fail (and thereby promulgate unabridged 'unethical' politics); or moreover, is merely a tool for political intrigue. Skilled policy-makers can use guiding principles of proceduralism, such as transparency, accountability, and consistency, to make deliberation fair and accessible, just as well as they can manipulate them for disingenuous ends.[70] This charge is not particular to proceduralism; in any high stake circumstance — including in the 'business' of bioethics — there is scope for pacts, tradeoffs, deceit, insincerity, and duplicity.

A more profound anxiety, however, is found in the second objection: political aspirations cannot be taken beyond their contextual limits, because they are achieved by forgoing rigorous ethical argumentation.[71] Ultimately, therefore, they must be rejected as ideas of *ethical* regulation. Richard Ashcroft suggests that the exclusion of ethical debate does little to reassure the 'public that the issues have been thought out, or that this has been done in a reasonably just or ethical way'.[72] Moreover, proceduralism cannot meet the 'high calling of ethics', because it fails as a 'litmus [test] to tell us which political acts are legitimate (respect-worthy, even if wrong) and which are not'.[73] It is, therefore, a politically disingenuous way to ignore the conflict to be found at the heart of modern pluralistic democracies; it merely '...hopes to vault people past their real,

---

[70] B. Capps. Authoritative Regulation and the Stem Cell Debate. *Bioethics* 2007; 22: 43–55.

[71] It is easy to achieve a desired outcome by establishing the pre-agenda; see, for example: House Committee on Oversight and Government Reform, *Political Interference With Climate Change Science Under The Bush Administration* at (Dec. 2007) (revealing that 'the Bush Administration has engaged in a systematic effort to manipulate climate change science and mislead policymakers and the public about the dangers of global warming'); G. Harris. White House is Accused of Putting Politics Over Science. *N.Y. TIMES*. 10 Jul 2007 (reporting claims by former Surgeon General Richard H. Carmona that 'top officials in the Bush administration repeatedly tried to weaken or suppress important public health reports because of political considerations'); and E. Blackburn. Bioethics and the Political Distortion of Biomedical Science. *New England Journal of Medicine* 2004; 350: 1379–1380 (who alleges the stacking of the President's Council on Bioethics by the Bush Administration in 2001 to silence pro-embryo research voices).

[72] R. Ashcroft. Fair Process and the Redundancy of Bioethics: A Polemic. *Public Health Ethics* 2008; 1: 3–9, p. 7.

[73] Michelman, *op. cit.* note 69, p. 6.

unliquidated disagreements'.[74] These arguments focus on the legitimacy of these endpoints; and they raise doubts about whether an adequate ethical justification is forthcoming from a purely procedural approach — even if it is legitimate. *Fair* procedures, on their own, cannot create *just* endpoints; nor can they say anything creditable about the ethics of public policy.

The procedural turn is about instituting coherent sociality. This is achieved by legitimising regulatory policies which, it is argued, generate an idea of mutual public recognition (we all support a given policy because we were all part of its establishment). Moreover, procedural ethics considers that it is possible to do this without destabilising the local (or even international) community. Justifying this approach can be achieved by locating it in an idea of 'public ethics'; or specifically, a moral theory that purports to show how *community values* can *transcend pure self-interests* when considered within a system of public policy.[75]

The *legitimacy* of proceduralism is found within a theory that bridges private and public.

'The public', in this sense, refers to a collection of private individuals who may or may not be congruous in their collective goals; each member represents a sovereign agent with powers of self-determination and governance. This is the source of democratic plurality and the inevitable conflict of interests. Private ethics begins with the opinions, viewpoints, convictions and beliefs of an agent's dialectic rationality; they are often then to be aired only within private dialogue or the cosy theatres of bioethics. It is an ethics which signifies 'integrity, gentleness, disposition to sympathy, a fastidious sense of honour'.[76] Public ethics, however, concerns ideas which are grounded in the circumstances created by communities and public life. It is about: 'tenacity and resolution... largeness of design and purpose ...habits of leadership'.[77] Public

---

[74] Ibid: 7–8.

[75] Capps, *op. cit.* note 70.

[76] Hampshire, *op. cit.* note 63, p. 177.

[77] Ibid.

decisions are often expedient and extensive, and not always popular or welcome, meaning that often they are only possible where there is a dis-association between 'the public interests' and personal beliefs or sentiments. The latter cannot be definitive of public policy, since we cannot *expect* others to share them, nor can the agent's approbation or affirmation of a set of relevant facts be a measure of the appropriateness for public policy. Personal ethics may be specifically directed to private gain or goals, sometimes reprehensible or unintelligible, and which are often parochial with respect to those who share a close existence. They are based on our approval of facts that we are comfortable with, which often lacks considerations of justice or reflectivity of public purposes; and sentiments that we are used to, rather than those which are remote, unfamiliar, and 'public'. This is not an abandonment of ethics (it is, however, a rejection that private ethics is a suitable endpoint for public policy), but an ethics suited to the expedient political world. 'The public interest' concerns the obligations of collective and impersonal choices which are necessary for the governance of the state — grounded in, what one might call, *political instinct*.

But, this does not sanction a Machiavellian 'princely fox', unable to uphold the virtues of a good citizen if he is to do his political duty; not least because his moral obligations are tainted by a desire to avoid dishonour — a seat of glory that requires the fox to maintain the dignity of office by cover-ups and corruption.[78] But nor does it seem wise to turn to the 'saintly' to make such decisions: they are naive and inexperienced of the demands of office, finding solace in provincial interests and relying on skills honed in the familiar surroundings of academic debate. The capable public official is aware of his or her own conviction, and accomplished in the political virtues. However, policy-makers are, at the same time, private individuals and public officials; and their interests in one will inevitably influence and overlap with the other (and there is nothing to oppose private virtues informing public dealing too). But the subjectivism that this entails means that the public have to be confident in the *authority of reason*, and specifically, a theoretical con-

[78] M. Hollis. 1996. *Reason in Action*. Cambridge NY: Cambridge University Press: 139.

struction of *reasonable* public decision-making.[79] The role of the public official is one open to the elements of public criticism: their public decisions cannot be made for personal advantage. To justify public decisions, and thus impart a public moral obligation, evidence, opinions and judgement must meet rigorous scientific authentication and ethical scrutiny. Officers are licensed to do a certain job (and the privileges that go with this), but the public expect checks and balances — that procedures are in place to scrutinise their public conduct. Furthermore, procedural mechanisms, which grant individuals privileges and entitlements to make policy, also require that individuals have rights to take part in the debates of their choosing and to be listened to; thus, it ensures that all members of the community are under the same ethical obligations to exercise their rights so as not to deceive or wilfully misrepresent information to insidious ends.

The Notion of Respect and Global Values

The next four papers document how individual countries have implemented regulations in stem cell research. There appear to be a number of common ideas which can be found in both Asian and Western bioethics arguments; principally, this is a symptom of a procedural way of conducting deliberative bioethics.

We begin with the recent developments in the UK. The UK is one of the few countries that have found it necessary to review existing statutory laws, because they have become increasingly disconnected from scientific developments. The *Human Fertilisation and Embryology Act 1990* brought embryo research under comprehensive oversight — the problem, which has become increasingly evident as a result of persistent legal challenge, is that novel technologies have strained the operation of the Act. This detachment has been compensated through a number of interpretive measures. Notably, in *Royal College of Nursing of*

[79] Seymour Martin Lipset argues that government legitimacy 'involves the capacity of a political system to engender and maintain the belief that existing political institutions are the most appropriate and proper ones for the society'. *Political Man: The Social Bases of Politics*. London: Heinemann: 2nd edition, 1983: 64.

the United Kingdom v Department of Health and Social Security, Lord Wilberforce made a seminal speech on purposivism,[80] which has been subsequently used to reattach Parliament's policy or intention at the time of drafting the Act, to current issues outside current law.[81] But purposivism has a tendency to become a tool for the presiding legislative tilt: that it will be interpreted in terms of the current political leaning, rather than that of the time of drafting. As Brownsword writes, 'what constitutes gap-filling and second guessing [of Parliament's intention] largely hinges on whether the present case can be subsumed under the same genus of the covering policy, which in turn depends on whether the court judges that a liberal or restrictive approach is called for'.[82] The precarious stability and need for constant reattachment gathered momentum, resulting in the review of 1990 Act.[83]

Natasha Hammond-Browning and Søren Holm discuss the review of the 1990 Act in respect of the prospect of creating hybrid embryos. The 2008 Act, unlike its predecessor, explicitly mentions 'human admixed embryos', which refers to the 'human end' of chimeric entities (entities with a predominantly human genetic content and not created by fertilisation nor intended for postnatal life).[84] Hammond-Browning & Holm suggest that such a term is misleading: 'The *legal* name for such embryos does not truly acknowledge the animal contribution, however small that may be, since it does not make it clear what the human is "admixed" with' [386]. They further note that the legislation now requires chimera research to be 'necessary and desirable' for the purposes of licensing by the *Human Fertilisation and Embryology Authority*; and that the Act will not justify the issuing of licences for hybrid embryo research where a viable

---

[80] [1981] AC 800.

[81] See: R. v Secretary of State for Health ex parte Quintavalle (on behalf of the Pro-Life Alliance) [2001] EWHC 918 (Admin) (Crane J), [2002] EWCA Civ 29, [2003] UKHL 13.

[82] Brownsword, *op. cit.* note 9, pp. 172–173.

[83] Department of Health. 2006. *Review of the Human Fertilisation and Embryology Act*. Cm 6989.

[84] Lord Darzi of Denham 15 Jan 2008. House of Lords Hansard (Debates) Vol. 697, Col 1195 HL. Such embryos cannot be implanted in a woman's or animal's womb. 'True chimeras' can be legally created by the mixing of hamster sperm with human oocytes for fertility purposes, and not research.

alternative exists. Looking to the future, the authors raise the issue that 'whilst it may be desirable and necessary to use hybrid embryos for research, it is debatable whether it is desirable to use such embryos for use in *human* clinical trials or treatments' [389]. With the advent of iPS cells — which do not involve gametes or embryos in the derivation process, and their derivation is therefore outside of the remit of the HFEA — the answer is possibly not. Chimera-derived cells to be used in clinical implantation will face similar concerns as those voiced in debates on xenotransplantation: safety concerns, inefficiency, and less contentious alternatives may make hybrid research in the clinical contexts obsolete. However, while the UK's Act does cover the derivation of chimera cells, there is little said in respect to their clinical use.[85]

In their contribution, Renzong Qiu and Xiaomei Zhai describe how the 'cloning and stem cell debate in China is taking place at a time when the country is in transition from a monolithic society to a more or less pluralistic civil society' [396]. This creates a complex regulatory response, which assimilates China's historical cultures with periods of adaptation to external philosophies and its modern integration into the international community. The commitment to investment in the biotech industry has concurrently initiated a need to address the ethical, legal and social implications of the scientific discovery; and this has resulted in a number of regulations to protect the interests of human participants in research and

[85] The EU Tissue and Cells Directive, as transposed into UK law by the *Human Tissue (Quality and Safety for Human Application) Regulations 2007* 'sets standards of quality and safety for the donation, procurement, testing, processing, storage and distribution of human tissues and cells'. While this sets high standards for *human* cells, there may be concerns that the animal content of may disqualify chimera cells from this oversight. Clinical use will come under the remit of *Regulation on Advanced Therapies* (Regulation (EC) 1394/2007). This regulation recognises the unique character of stem cell-derived therapies; and that they lie at the border of the traditional pharmaceutical area and other fields (e.g. medical devices). The inclusion of animal engineered components in human cells is covered, but the effectiveness and extent of this has been questioned; see: European Commission. 2005. *Tissue Engineering and Beyond: Summary of the 2005 Public Consultation on the Draft Proposal for a Regulation on Advanced Therapies.* Enterprise and Industry Directorate-General; Consumer Goods; Pharmaceuticals. Brussels. European Commission. November.

patients in clinical practice. In respect to stem cell research, there has been a distinguishing permissive tilt strongly influenced by a Confucian pro-life precedent that saving lives (*renzheng,* or humane policy) is an ethical imperative: the peoples' *minsheng* (well-being) is the driving force justifying the acceptability of embryo research and therapeutic cloning. The authors trace the political solution to the embryo question in China by reference to the 'spirit' of graduated priority, which may be found in Confucian thought: the person is formed from their achievements and by fulfilling certain roles. The embryo, accordingly, appears at the beginning of this process — and is considered as a potential or proportional person to be extended respect according to the distance and difference between their ontology and actual persons.[86] Given the benefits of research, it is justifiable to use such embryos to derive stem cells. *Rén* (benevolence) may be shown to the embryo, even if it is used is research, by showing it respect; this may include a proper committal subsequent to use.

The Chinese government explicitly banned reproductive cloning in 1998. It is a country that has enthusiastically embraced stem cell research, and the '*Ethical Guiding Principles*' from December 2003, issued by the *Ministry of Science and Technology*, permit research on human embryonic stem cells, embryo research up to 14 days, therapeutic cloning, human foetal research and induced parthenogenesis. The Guidelines also reaffirm that gametes and tissues must be voluntarily donated in accordance with the principle of informed consent; and that research institutions proposing to experiment with human embryonic stem cells must establish an ethical committee to review the research, prohibit the implantation of human embryos used in stem cell research, and prohibit the buying and selling of human eggs, sperm, embryos and foetal tissue. The Guidelines address an oversight, which was revealed when a reputable Shanghai team announced that it had generated stem cells by transferring nuclei from human skin into rabbit eggs.[87] These Guidelines, according to Qiu & Zhai, lack legal clout; and moreover, there is no system for

[86] Cf. D. Tsai. Human Embryonic Stem Cell Research Debates: A Confucian Argument. *Journal of Medical Ethics* 2005; 31: 635–640.

[87] The goal was to develop a way of generating embryonic stem cells that did not require scarce human ooyctes; Chen, *op. cit.* note 31.

overseeing compliance with the Guidelines or for inspecting stem cell research facilities. China's policy of well-being has led to further regulations that came into effect on the 1st of May, 2009, and that designate all forms of stem cell therapy as 'category three' medical technologies: those deemed 'ethically problematic', 'high risk' or 'still in need of clinical verification', and thus under Ministry oversight (including the requirement for submitting clinical-trial protocols).

Satoshi Kodama and Akira Akabayashi describe the circumstances in Japan which led up to the *Law Concerning Regulations Relating to Human Cloning Techniques and Other Similar Techniques,* enacted on 6th June 2001. Once again, the idea that the human embryo is morally distinct from a person is central to a permissive tilt. The embryo is described as the 'sprout of human life', thus suggesting its *potential* to become a moral being: 'the harm in violation of embryos that are no more than a sprout of life is minute relative to that of foetuses or humans'.[88] In expanding this concept, Ryuichi Ida is quoted in the chapter as remarking:

> 'an embryo is not just a "thing" either; if it divides, it will naturally become a person. This is why we used the expression "sprout of human life", and thus in a sense it describes an intermediate stage on the way to becoming a person... If the embryo was deemed to be human life, then to take it to an extreme, these researchers would be committing murder' [432].

The 2001 law has two roles: it specifically bans reproductive cloning; and it required the *Ministry of Education* to produce national guidelines for the creation of 'Specified Embryos' for research purposes. On 23 July 2004, Japan's *Council for Science and Technology Policy*, the Government's eminent science and technology policy body, approved the final report of its *Bioethics Expert Panel* on human embryo and stem cell research. The report recommended a change in Japanese policy to allow the creation of human embryos using therapeutic cloning techniques.

---

88 From Kodama & Akabayashi, this volume [430].

The Potentiality Argument

The gradualist idea that appeared in both China and Japan is common in Western political ideas of embryo status as well; and has been seen as the 'compromise' position between 'pro-life' (the embryo has full moral status) and 'pro-choice' (the embryo has no moral status sole by virtue of its own characteristics) positions. Gradualist arguments in the Western context have tended to come under criticism because they must rest on the metaphysical ideas of potentiality and proportionality. These have been seen variously as vulnerable to *reductio ad absurdum* arguments: that potentially reaches back to limitless 'what ifs'. Far more difficult is the challenge that *mere* potentiality cannot be morally relevant because a being's status at a certain time depends on the being's properties *at that time*; properties that the being has yet to actualise cannot matter in a morally relevant way and cannot serve as a surrogate for actuality. If a being has full moral status by virtue of being a person, then a potential person can only have potential moral status, not actual moral status. Proportion, on the other hand, opens up the propositional risk that agents can have degrees of *higher* status, and this suggests a distinctly un-egalitarian idea of moral status.

This, at first, appears to be very different from the Confucian understanding of potentiality and proportionality. The latter suggests the relational aspects of *becoming a person*, and these are observations which are far more accessible to Confucian cultures than Western epistemology. Moreover, in Kodama & Akabayashi's paper, the Western idea of dignity is seen as being 'out of place when considered from an Asian, or Japanese, perspective'.[89] (But the authors themselves conceive that: 'Accepting the Western idea of human dignity and at the same time making ambiguous the Western dichotomy of things and persons, the *Committee* made it possible for ethics and science to reconcile with each other, at least for the time being' [439].)

However, within the Confucian approach we see that relating ideas to personhood leads to a concept of 'respect'. In Japanese law, practices which contradict the prescription that 'All people shall be respected as

[89] From Kodama & Akabayashi, this volume [427].

individuals' are prohibited — but, this does not rule out embryo research — embryos 'require careful handling, but they are still at a different stage than foetuses or post-natal humans' [430]. This idea — that the embryo does not meet the criteria of a full 'person' — is found in Western thought; as is the notion that such being may still be respected. Thus, the idea of respect may be surmised as the *use* of the human embryo so that it does not become an object or mere thing, but as a locus of diminished, but important moral value. The *respect* is not so much shown in what the embryo *is*, but what we do to it. This means that it ought to be treated in a certain way, and even, if appropriate, afforded some legal protection.[90] Thus, working back, when such protection is translated into an idea of 'respect', it requires that research is subject to strict oversight and that certain limits are in place (supported by criminal sanctions).

However, some critics focus on the fact that 'protection' is ill defined, and is ultimately vacuous because it inevitably results in the destruction of the embryo. Qiu & Zhai articulated an idea of respect to suggest that it could be shown if research is performed only when there are laudable scientific goals.[91] Likewise, Kodama & Akabayashi quote the Japanese *Subcommittee on Human Embryo Research*, which states: stem cell research requires 'a swift response in Japan and is the source of high hopes for regenerative medicine'.[92] Moreover, the call for strict rules for conducting research also suggests a level of respect towards embryos; essentially confirming that they cannot be used except under certain specific conditions.

It is perhaps remarkable that the stories of regulative struggle in China and Japan, as given here, have been preceded by similar struggles elsewhere, especially where the legislative tilt has been permissive; and it is likely that states lacking regulation in this area, and willing to make the same legislative step, will face similar difficulties. The problem for international law, as skilfully shown in the chapter of Cutas & Munthe, is where

[90] M. Warnock. 1985. *A Question of Life: The Warnock Report on Human Fertilisation and Embryology.* Oxford: Basil Blackwell Limited: 62.
[91] Cf. House of Lords Select Committee (Sel Com.). 2002. *Stem Cell Research.* HL Paper 83(i) London: HMSO, February.
[92] From Kodama & Akabayashi, this volume [431].

different legislative tilts (permissive and prohibitive) come into contact. While this idea of respect has been used to move forward from national debates to regulatory action, it remains to be seen whether 'respect' can be taken into multinational fora, and where regulatory progress in regard to these controversies is notably absent. To illustrate this point further, the Singapore *Biomedical Ethics Advisory Committee* stated that 'respect' is about allowing different views to be expressed (given the multicultural circumstances of the city-state), and for due consideration to be given to them.[93] In the end, a global policy may be about a position which may be tolerated in a pluralistic world, created by 'considered weighing and balancing of the spectrum of views held'.[94] Although the BAC were writing about the pluralism within Singapore itself, in many areas — notably human rights — the weighting of interests has been successful to a degree; and an international balance, promulgated by regional groups such as the EU, and the wider influence of the UN, has been achieved.

But it is noticeable that many appear unconvinced that an adequate level of harmonisation at this level is possible[95]; others lack confidence in those who are responsible for the international community's advocacy of rights are able, or even willing, to assert themselves properly. We also are also mindful that a concept of 'respect' will probably creep into the same unhelpful niches of our human rights frameworks as has dignity; but by foreknowing the difficulties that a vague and inconsistent use of dignity has caused, can we avoid such indeterminacy happening again? Can we in fact respect individuals, as rights holders, while leaving the embryo question to one side? (In this regard, it was perhaps a mistake to include the embryo in the Council of Europe's *Convention for the Protection of Human Rights and Dignity of the Human Being with Regard to the*

---

[93] C. Ho, B. Capps & T.C. Voo (in press). Stem Cell Science and Its Public: The Case of Singapore. *East Asian Science, Technology and Society: An International Journal.*

[94] Bioethics Advisory Committee, Singapore. 2002. *Ethical, Legal and Social Issues in Human Stem Cell Research, Reproductive and Therapeutic Cloning*. Jun. Singapore: BAC: 21.

[95] I. De Melo-Martin. Forthcoming. Human Dignity in International Policy Documents: A Useful Criterion for Public Policy? *Bioethics* (online early) 10.1111/j.1467–8519.2009.01737.x.

Application of Biology and Medicine, given all but one of the Articles referred to agent-relevant capacities.) Can a weakened idea of respect be sensitive to variations in cultural values, or flexible enough to allow rudimentary progress in international law? Now, of course, we are at risk of embarking on an equally difficult task, and too ambitious one for this introduction, of spelling out what we mean by 'rights' (and what it means to be respected in having one's rights claims recognised) — but given the almost universal assent to documents which are unambiguous in their agent targets (such as the Declaration of Helsinki and the conditions of volunteering for research), this might be an opportunity to explore at another time. A conceptual idea of 'respect' is unlikely to supplant dignity in our international language, as it is deeply ingrained and would require the onerous task of reorganising current institutions. Many would be unwilling to abandon our current intentional framework given its achievements in some areas; others would dismiss this as reinventing the wheel, and it is likely to be seen by some as further muddying of the conceptual water of international law. While it is unlikely that any core concept — no matter how well, or even intentionally vaguely, defined — will reach out to all cultures and all corners of the globe, we speculate that, just maybe, and with hard work, a breakthrough may be found.

The Complexity of National Legislation

Peter Sýkora considers the unusual case of two closely related countries developing very different regulatory approaches: Slovakia, in which embryo research is banned; and the Czech Republic, where it is permitted. Sýkora analyses the reasons for the juxtaposed biopolicies. The two countries have employed different strategies to address the then 'bioethical deficit' in their healthcare legislation. The reason for this may not be merely different religious and secular developments, because, as the author argues, a probable key factor was the impact of national research lobbies.

Slovakia has prohibited stem cell research using human embryos through general and criminal provisions. The origins of the prohibition stemmed from the *Health Care Law*, which, Sýkora argues, was used to protect the embryo as a 'vulnerable' person, including it in a list of excluded populations from research. Sýkora adds that at the time, and subsequently, there has been little explanation or comment on the issues in the health care reforms; and indeed, more weighty issues — health care reform itself and criminal jurisprudence — overshadowed any potential attempt to engage in bioethical debate. Thus, the *in vitro* embryo is protected as a vulnerable person (the embryo lacks any definition in Slovak law), and despite the law not actually recognising such a status (as stated by the Slovak Constitutional Court). The *Penal Code* (2006) further strengthens the prohibition on embryo research by listing a number of banned activities, including any human cloning. Furthermore, the *Code* makes a prohibitive extraterritorial claim (a first in Slovak history) on Slovakian researchers, effectively ruling out any international collaboration that involves human embryos. Within the European Union, Slovakia has continued to formally support 'anti-embryo' initiatives.

The Czech Republic, in stark contrast, adopted legislation in 2006 which permitted the procurement of human embryonic stem cells from surplus embryos. It prohibited the creation of research embryos, reproductive cloning and chimera/hybrid research; and outlined in some detail the definitional aspects of embryo research (including defining the embryo). Unlike Slovakia, the law was passed after direct parliamentary debate, with an argument that prohibition would mean the 'continuation of [the Czech] excelling reputation in this research field would end' [456].

The reasons for these divergent policies, Sýkora argues, were not only about the religious circumstances of each country ('Catholic Slovakia' and 'atheistic Czech Republic' [457]): he also points to a more obvious pro-science culture in the Czech Republic, and one which was organised into an effective lobby to promote research and the use of hES cells. (These issues, Sýkora suggests, were for the most part ignored by the major scientific groups in Slovakia; and in general there was a lack of awareness or interest shown by the public). Furthermore, the Czech Republic had earmarked considerable funding for biotech industry, and it was not going to be prevented from injecting capital into promising embryonic stem cell research. This pro-science environment was, Sýkora argues, instrumental in pushing a pro-embryo research agenda. (And quoting Michael Mulkay's *The Embryo Research Debate*, he suggests that the pro-science lobby groups — which overcame a prominent anti-abortion sentiment — were an essential component of passing the UK's permissive *Human Fertilisation and Embryology Act*, and again were important in the revision of the Act in 2008; this time, overcoming opposition to chimera/hybrid research.)

Peter Sýkora's chapter highlights an important aspect of a country's legislative tilt: that a developed and organised scientific organisation has a major role in centralised policy. His contribution is further evidence that understanding the legislative tilt of a country — a necessary step in reconciling international harmonisation — requires a careful analysis of the complexity of background details informing that position. One can see, for example, how a particular pro-science environment was created in Singapore: the need to establish a legal and regulatory climate that enabled this relatively new investment initiative to flourish was identified early on in the policy process, and the involvement of leading scientists on high-level advisory bodies was actively pursued to this end.[96] One can also see how a country's particular circumstances can dampen scientific enthusiasm: Germany, for instance, despite having a highly-developed scientific infrastructure, was unable to support the controversial aspects of stem cell science — the reasons for this may be as a result of a pre-existing conservative ruling thesis (that protects the human embryo as a human being), and which takes precedence over the freedom of research due to reservations still engrained from past scientific atrocities.[97] While it is relatively easy to characterise the two main 'permissive' and 'prohibitive' countries in the stem cell debates, we do disfavour to their history and culture if further contextual elements are lost in 'the vote'.

CLOSING REMARKS

During the editing of this volume, it became clear to us that the final text would be much more than a rehearsal of the familiar aspects of the

---

[96] K. Wong & T. Bunnell. 'New Economy' Discourse and Spaces in Singapore: A Case Study of One-North. *Environment and Planning A* 2006; 38: 69–83.

[97] D. Beyleveld & S. Pattinson. 2001. Embryo Research in the UK: Is Harmonisation in the EU Needed or Possible. In: *Embryo Experimentation in Europe: Bio-medical, Legal, and Philosophical Aspects. Bad Neuenahr- Ahrweiler GmbH: Europäische Akademia zur Erforschung von Folgen wissenschaftlich-technischer.* M.B. Friele, ed. Entwicklugen: Gray Series: 58–74.

'embryo question'. In this comprehensive critical introduction, we have attempted to draw together the several issues beyond the dualistic 'yes' or 'no' solution to stem cell research; in this book, the reader will find original articles considering translational issues, which — of foremost concern — are about the possibility of scientific and medical advancement which could eventually save lives. But, let us not forget the complex relationships that develop as a consequence of this shift, such as the possible threat to the integrity of transactions between scientists and donors, as well as questions about the reputation of scientists and clinicians. In particular, one will find nuanced scrutiny of the root causes behind regulatory tilts in the respective countries, and how these could in turn affect international harmonisation efforts in stem cell science. Importantly, one will appreciate how culture (such as the pro-science Czech republic) and philosophy (China and Japan), as well as history (Germany), and even public assessment of the scientific community as the 'benchmark' of evidence for parliamentary uses, can shape policies regarding stem cell science. We conclude on a general note on the place of contention in bioethics and biotechnology.

The stem cell debates have persisted throughout a particularly intense period in growth of innovative biotechnology and global bioethics. The future for stem cell regulation will depend in part on how the disparate disciplines found in 'bioethics' — law, philosophy, social science — influence the course of governance development in the stages of translational medicine. All the while, scientific endeavour and market forces will be pulling regulators in diverse, sometimes conflicting, directions. The legitimacy of bioethics has extensively permeated zones of governance; it is no longer the case that bio-medical controversy can be negotiated within specific cultural and political contexts of the state, because each nation's position within a regional and global economy, ensures that they cannot operate independently. The creation of complex international networks has created a need for greater integration and harmonisation; but while questions still hang over the competency and effectiveness of institutions of global governance, the push to reform has predominantly come from meeting the standards of the global markets, rather than universal ethical norms.

The papers in this volume should initiate a sustained, focused and forward looking debate about aspects global governance; and we think that they are a valuable contribution to redressing the balance between the economic imperatives of stem cell science, and the contemporary social and ethical thought about the best conception of an ordered and just global community. Moreover, the unique international perspectives presented in this book provide a snapshot of where global regulation might be heading.

We would like to thank Alvin Chew Kiah-Sian and Theodora Kwok Hui Xuan for assistance in the preparation of the manuscript for publication. Alvin also edited the abstracts for the chapters. Both scholars were meticulous and industrious in the tasks asked of them, and they proved to be astute judges in their own assessments of the contributions.

Our sincere gratitude also goes to the contributors to this volume, who spent their time and effort in the careful preparation of their papers. Each author was a pleasure to work with, and wrote a thoughtful essay for this volume. In this introduction, we have begun a critical analysis of the contributions, and with the intention of this representing the beginning of further debate, we look forward to responses and further discussion with the authors. We hope our readers will also find in this rich collection of papers a stimulus to further thought about the complexities of the stem cell controversy.

Benjamin Capps and Alastair V. Campbell
Centre for Biomedical Ethics
Singapore
31 September 2009

Part One

CONTESTED CELLS: UNDERSTANDING THE ETHICAL CONTROVERSY

(a) The Problems of Regulation

1

A CASE STUDY OF EXPERIMENTAL STEM CELL THERAPY AND THE RISKS OF OVER-REGULATION

Anthony Hollander

One Sunday afternoon in March 2008 whilst out to lunch with my family, I received a telephone call from my colleague at the University of Bristol, Professor Martin Birchall, a surgeon and clinical scientist specialising in diseases of the upper airway. I remember the call well because he started our conversation with the statement 'Anthony, there is a patient in Spain who is going to die and we want you to help us grow her a new trachea'. He certainly knew how to get my attention! He explained to me that his surgical colleague in Barcelona, Professor Paolo Macchiarini, had a young lady patient who was seriously ill following a prolonged tuberculosis infection that had damaged her left bronchus. Removing her left lung was the only remaining conventional option and that would carry a high risk of death and (if she survived) would severely impair her quality of life. These two surgeons had decided that this was a perfect case in which to attempt reconstruction using an engineered segment of tracheal tissue. They had already been working with two research teams in Italy on some techniques that could be used. Dr. Sara Mantero in Milan had developed a bioreactor (an incubator designed to ensure effective delivery of nutrients to a growing tissue) for the growth of vascular tissue[1] and she was

[1] C. Arrigoni *et al.* Rotating versus Perfusion Bioreactor for the Culture of Engineered Vascular Constructs Based on Hyaluronic Acid. *Biotechnology and Bioengineering* 2008; 100(5): 988–997.

now developing an equivalent bioreactor specifically for the culture of a cylindrical segment of trachea. Dr. Maria-Teresa Conconi in Padua was independently developing a method for removing all the cells from cadaver trachea, leaving a mechanically competent cell-free matrix that could act as a scaffold from which to construct a new trachea.[2] In the meantime in Bristol my team had been developing methods for culturing bone marrow mesenchymal stem cells and turning them into cartilage cells (chondrocytes) whilst avoiding the formation of a calcified bone-like tissue.[3] Finally, Martin Birchall had been culturing airways epithelial cells which normally line the inside (lumen) of the trachea and produce a mucosal surface which acts as a barrier to infection.[4] So there was a clear logic to bringing each of these techniques together in the hope of creating a new segment of tracheal-like tissue that was 'personalised' by using the patient's own stem cells and epithelial cells.

I was initially resistant to the idea of putting together a tissue engineering method in a very short space of time, with no grant application, no pre-clinical testing and no regulatory validation. As a scientist I have been trained to pay attention to every detail, make no assumptions, test every theory to the limit of technical capability and even then to be aware that my hypotheses may be wrong. What I was being asked to do was ignore many details, make numerous assumptions, work on the basis that my current theoretical knowledge was sound and find a way to proceed despite the regulatory hurdles. In other words I was being asked to behave in a quite unscientific way. On further consideration I realised that: a) we

[2] M.T. Conconi *et al.* Tracheal Matrices, Obtained by a Detergent-Enzymatic Method, Support *in Vitro* the Adhesion of Chondrocytes and Tracheal Epithelial Cells. *Transplant International* 2005; 18(6): 727–734.

[3] W. Kafienah *et al.* Three-Dimensional Cartilage Tissue Engineering Using Adult Stem Cells from Osteoarthritis Patients. *Arthritis and Rheumatism* 2007; 56: 177–187; W Kafienah *et al.* Pharmacological Regulation of Adult Stem Cells: Chondrogenesis Can Be Induced Using a Synthetic Inhibitor of the Retinoic Acid Receptor. *Stem Cells* 2007; 25: 2460–2468.

[4] L.E. Rees *et al.* The Isolation and Characterisation of Primary Human Laryngeal Epithelial Cells. *Molecular Immunology* 2006; 43(6): 725–730; L.E. Rees *et al.* Campylobacter and IFNGamma Interact to Cause a Rapid Loss of Epithelial Barrier Integrity. *Inflammatory Bowel Diseases* 2008; 14(3): 303–309.

would probably never get funding for such a complex proposal; but, b) we might, just might, make a real difference to this lady's life and surely it was worth trying. The European scientific team met in my home one evening to figure out some of the details. In this informal setting we had to make a series of technical decisions that would collectively determine the success or otherwise of our strategy. The scientific staff went back to their laboratories, each to work on their contribution to the process. The two surgeons worked on the process of getting regulatory permission and transporting cells from Barcelona to Bristol and back again without delay. That part of the plan nearly failed when Martin Birchall took the cells cultured in Bristol to the airport for transport back to Barcelona. The airline concerned, despite numerous preparatory telephone calls, refused to allow the cells onboard because the volume of culture medium was way in excess of the regulatory maximum of 100 ml. The situation was looking catastrophic; we had grown the patient's cells and had to have them in Barcelona within a few hours to seed onto the tracheal scaffold before they lost viability. After a series of telephone calls Martin arranged for a German thoracic surgeon who had a pilot license, to fly a small private plane from Germany to Bristol and then on to Barcelona at the cost of about €14,000 (the bill was subsequently paid by the Vice-Chancellor of the University of Bristol). On 12th of June 2008, the engineered trachea was implanted in Claudia Castillo and the scientific report of the tissue engineering method, surgical technique and follow-up of the patient was published after three months' follow-up.[5] Since the operation the patient has been trouble-free with no signs of immune rejection and a fully functioning airway. Given the initial prognosis, the improvement to her health of this experimental procedure has been exceptional; and furthermore, she is no longer drawing on the resources of her country's health care system. This illustrates the potential power of stem cells and tissue engineering to remove a disease from a patient's life altogether (unlike most pharmaceutical therapies, which manage systems over many years).

Almost every aspect of our project required us, under guidance from the authorities concerned, to side-step the *normal* regulatory rule-book.

[5] P. Macchiarini *et al.* Clinical Transplantation of a Tissue-Engineered Airway. *Lancet* 2008; 372(9655): 2023–2030.

For example: (i) In the UK we should have been growing the cells in a laboratory facility licensed by the Human Tissue Authority (HTA) in order to comply with the Human Tissue Act 2008. For practical reasons we were not able to do this; and it was necessary for us to get special permission from the HTA to grow these cells in an unlicensed laboratory for this one case. (ii) We should have been growing our cells in a laboratory working to 'Good Manufacturing Practice' (GMP) standards with guaranteed procedures for ensuring sterility and for tracking the cultures. This was simply not possible in the time-frame available to us. However the Spanish transplantation authority was prepared to allow this as an exception. (iii) Our tissue engineered product should have been shown to be effective in an animal model. The Barcelona team did have some animal model data.[6] However the method used to treat Claudia was significantly different from this original demonstration of the approach. Nevertheless this was allowed as an exceptional case by the Spanish authorities. Even though there was no direct evidence that our proposed approach would work. (iv) The decellularised scaffold had to be free of donor cells to avoid immune rejection. The process for producing the cell-free scaffold should have been regulated and the material should have been CE marked for human use. Again, the Spanish transplantation authorities allowed this as an exception.

In January 2009 the European Union brought into force the 'Advanced Therapy Medicinal Products' (ATMP) Regulation, providing a new regulatory framework for development of cell therapies. In order to turn a cell therapy into a product that can be made available to large numbers of patients the production process has to be validated and finally approved by the European Medicines Agency (EMEA). A further layer of regulation is involved if the cells being used for a therapy have had a gene inserted. In the UK, permission for a clinical trial for a gene and cell therapy must come from the Gene Therapy Advisory Committee (GTAC) in addition to the 'Medicines and Healthcare Products Regulatory Agency' (MHRA)/EMEA. The UK Department of Health, recognising the complexity of the

---

[6] T. Walles *et al.* Experimental Generation of a Tissue-Engineered Functional and Vascularized Trachea. *The Journal of Thoracic and Cardiovascular Surgery* 2004; 128(6): 900–906.

existing situation, has produced a draft UK Regulatory Route Map for Stem Cell Research and Manufacture[7] to help those of us working in the field navigate our way around an otherwise quite incomprehensible legislative framework. This new regulatory environment is potentially of benefit if it provides a robust, single process that allows new cell therapies to be used in all EU countries. However there is a serious risk that the regulations will be interpreted by the authorities with minimal flexibility and that will make it essentially impossible to exploit this new technology effectively.

An unregulated health care industry is unthinkable. Protecting patient safety must be paramount in our planning and procedures. The current raft of legislation is designed to minimise risk to patients and to measure what happens if things go wrong. However there is another risk that is not routinely quantified by the regulators. It is the risk that some therapies will never reach clinical trial or commercial exploitation because the burden of meeting regulatory requirements is so heavy that resources will not be available. Patients may continue to suffer and some may die because a new treatment could not be exploited. The challenge is to measure this outcome effectively. If a cell therapy does not get the backing of investors to be developed in line with regulatory requirements, then it will be impossible to know how effective it would have been in treating patients. How do you measure the negative effects of over-regulation on the number of useful treatments? As a scientist working with stem cells my aim is to bring as many new therapies into clinical reality as possible so that they can benefit the largest number of patients. Minimising the very real and partially quantifiable risks of side effects from new treatments must surely be balanced against the equally real, but impossible to quantify, risks of failing to develop treatments because of excessive or inflexible regulation. Without this balanced approach the regulatory system will be guilty of the bureaucratic equivalent of walking by on the other side of the road. In Claudia's case this balance was achieved by making her well aware of the early stage of development of the procedure. Indeed at one point in her

[7] Department of Health UK, Gene Therapy Advisory Committee. 2009. *UK Regulatory Route Map for Stem Cell Research and Manufacture.* Available at: http://www.advisorybodies.doh.gov.uk/genetics/gtac/InterimUKSCroutemap120309.pdf [Accessed 09 Jul 2009].

decision-making process she asked to see some of the pigs that had been implanted with an experimental trachea. What was good enough for them was good enough for her!

I raise these issues in a frank way to stimulate further ethical discussion: and I hope that the example given here emphasises that the issues discussed in this book are very real and have a human face. There are of course many reasons not to do things; not to take risks. But at some point we have to cross over the road and plunge headlong into helping those who are suffering. Regulators have no choice but to work within the regulatory framework that has been established in law. There may some degree of flexibility of interpretation but otherwise there can be no questioning of the procedures that must be followed. I am bound by the law, but unlike the regulators I am also free to question the law and how it operates. As a scientist directly involved in therapeutics, I plead with my colleagues who are experts in ethics to grapple with these complex issues and help us to find a way forward that protects the patient both from the harm of doing too much and the harm of doing nothing at all.

2

STEM CELL TECHNOLOGY: FROM RESEARCH REGULATION TO CLINICAL APPLICATIONS

Donald Chalmers

INTRODUCTION

Stem cell science has received widespread international coverage since two important breakthroughs in the 1990s. Firstly, the cloning of Dolly the sheep in 1996 — the first mammal to be created using somatic cell nuclear replacement — showed that somatic nuclei could be reprogrammed to a pluripotent state.[1] Secondly, the isolation and culture of human embryonic stem cells in 1998, demonstrated that human pluripotency was possible.[2] The benefits for regenerative medicine were potentially revolutionary for therapeutic applications. In fact, stem cell technology dates back much further. Bone marrow transplants have been established treatments in clinical cancer care for many years. This procedure relies on the same underlying premise of other stem cell technologies; namely, the regenerative properties of stem cells. In the treatment of leukaemia, for example, the cancerous forming bone marrow of the recipient is destroyed, before being replaced with the healthy bone marrow of a matched donor. The healthy marrow contains haematopoietic stem cells, which readily regenerate a functional

---

[1] I. Wilmut *et al.* Viable Offspring Derived From Fetal and Adult Mammalian Cells. *Nature* 1997; 385(6619): 810–813.

[2] Potency — the capacity to differentiate into specialised cell types — is discussed in more detail below. J. Thomson *et al.* Embryonic Stem Cell Lines Derived from Human Blastocysts. *Science* 1998; 282: 1145–1147.

blood system. These stem cells, however, are multipotent, and limited to becoming progeny found in the blood system niche.

The breakthrough with human pluripotent stem cells in 1998 — that is cells which are not limited to any cell lineage — has been followed by a massive research and investment effort by the private and public sectors in stem cell technology and specialised facilities. Stem cell research has become an area of intense international competitiveness.[3] The reason for this excitement is the prospect of finding cures for novel disease targets, and for developing therapies for previously untreatable cell, tissue and organ damage. Stem cells are also a valuable tool for basic science, shedding light on the processes of embryogenesis, normal growth and disease development.[4] Some of this research is translating into early phase clinical trials. The US National Institutes of Health (NIH) lists over 2400 stem cell trials, some of which have been completed, but many are active and recruiting.[5] More concerning, a few offshore clinics and companies operating out of various low regulation countries, are offering dubious, unpublished and unconfirmed stem cell 'treatments'.[6]

This paper aims to set the stage, and introduce some of the themes of this book. The paper also examines the current stage of experimentation in stem cell technology, the regulatory frameworks established for the derivation of stem cells, particularly those derived from human embryos, and the protections and procedures for the applications of stem cells generally in clinical practice. The paper concludes with an analysis of the important *International Society for Stem Cell Research Guidelines*, and assesses

[3] D. Sipp. Stem Cell Research in Asia: A Critical View. *Journal of Cellular Biochemistry* 2009; Ahead of Print: doi: 10.1002/jcb.22160.

[4] J. Thomson. 2001. Human Embryonic Stem Cells. In *The Human Embryonic Stem Cell Debate: Science, Ethics, and Public Policy*. S. Holland, K. Lebacqz and L. Zoloth, eds. Cambridge, Massachusetts: Massachusetts Institute of Technology: 15–26.

[5] The United States National Institutes of Health clinical trials website. Available at: http://clinicaltrials.gov/ct2/results?term=stem+cell+trials [Accessed 15 March 2009, with 2452 trials listed].

[6] S. Kiatpongsan and D. Sipp. Monitoring and Regulating Offshore Stem Cell Clinics. *Science* 2009; 323: 1564–1565; and M. Enserink. Selling the Stem Cell Dream. *Science* 2006; 313: 160–163.

whether these represent an acceptable, best-practice model for the future development of international policies and national regulation of stem cell research as it translates to clinical applications.

THE DERIVATION OF STEM CELLS AND THE CURRENT SCIENCE

Much of the heightened public coverage of stem cells dates from the Dolly report of a somatic cell nuclear transfer procedure undertaken at the Roslin Institute in Scotland in 1997. This 'cloning' procedure built on earlier research work in animal studies.[7] The experiments showed that differentiated somatic cells could be reset by transferring them to an enucleated oocyte, and thus suggesting that any adult cell could be changed back to a premature pluripotent state (a process called Cell Nuclear Replacement or CNR, sometimes also referred to as Somatic Cell Nuclear Transfer).[8] But the Dolly research also extended to discussion of stem cell technology in humans: a year later, Thomson *et al.*'s work showed that a human pluripotent state was present in human blastocysts; and in 2001, the first human cloned embryo was reported.[9] The latter experiment showed that any human somatic cell — given the conditions provided by a human or animal ooctye — could be reprogrammed to a pluripotent state. Later, in 2008, the factors necessary for reprogramming somatic cells were characterised, and were used to induce human skin cells to a pluripotent-like state.[10] Together, these advances in the understanding of human pluripotency create a vision of regenerative medicine — prospectively allowing the clinical replacement of any cells, tissues and organs genetically compromised, or

---

[7] The isolation of embryonic stem cells from mouse embryos was reported as early as 1981. G. Martin. Isolation of a Pluripotent Cell Line from Early Mouse Embryos Cultured in Medium Condition by Teratocarcinoma Stem Cells. *Proceedings of the National Academy of Science* 1981; 78: 7634; M. Evans and M. Kaufman. Establishment and Culture of Pluripotential Cells from Mouse Embryos. *Nature* 1981; 292: 154.

[8] Wilmut *et al., op. cit.* note 1.

[9] J. Cibelli, R. Lanza and M. West. 2001. The First Human Cloned Embryo. *Scientific American*. 24 November.

[10] K. Takahashi *et al.* Induction of Pluripotent Stem Cells from Adult Human Fibroblasts by Defined Factors. *Cell* 2007; 131: 861–872; J. Yu *et al.* Induced Pluripotent Stem Cell Lines Derived from Human Somatic Cells. *Science* 2007; 318: 1917–1920.

damaged by diseases or accidents. What is more, these transplants may be engineered to be compatible with the recipient's immune system.[11]

The unique properties of stem cells are their capacity for '... prolonged proliferation with retention of their undifferentiated form ... together with a stable developmental potential to give rise to derivative cells'.[12] A UK Report described a stem cell as:

> '...an unspecialised cell at an early stage of development. Under certain conditions, stem cells can divide and differentiate into a large number of cell types that make up the tissues and organs of the body. In addition, they can undergo self-renewal, a process by which an unspecialised stem cell divides to produce two further unspecialised stem cells. The ability of stem cells to self-renew in this way means that a relatively small number of stem cells can be grown in the laboratory into the very large number of stem cells that would be needed for clinical applications'.[13]

---

[11] Pluripotent stem cells appear to induce a limited immune response; although whether this is the same for larger tissues and organs remain to be seen. Induced Pluripotent Stem Cells will be derived from the recipients own cells, and thus are recognised as autologous (self-) transplants (discussed below). Likewise, embryonic stem cells can be derived from embryos created by CNR techniques (using an embryo to reprogramme the potential recipients own somatic DNA). See: A. Kind and A. Colman. Therapeutic Cloning: Needs and Prospects. *Cell and Developmental Biology* 1999; 10: 279–286. The term 'therapeutic cloning' was used as a synonym for stem cell research in the late 1990s. Although the term is considered as misleading by some, it is the prevailing term used to distinguish cloning techniques for the derivation of stem cells from those used for reproductive cloning. See criticisms of the term in the Report of the Human Genetics Advisory Commission and the Human Fertilisation and Embryology Authority. 1998. *Cloning Issues in Reproduction, Science and Medicine*. Available at http://www.advisorybodies.doh.gov.uk/hgac/index.html [Accessed 12 May 2009].

[12] See: Australian Health Ethics Committee. 1998. *Scientific, Ethical and Regulatory Considerations Relevant to Cloning of Human Beings A Report to the Commonwealth Minister.* Canberra: NMMRC: para 2.17. Available at http://www.nhmrc.gov.au/publications/synopses/e45.htm [Accessed 12 May 2009].

[13] Department of Health. Chief Medical Officer's Expert Group. 2000. *Stem Cell Research: Medical Progress with Responsibility.* UK: Department of Health: 17; see also: UK Government. 2000. *Government Response to the Recommendations Made in the Chief Medical Officer's Expert Group Report 'Stem Cell Research: Medical Progress with Responsibility' Cmd 4833.*

Researchers are endeavouring to develop and improve procedures for the derivation of human stem cells by culturing and maintaining undifferentiated cells derived from human tissue, including bone marrow, certain adult organs,[14] the umbilical cord and placenta, but also, more controversially, foetal tissue[15] and early-stage human embryos.[16] Some stem cells have greater potential for proliferation; and the gold standard is generally recognised as those obtained from early embryos (at seven to eight days development of the blastocyst).

Stem cells which can derive an entire mature being — including the extra-embryonic support tissue — may be referred to as being *totipotent*: having the potential to differentiate into *all* cell types, including the placenta. This state of potency is limited to the zygote — the pre-blastocyst stage of embryonic development. At the blastocyst stage, the stem cells are referred to as being *pluripotent*, having the potential to differentiate into all the body cells of the organism it is developing into.[17] Later still are multipotent stem cells, which can become a wide range of different cell types, but which are limited to certain cell lineages (and cellular systems, such as the haematopoietic blood system). Others, particularly those derived from adult cells, appear to be more limited in their potency to differentiate and proliferate into multiple cell types. CNR, however, showed that adult cells could revert to a pluripotent state given the conditions of an enucleated oocyte. Furthermore,

---

[14] Including brain, blood, skeletal muscle, pancreas, liver, skin, the eye and the lining of the gastrointestinal tract. See: National Academies Committee on the Biological and Biomedical Applications of Stem Cell Research. 2001. *Stem Cells and the Future of Regenerative Medicine.* Washington DC, US: National Academies Press.

[15] Including neural stem cells, neural crest cells, haemopoietic (blood) stem cells and progenitors of pancreatic islet cells. See: Department of Health. Chief Medical Officer's Expert Group, *op. cit.* note 13, p. 9; and National Academies Committee on the Biological and Biomedical Applications of Stem Cell Research, *op. cit.* note 14, pp. 17–29.

[16] Wilmut *et al., op. cit.* note 1.

[17] Although there was a flurry of interest in the distinction between *totipotency* and *pluripotency* there now seems to be a preference for the term *pluripotency* in the lexicon. This is partly because although the totipotent state may be considered as absolute potency — being able to form the embryo independently and *de novo* — it is unlikely to be an exploitable area for research and future therapies.

recent evidence suggests that a pluripotent state may be induced by altering specific genes in somatic cells to create induced Pluripotent stem cells (iPS Cells).[18] iPS cells, some expect, will sidestep the ethical barriers of embryonic and foetal research.[19]

The Promise and Hype of Stem Cells

Stem cell technology is another chapter in the continuing search for reliable sources of regenerative tissue for medical treatments. The excitement about stem cell research derives principally from two facts: their *proven* and successful use for some blood disorders (e.g. whole blood transplants);[20] and their ability to fix complex diseases, often within intricate systems (such as the spinal cord or brain). The technology is being promoted, like foetal tissue before, as a potential treatment for degenerative brain diseases, which are often associated with ageing, such as Parkinson's disease and Alzheimer's disease. Unsurprisingly, many of the current disease targets for stem cells are those affecting the ageing demography of most OECD countries. These disease targets are also where resources are available to invest in this high-tech, and expensive area. Stem cell therapy is also targeting treatment for diabetes,[21] heart disease, spinal cord injury and some cancers.[22] Stem cell therapies may eventuate in a range of transplantation procedures, including stem cell therapy for nerve, muscle, various blood cell types, liver, pancreas and heart diseases.[23] There is also conjecture about the prospect of engineering multi-cell organs.[24] CNR (with respect to

---

[18] Discussed below. For an overview of the science, see: S. Yamanaka. A Fresh Look at iPS Cells. *Cell* 2009; 137: 13–17.

[19] Cf. J. Meyer. The Significance of Induced Pluripotent Stem Cells for Basic Research and Clinical Therapy. *Journal of Medical Ethics* 2008; 34: 849–851.

[20] J. Hows. Status of Umbilical Cord Blood Transplantation in the Year 2001. *Journal of Clinical Pathology* 2001; 54: 428–483.

[21] Treated stem cells may enable patients to avoid insulin injections, see: Juvenile Research Foundation International at http://www.jdrf.org/index.cfm.

[22] Department of Health, *op. cit.* note 13, p. 5.

[23] Ibid: 16–17.

[24] P. Bianco and P.G. Robey. Stem Cells in Tissue Engineering. *Nature* 2001; 414: 118–121.

creating embryonic stem cells) and cell inducement (to modify somatic cells) techniques would additionally mean that autologous cell lines are possible, thus avoiding the problems of allogeneic transplants and immune-rejection.

There is much optimism, and a degree of hype, about the promise of stem cell research. The technology has been claimed to be 'the greatest and most exciting medical breakthrough' and 'one of the biggest breakthroughs in human medicine', promising 'very great potential benefits'.[25] In the same vein, a US Report stated that: '[s]tem cell research offers unprecedented opportunities for developing new medical therapies for debilitating diseases and a new way to explore fundamental questions of biology'.[26]

Adult and Embryonic Stem Cell Lines

Stem cells derived from human tissue, other than human embryos, have generally met with little controversy since they involve minimal invasive techniques. That is not to say, however, that an ethically robust framework of property and ownership rights currently exists, and which represent ongoing complexity in the procurement and commodification of human cells.[27] On the other hand, embryonic stem cells have been surrounded with great ethical controversy because they are, and have been, sourced from 'surplus' (excess to the needs of the couple) embryos in Assisted Reproductive Technology (ART) programs, or created by CNR techniques, specifically for research.[28] The use of

[25] See: generally, the House of Representatives Standing Committee on Legal and Constitutional Affairs. 2001. *Human Cloning: Scientific, Ethical and Regulatory Aspects of Human Cloning and Stem Cell Research*. Canberra: AGPS: paras 3.23–3.34.

[26] National Academies Committee on the Biological and Biomedical Applications of Stem Cell Research, *op. cit.* note 14, p. 1.

[27] See: MacKenney and Capps, this volume.

[28] The National Research Council Institute of Medicine of National Academies, Human Embryonic Stem Cell Research Advisory Committee. 2008. *The National Academies' Guidelines for Human Embryonic Stem Cell Research*. Washington US: National Academies Press.

human embryos raises profound issues about the moral status of the human embryo and its use as a means to an end.[29] From a scientific point of view, however, most advocate research on both embryonic and adult stem cells as it is not yet possible to conclude which are most clinically suitable. For example, embryonic stem cells may possess greater potential levels of plasticity than stem cells isolated from adult tissue.[30] Embryonic stem cells, however, also raise scientific questions. For example, the *Stem Cells and Regenerative Medicine* Report noted that embryonic stem cell lines may be unstable, exhibit and accumulate genetic mutations as a consequence of continual expansion and differentiation,[31] and raise the possibility of tumour development; concluding that: '[m]ajor questions remain about the genetic or environmental factors…that control the fate of ES [embryonic stem cells] and about the…various stages of cell differentiation'.[32]

Recent Developments in Alternatives to Embryonic Stem Cells

Some procedures for the creation of stem cells were proposed that attempted to avoid the use of human embryos or human embryo derived stem cell lines. Various proposals emerged, particularly during 2004. In the United States, the US President's Council on Bioethics considered one that appeared to circumvent human embryos by engineering embryos that fail to develop the trophectoderm (from which the placenta

[29] R. Deech. Playing God: Who Should Regulate Embryo Research? *Brooklyn Journal of International Law* 2007; 32: 321–341; and D. Chalmers. Professional Self-Regulation and Guidelines in ART. *Journal of Law and Medicine* 2002; 9: 414–428. See also: L. Andrews. The Legal Status of the Embryo. *Loyola Law Review* 1992; 32: 357; and A. Eser. The Legal Status of the Embryo in Comparative Perspective. *International Journal of Medicine and Law* 1992; 11: 579.

[30] Y. Qi-Long *et al.* The Ground State of Embryonic Stem Cell Self-Renewal. *Nature* 2008; 453: 519–523.

[31] National Academies Committee on the Biological and Biomedical Applications of Stem Cell Research, *op. cit.* note 14, p. 27.

[32] Ibid. 23.

normally develops).[33] This particular proposal was treated with skepticism and was scientifically criticised.[34] Other reports emerged around this time about 'embryoid' (embryo-like) bodies and protein injection to human eggs to stimulate a parthenogenetic blastocyst development that could produce a source of cells without creating a 'normal' embryo.[35]

The research effort has also focussed on attempts to create a reliable supply of cells that have the same genetic makeup as the patient with the specific disease. In this respect, much effort has been devoted to CNR procedures that attempt to create stem cell lines of specific disease conditions for study. In turn there are efforts to manipulate stem cell lines from the patient and to use these cells to combat the particular patient's disease (often in combination with other drugs).[36]

There has been a significant development with the simultaneous publication of two reports of the creation of iPS cells from human fibroblasts: one

---

[33] Dr. William Hurlbut, at Stanford University, proposed using 'altered nuclear transfer' to create entities in which a *Cdx2* mutation would be introduced *in vitro* into a human (skin) cell that would then be used as a nuclear donor to obtain embryonic stem cells by nuclear transfer. In this way the CNR entity could never become a viable embryo, and would thus represent an ethically uncontroversial source of human embryonic stem cells. W.B. Hurlbut. 2004. *Altered Nuclear Transfer as a Morally Acceptable Means for the Procurement of Human Embryonic Stem Cells.* Washington US: The President's Council on Bioethics. Available at: http://www.bioethics.gov/background/hurlbut.html [Accessed 12 May 2009].

[34] Dr. Charles Jennings, of the Harvard Stem Cell Institute, argued the Cdx2 gene will not work in humans as it does in mice; D. Melton, G. Daley and C. Jennings. Altered Nuclear Transfer in Stem Cells: A Flawed Proposal. *New England Journal of Medicine* 2004; 351: 2791–2793; with reply from C. Hurlbut, in *New England Journal of Medicine* 2004; 352: 1153–1154.

[35] See: H. Mertes, G. Pennings and A. Van Steirteghem. An Ethical Analysis of Alternative Methods to Obtain Pluriopotent Stem Cells Without Destroying Embryos. *Human Reproduction* 2006; 21: 2749–2775; see also: K. Devolder. What's in a Name? Embryos, Entities, and ANTities in the Stem Cell Debate. *Journal of Medical Ethics* 2006; 32: 43–48.

[36] D. Dimos *et al.* Induced Pluripotent Stem Cells Generated from Patients with ALS Can Be Differentiated into Motor Neurons. *Science* 2008; 21: 1218–1221.

in Japan;[37] and the other in Wisconsin, USA.[38] More recently, researchers have for the first time reprogrammed mouse skin cells into an embryonic-like state using proteins alone; and this avoids the use of potentially carcinogenic viruses, which were used in earlier experiments.[39] iPS cells show many similarities to pluripotent stem cells; and importantly, they appear to proliferate indefinitely and to differentiate into functional daughter cells across cell lineages. Importantly, these iPS cells are not derived from human embryos. Equally, because they can be derived from skin cell biopsies, autologous transplant techniques would avoid using enucleated human (or animal) eggs for the creation of immunological matched embryonic stem cells using CNR. It has been widely suggested that this procedure removes much of the moral objection to the use of excess embryos for the production of stem cells. Not only does it avoid using human embryos, but additionally it curtails the demand on women to donate oocytes for research, and negates the supposed needs to create animal occyte-human chimeras. However, much research work lies ahead in the characterisation of the respective qualities of embryonic, CNR and iPS stem cells.[40]

REGULATION OF STEM CELL RESEARCH

Stem cell research that does not involve the use of surplus ART (which is specifically using *in vitro* fertilisation techniques) embryos has generally not created any great conundrums for legislators, since this type of

---

[37] K. Takahashi *et al.* Induction of Pluripotent Stem Cells from Adult Human Fibroblasts by Defined Factors. *Cell* 2007; 131: 861–872; K. Takahasi and S. Yamanaka. Induction of Pluripotent Stem Cells from Mouse Embryonic and Adult Fibroblast Cultures by Defined Factors. *Cell* 2006; 126: 663–676. See also: B. Goldman. 2008. Embryonic Stem Cells 2.0. *Nature Reports Stem Cells* 1 May. doi: 10.1038/stemcells.2008.67.

[38] J. Yu *et al.* Induced Pluripotent Stem Cell Lines Derived from Human Somatic Cells. *Science* 2007; 318: 1917–1920. This paper was co-authored by the leading scientist, Professor J.A. Thomson.

[39] H. Zhou *et al.* Generation of Induced Pluripotent Stem Cells Using Recombinant Proteins. *Cell Stem Cell* 2009; 4: 381–384.

[40] On the comparison of iPS embryonic stem cells and CNR stem cells, see: S. Nishikawa *et al.* The Promise of Human Induced Pluripotent Stem Cells for Research and Therapy. *Nature Reviews Molecular Cell Biology* 2008; 9: 725–729.

research has traditionally proceeded under the umbrella of national guidelines for human research, particularly those dealing with human tissue research.

Whether legislation or guidelines are introduced, regulation has a similar effect in substance rather than form. Legislation and guidelines in countries that permit human embryo research to develop stem cell lines endorse, what Professor Brownsword has described accurately, a 'restrictive tilt'. This includes:[41]

- only surplus ART embryos may be used in research;
- the consent of the parties creating the embryos is required, both ensuring that the embryos are 'surplus' and that permission is given from them to be used in research;
- the purposes of the research are generally limited and require careful justification;
- the research must be approved by Research Ethics Review Committees;
- the research results are often required to be published; sometimes the material (such as stem cell lines) must be deposited in a public bank;
- national licensing or approval agencies may impose conditions on the research.

Restrictions are usual in relation to the purpose of the human embryo research. No country has allowed, as yet, unlimited research on embryos (where national legislation is lacking, 'soft law' — usually that concerning professional regulation and ART clinics — fills the void.) There are important differences in some states (see tables 1 and 2) — for example, some countries allow the creation of embryos by any means (UK), others permit ART techniques only, and others allow CNR only (Sweden). In countries that prohibit embryo research, there may be permission for stem cell lines derived elsewhere (under the conditions above) to be used.[42]

---

[41] R. Brownsword. Regulating Human Genetics: New Dilemmas for a New Millennium. *Medical Law Review* 2004; 12:14–39. See also: D. Chalmers. The Regulation of Embryo and Stem Cell Research in Australia: Licensing with a Restrictive Tilt. *Journal of International Biotechnology Law* 2008; 5: 177–185.

[42] R. Green. Benefiting from Evil: An Incipient Moral Problem in Stem Cell Research. *Bioethics* 2002; 16: 544–556.

Table 1: Current Regulation — European Union[43]

Permits Research[i]	Not Clear	No Law	Prohibits Research
Belgium[C, T,]	*Cyprus*	Luxemburg	*Austria**
Czech Republic (see: Sykoria, this volume)	*Bulgaria* *Portugal* Romania	Malta	*Germany** (imported lines created before 1 May 2007)
Denmark	*Slovak Republic* (see: Sykoria, this volume)		*Ireland*
Estonia			*Italy**
Finland[C?]			Lithuania
France			*Poland*
Greece			
Hungary			
Latvia			
Netherlands			
Slovenia			
Spain			
Sweden[C,T]			
UK[C, T, HA] (see: Holm and Hammond-Browning, this volume)			

KEY

[i] = On supernumerary embryos

Italics = ratified European Convention on Human Rights and Bioethics

[C] = Allows creation of embryos

* = Allows import of ES cells

[T] = Allows CNR

[HA] = Allows creation of human-animal chimeras

However, stem cells derived from human embryos have created conundrums for national legislators struggling to find the right regulatory balance between freedom to pursue this promising and lucrative research, and 'respect' for the profound ethical concerns in some sectors of society about the moral status of the human embryo, whether surplus to reproductive

[43] See: B. Capps. 2005. The Human Embryo, Stem Cell Research, and the European Union. In *Crossing Borders: Cultural, Religious, and Political Differences Concerning Stem Cell Research: A Global Approach.* W. Bender, C. Hauskeller and A. Manzei, eds. Münster: Agenda Verlag: 435–467. Updated for this chapter.

Table 2: Current Regulation — Global[44]

Permits Research on Spare Embryos, Creation of Embryos and CNR	Moratorium Lifted	Spare Embryos Only	Prohibits Derivation, Allows Import/Use of Cell Lines
Australia (see: Kerridge and Lysaght, this volume)	South Korea[45]	Brazil	Norway
		Canada[46]	USA Federal (see: Lomax, this volume)[47]
		India	
P. R. China (see: Qiu and Zhai, this volume)		Switzerland (approved in national referendum, 2004)	
Israel[48]			
Japan (see: Akabayashi and Kodama, this volume)		Taiwan	
Mexico			
New Zealand[49]			
Russia			
Singapore [HA,50]			
Saudi Arabia			
South Africa			
USA: Seven states have permissive laws[51]			

KEY

[HA] = Allows creation of animal-human hybrids.

[44] Unless otherwise stated, this information is from a number of verifiable sources to be found on the University of Minnesota's MBBNet website: http://www.mbbnet.umn.edu/scmap.html [Accessed 12 May 2009].

[45] A three-year ban on embryo research was lifted in 2009; South Korea to Lift Ban on Human Stem Cell Research. *The Washington Post* (The Associated Press). 29 April 2009. Chimera/hybrid research was banned in 2008; Anon. 2009. South Korea Re-enters Human Stem-cell Research. *Nature* 459: 23.

[46] The *Assisted Human Reproduction Act* 2004 establishes a federal agency (the AHRC Assisted Human Reproduction Canada) to regulate ART and the Act essentially bans human embryo research.

needs or not. As Professor Pellegrino has aptly stated: 'How in essence do we place biotechnology within ethical constraints without losing its therapeutic potential? How do we do so in a democratic, morally and pluralistically divided society, driven equally by market forces and a yearning for immortality through technology?'[52]

While there is no international consensus on the status of the embryo, there has been some headway in establishing minimum standards with respect to research using embryonic stem cells derived from human embryos. This is typified by the approach taken in the European Union's

---

[47] The restrictive policy of President Bush, limiting funding to 22 cell lines existing before August 2001, was repealed by an executive order by President Obama on 9 March 2009. The Dickey-Wicker amendment signed on 11 March, however, prohibited any federal funding for research which destroys human embryos. Federal research must use cell lines created by other scientists from spare embryos, and not use those from CNR or chimeras. The NIH Guidelines (effective on) 7 July 2009 are available at: http://stemcells.nih.gov/policy/2009guidelines.htm; see also: 2009. *Part IV Executive Order 13505 — Removing Barriers to Responsible Scientific Research Involving Human Stem Cells.* 9 Mar. Federal Register. On the Policy of George Bush, see: Green, *op. cit.* note 42; also: Australia Parliament House of Representatives Standing Committee on Legal and Constitutional Affairs. 2001. *Human Cloning: Scientific, Ethical and Regulatory Aspects of Human Cloning and Stem Cell Research.* Canberra: AGPS: para 10.72.

[48] J. Schenker. Legal Aspects of ART Practice in Israel. *Journal of Assisted Reproduction and Genetics* 2003; 20: 7.

[49] *Human Assisted Reproductive Technology Act* 2004 also allows regulated research.

[50] See: Ministry of Health, Singapore. *Research Involving Human Embryos Act* and *Prohibition of Human Cloning Act*, which was based on the Australian State of Tasmania's legislation. Available at: http://www.moh.gov.sg/mohcorp/legislatios.aspx?id=7084 [Accessed 12 May 2009].

[51] As a result of Bush's policy, embryonic research passed to the private sector; but taking on the responsibility of regulating such research, many of the states enacted their own legislation to either permit or prohibit such research. Although it is clear that two States prohibit research, the rest vary from being restrictive, unclear, and 'supportive' of human embryonic stem cell research; see National Conference for State Legislatures: http://www.ncsl.org/programs/health/Genetics/embfet.htm.

[52] E. Pellegrino. Balancing Science, Ethics and Politics: Stem Cell Research, a Paradigm Case. *Journal of Contemporary Health Law and Policy* 2002; 18: 591. See also: A. Capron. Stem Cells: Ethics, Law and Politics. *Biotechnology Law Report* 2001; 20: 678.

Tissue Directive, which states, in aiming to establish minimum standards in aspects of stem cell research, that:[53]

> 'This Directive should not interfere with decisions made by Member States concerning the use or non-use of any specific type of human cells...including embryonic stem cells [see also: Article 4(3)]. If...any particular use of such cells is authorised in a Member State, this Directive will require the application of all provisions necessary to protect public health... (Recital 12)'.

Public health, in this sense, referred to the interests of donors and patients involved in research; and intentionally it excludes any interests of the embryo.

Research using cells from non-embryonic sources has generally been covered by the established international standards for medical research. As the tables above indicate, there is a diversity of national policies in relation to human embryo research, including research to derive stem cells and cloning techniques.[54] This diversity reflects the multiplicity of regulatory schemes on ART in the various countries.[55] Broadly, national regulation on human embryo research and the derivation of stem cells can be classified into three categories of *strict* (with a predominant prohibition), *licensing* (to allow limited research), or *guideline* schemes (denoting 'soft' professional regulations).[56]

---

[53] Directive 2004/23/EC of the European Parliament and of the Council of 31 March 2004 *on setting standards of quality and safety for the donation, procurement, testing, processing, preservation, storage and distribution of human tissues and cells*. See: Capps, *op. cit.* note 44.

[54] R. Isasi *et al.* Research Ethics: Legal and Ethical Approaches to Stem Cell and Cloning Research: A Comparative Analysis of Policies in Latin America, Asia and Africa. *Journal of Law, Medicine and Ethics* 2004; 32: 626–640.

[55] I. Bleiklie, M. Goggin and C. Rothmayr. 2003. *Comparative Biomedical Policy: Governing Assisted Reproductive Technologies*. London: Routledge.

[56] S. Halliday. A Comparative Approach to the Regulation of Human Embryonic Stem Cell Research in Europe. *Medical Law Review* 2004; 12: 40–69. In this paper, Halliday suggests there are, essentially, either prohibitive bans or permissive licensing.

Strict Regulation

The German legislative framework reflects an attitude that is highly protective of human embryos;[57] and provides a clear legislative example of the deployment of strict regulations in embryo research. The German *Embryo Protection Act* (*Embryonenschutzgestz*) 1990 introduced severe criminal penalties for unsanctioned attempts to fertilise eggs or cause pregnancies.[58] These criminal penalties set limits on the type of activity, which could be undertaken in ART facilities, and specifically it is an offence to create, or destroy any embryo, for the purpose of research. In 2002, via a new Act, the German Parliament allowed embryonic stem cell research, but only on imported lines, and whilst maintaining its strict prohibition on all forms of human cloning.[59] The law created a cut-off date, after which any embryonic cell line created could not be used. Subsequently, this date was extended.[60] Other countries maintain bans on all embryo research, such as Austria, Ireland and the Philippines. Italy has moved from the unregulated to the strict regulation category. In 2003, Italy introduced *Law 40*, which limited ART to heterosexual couples of childbearing age and placed strict prohibitions on research that involves the destruction of an embryo.[61]

---

[57] H. Gottweis. Stem Cell Policies in the United States and Germany: Between Bioethics and Regulation. *Policy Studies Journal* 2002; 30: 441. See also: H.-G. Dederer. Regulation of Human Embryonic Stem Cell Research in Germany. *Journal International Biotechnology Law* 2006; 3: 63–71; and J. Robertson. Reproductive Technology in Germany and the United States: An Essay in Comparative Law and Bioethics. *Columbia Journal of Transnational Law* 2004; 43: 189–203.

[58] *Embryo Protection Act* 1990; Gesets zum Schutz von Embryonen [Embryonenschutzgesets] translated in *Bulletin of Medical Ethics* Dec 1990 at 9–11.

[59] T. Heinemann and L. Honnefelder. Principles in Ethical Decision-Making. *Bioethics* 2002; 16: 541. The *Stem Cell Act* ('Bill Guaranteeing Embryo Protection in the Context of Importation and Use of Human Embryonic Stem Cells'; 'Stammzellgesetz' — StZG) 2002.

[60] N. Stafford. Germany Liberalises Law on Stem Cell Research. *British Medical Journal* 2008; 336: 851.

[61] *Legge 19 Febbraio 2004,* No. 40 'Norme in material di procreasione medicalmente assistita' Article 11. Italy was one of the last European countries to pass such laws. *Law 40* rejected the recommendations of the Nobel Prize winner Renate Dulbecco, whose Commission had recommended stem cell research on surplus embryos. See: M. Rechlin. Bioethics in Italy: Two Reasons of Discontent. *Journal International de Bioethique* 2004; 15: 173–185. Available at www.cairn.info/load_pdf.php?ID_ARTICLE=JIB_152_0173 [Accessed 12 May 2009].

Licensing Schemes

Australia has a national licensing scheme, under the *Research Involving Human Embryos Act* 2002,[62] for research on surplus ART human embryos and CNR. This Act creates a Licensing Committee, within the *National Health Medical Research Council*, which overseas embryo research in the private *and* public sector. The Act allows the use of '*excess* ART (IVF) embryos' to carry out approved research. Criminal offences apply when excess ART embryos are used *without* a valid licence.[63] A Legislation Review recommended the introduction of licences for CNR and the legislation was amended to this effect in 2005.[64] Embryo research is permitted when the licence applicant demonstrates, amongst other matters, that the embryo research project: (a) restricts the number of ART embryos to the number *necessary* to achieve the goals of the project and (b) demonstrates a likelihood of significant advance in knowledge or improvement in technologies for treatment, which could not reasonably be achieved by other means. These two considerations have been described by Brownsword (in respect to UK regulations) as the principles of proportionality and necessary purpose.[65] In practice, the Licensing Committee's deliberations have often focused on these two considerations[66]

---

[62] See: Chalmers, *op. cit.* note 41; and D. Chalmers. 2006. The Regulation of Cloning and Stem Cell Research. In *Disputes and Dilemmas in Health Law*. I. Freckelton and K. Petersen, eds. Sydney: Federation Press: Chap. 12: 237–256.

[63] On stem cells and regulation. See: D. Chalmers and D. Nicol. Embryonic Stem Cell Research: Can the Law Balance Ethical, Scientific and Economic Values. *Law and the Human Genome Review* 2003; 18: Part 1 at 43–53 and Part 2 at 91–108; and D. Nicol *et al.* Regulating Biomedical Advances: Embryonic Stem Cell Research. *Macquarie Law Journal* 2002; 2: 31–59.

[64] Australian Government Legislation. 2005. *Review of the Prohibition of Human Cloning Act 2002 and the Research Involving Human Embryos Act* 2002 *Report*. Canberra: AGPS (Chair Justice Lockhart). See: D. Cooper. The Lockhart Review: Where Now for Australia? *Journal of Law and Medicine* 2006; 14: 27–44.

[65] R. Brownsword. Stem Cells, Superman, and the Report of the Select Committee. *Modern Law Review* 2002; 65: 568–587.

[66] NHMRC Licensing Committee. 2004. *Report to the Parliament of Australia*. Period 1 April to 30 September 2004, at 8.

in the 12 licences issued,[67] with three applications for CNR licences pending.

The United Kingdom was the first country to introduce a licensing scheme with the Human Fertilisation and Embryology Authority (HFEA),[68] (following the first ART legislation enacted in Victoria, Australia). Essentially, the HFEA licenses ART clinics and regulates their procedures of gametes collection and storage, clinical use and monitoring. The licensing controls extend to laboratories involved in embryo research. Rules for embryo research include 14-day research limits and standards of consent. The 1990 Act originally set out research purposes which related principally to understanding the causes of infertility, miscarriages, genital diseases, contraception and chromosome abnormalities. These purposes were expanded in 2001 to include research for the purposes of understanding the development of embryos, increasing knowledge of serious disease and the treatment of those diseases.[69] The 2002 amending legislation allows the creation of embryos by CNR, if conditions are met, to obtain embryonic stem cells.[70] The first license was granted in 2004.[71] This is a step beyond many other EU countries.[72]

---

[67] Details of these licences can be seen in the quarterly Reports to Parliament that can be accessed on line at the NHMRC site: http://www.nhmrc.gov.au/research. The Licensing Committee has authorised a number of embryos (2015) for use but the embryos actually used is much less (443). Concerns were expressed during the Parliamentary debates that the numbers in storage and available for research were around the 70,000 figure; see: House of Representatives Standing Committee on Legal and Constitutional Affairs. 2001. *Human Cloning: Scientific, Ethical and Regulatory Aspects of Human Cloning and Stem Cell Research.* Canberra: AGPS.

[68] *Human Fertilisation and Embryology Act* 1990 c. 37. See: E. Nelson. Comparative Perspectives in the Regulation of Assisted Reproductive Technologies in the United Kingdom and Canada. *Alberta Law Review* 2006; 43: 1023–1048.

[69] 2001. Human Embryology and Fertilisation Act (Research Purposes) Regulations. UK.

[70] Halliday, *op. cit.* note 56.

[71] HFEA Grants the First Therapeutic Cloning Licence for Research. 11 August 2004. At: http://www.hfea.gov.uk/758.html [Accessed 12 May 2009].

[72] Note the UK has not signed the Council of Europe's *Convention on Biomedicine* (1997), which would preclude creating embryos for research purposes under Article 18. See: C. Romeo-Casabona. Embryonic Stem Cell Research and Therapy: The Need for a Common European Framework. *Bioethics* 2002; 6: 557–567. (The full title of the Convention is: *Convention for the Protection of Human Rights and Dignity of the Human Being with Regard to the Application of Biology and Medicine: Convention on Human Rights and Biomedicine* CETS No.: 164.)

Guidelines Regulation Schemes

Some jurisdictions continue to rely on 'soft law', such as professional self-regulation and guidelines. These regions of 'under legislation'[73] are less common. The United States has no national (i.e. federal) scheme for ART or human embryo research but has a range of NIH and Food and Drug Administration (FDA) regulations[74] for laboratory standards and Medicare and Medicaid Services supplemented by Department of Health and Human Services policies. There are also few regulations on embryo research[75] and only five states (New Hampshire, Pennsylvania, Louisiana, New Mexico and South Dakota) have regulatory schemes dealing with embryos in the context of ART. The US is following an 'individual-state' track, which follows principles of state sovereignty and federal separation of roles,[76] and has limited federal regulation to the restriction of public funds for existing cell lines (i.e. federal money cannot be used to derive stem cell lines). The President's Council on Bioethics has described the regulatory landscape as a 'patchwork, with authority divided among numerous sources of oversight'.[77] Similarly, the Japanese government has national guidelines for human embryonic stem cell research but has introduced legislation introduced to ban human cloning.[78] Other countries, including India,[79] China[80]

---

[73] An expression used by the Noelle Lenoir cited in: M. Casado. The Conflict Between Legal Interests in Clinical Genetics: Public Health Requirements and the Safeguarding of Human Dignity. *Law and the Human Genome Review* 1996; 4: 27–37.

[74] D. Adamson. Regulation of Assisted Reproductive Technologies in the United States. *Family Law Quarterly* 2005; 39: 727.

[75] A. Ouellette *et al.* Lessons Across the Pond: Assisted Reproductive Technology in the United Kingdom and the United States. *American Journal of Law and Medicine* 2005; 31: 419–446.

[76] See: Lomax, this volume.

[77] President's Council on Bioethics. 2004. *Reproduction and Responsibility: The Regulation of New Biotechnologies.* Washington US: 75.

[78] Japan has a mixed system with legislation banning cloning, the *Law for the Prohibition of Reproductive Cloning* 2000, and regulation for stem cells (Guidelines for the Derivation and Utilisation of Human Embryonic Stem Cells, 2001).

[79] M. Sleeboom-Faulkner and P. Kumar Patra. The Bioethical Vacuum: National Policies on Human Embryonic Stem Cell Research in India and China. *Journal of International Biotechnology Law* 2008; 6: 221–234.

[80] See: China and UK Could Lead World in Stem Cell Research. *BioNews* 17 January 2005; 292: 15–17.

and Spain have also followed the guidelines approach to regulation permitting research on surplus ART embryos.

TOWARDS THE CLINICAL USE OF STEM CELL TECHNOLOGY

It is accepted that a vast amount of basic research remains to be undertaken. Many challenges have to be overcome *before* the use of stem cell therapies become established procedures in the clinic. This is particularly important as some offshore clinics are opening and advertising costly stem cell treatments of unsubstantiated and unproven effectiveness,[81] with a high likelihood of exploitation of the very ill and vulnerable.[82] There is a developing stem cell therapy tourism, similar to the '*tourisme juridique et procreatique*'[83] of the ART business.[84] There have been some calls for monitoring and better regulation of these clinics.[85] There has clearly been some levelling-off of the early excitement about stem cell technology when rapid reporting of experimental results marked stem cell science. It is clear is that critical experimental work must continue and that the results will be much slower than originally expected. There is fundamental research to be done on comparisons between embryonic, adult and iPS stem cells; and this provides a strong, if pragmatic, argument for continuing all forms of research.[86]

---

[81] S. Kiatpongsan and D. Sipp. Offshore Stem Cell Treatments. *Nature Reports Stem Cells* 2008. 3 December. doi:10.1038/stemcells.2008.151.

[82] S. Kiatpongsan and D. Sipp. 2008. On Stem Cell Travel and the Need for Clinical Trials. *Genetics Policy Institute*: *World Stem Cell Report*. Available at: http://www.worldstemcellsummit.com/report_contents.html [Accessed 13 May 2009].

[83] M.-L. Revillard. 1986. Fecondation *in vitro* et Congelation D'embryons. In *Artificial Procreation, Genetics and the Law; Lausanne Colloquium 29–30 November 1985*. J. Stepan, ed. Zurich: Schulthess Polygraphischer Verlag.

[84] D. Spar. Reproductive Tourism and the Regulatory Maze. *New England Journal of Medicine* 2005; 352(6): 531–534; E. Morris. Reproductive Tourism and the Role of the European Union. *Chicago Journal of International Law* 2008; 8: 701–713.

[85] Kiatpongsans and Sipp, *op. cit.* 6.

[86] An argument made in the by the UK's House of Lords Select Committee. 2002. *Stem Cell Research — Report. HL 83(i)*. London: HMSO.

While there are a number of ongoing clinical trials, it will likely be a while before, for example, the current NIH listed experimental trials are subjected to proper scrutiny and assessment. Basic questions still need answers. For example, as yet there is no established standard for scientifically certifying whether an embryonic stem cell line is 'established' by reference to certain genetic tests and the number of times the lines should be able to be frozen, thawed and still demonstrate their capacity to replicate. There are continuing difficulties of both delivery and survival of introduced stem cells.[87] In addition, some stem cell lines have been cultured on murine feeder cells and are unsuitable for any clinical application on humans (restricting the use of any temporal limitation on stem cell lines, such as that of Germany). Furthermore, much of the promising research is still limited to animal models, and 'cannot be presumed to provide definitive evidence of the capabilities of human cells'.[88] Standards for Good Manufacturing Practice are a necessary pre-condition to the use of embryonic stem cells in a clinical setting as part of 'established' clinical practice.

Patient Safety in the Applications of Stem cells

The major ethical issues surrounding stem cells relate to the novelty and safety of the proposed applications. Some stem cell technologies, particularly those involving bone marrow, have been available as standard clinical care for many years. On the other hand, some of the new applications are untested and innovative. In this respect, issues of patient safety are critical. The proposed application must be carefully assessed for risk, that risk properly communicated to the patient and the risk involved in the application properly managed and addressed. Secondly, the application should be subject to independent scientific assessment and ethical review. Thirdly, as with all human research, the risks and benefits should be properly assessed by independent science and ethics review committees. Fourthly, the risks involved must be carefully communicated and

---

[87] Department of Health. Chief Medical Officer's Expert Group, *op. cit.* note 15, pp. 16–20.

[88] National Academies Committee on the Biological and Biomedical Applications of Stem Cell Research, *op. cit.* note 14, p. 22.

explained to the patient involved so that they can give voluntary consent to involvement in the trial. In view of the innovative aspect of the application, the benefits should not be overstated. These ethical issues, including quality control, pre-clinical work, ethical clinical trials, patient safety and ethical evaluation were uppermost in the guidelines looking towards clinical application, particularly those published by the International Society for Stem Cell Research (ISSCR).[89]

Clinical Trials and Combinatorial Therapy

Over the last few years, there has been a rapid escalation in not only in the funding for stem cell research but also clinical trials of the technology. The US NIH clinical trials register site lists 2452 trials that are completed, in progress, or recruiting.[90] Many of these trials are using autologous patient 'adult' stem cells and not controversial embryonic stem cells. This position is reflected in the 321 trials, mentioning stem cells, listed on the Australia and New Zealand Clinical Trial Registry.[91]

There have been some reports of instances of the use of stem cells in clinical therapy with some success. Heart disease is a major target for research effort. For example, in California stem cells were used to repair damaged heart muscles.[92] Cancer, in its many forms, is a major stem cell therapy target. The clinical trials currently in progress are also targeting combinatorial stem cell therapies for multiple sclerosis and other diseases of the immune system, HIV and stroke. A number of the stem cell trials,

---

[89] I. Hyun *et al.* New ISSCR Guidelines Underscore Major Principles for Responsible Translational Stem Cell Research. *Cell Stem Cell* 2008; 3: 607–609.

[90] See: http://clinicaltrials.gov/ct2/results?term=stem+cell+trials [Accessed 15 March 2009 with 2452 trials listed].

[91] See: http://www.anzctr.org.au/trialSearch.aspx [Accessed 12 May 2009], but most of these trials are conventional trials with minor stem cell components. None are listed as using embryonic stem cells. See: TGA. 2003. *Report on Information and Advertising Associated with Products Tested, Created or Manufactured Using Human Embryos or Human Embryonic Stem Cells*. Available at http://www.tga.gov.au/advert/stemcells.htm [Accessed 12 May 2009].

[92] National Academies Committee on the Biological and Biomedical Applications of Stem Cell Research, *op. cit.* note 14, p. 5.

particularly in cancer, rely on modern *Combinatorial Therapy* approaches. Combinatorial Therapy is an approach to treating diseases by using a variety of drugs simultaneously to eliminate or control the cause of the disease.[93] The expression can also be used when drugs are combined with other types of therapy, such as stem cell therapy.[94] There has also been a controversial reported use of adult stem cells in China to treat spinal cord injury, which is another major target.

Clinical Trials and the ISSCR Guidelines

The gradual introduction of stem cell therapies to relieve serious disabilities and diseases will take a number of years of pre-clinical and clinical research before they are approved. Some clinics, often in areas with lax or dubious regulatory structures, have been raising unrealistic hopes for seriously ill patients with promises of entirely novel and untested therapies. In response, the ISSCR has developed *Guidelines for the Clinical Translation of Stem Cells* (2008).[95]

The ISSCR is an independent, non-profit organisation established in 2002 to foster the exchange of information on stem cell research and other collaborations amongst stem cell researchers.[96] Concerned about the possibility of exploitation of vulnerable patients, the ISSCR decided to issue *Guidelines for the Clinical Translation of Stem Cells* with the aim of establishing guidance on the proper and responsible translation of stem

---

[93] P. Lu *et al.* Combinatorial Therapy with Neurotrophins and cAMP Promotes Axonal Regeneration Beyond Sites of Spinal Cord Injury. *Journal of Neuroscience* 2004; 24: 6402–6409.

[94] As examples the NIH clinical trials website lists Thiotepa-Clofarabine-Busulfan with Allogeneic Stem Cell Transplant for High Risk Malignancies; Treosulfan, Fludarabine, Total-Body Irradiation, and Donor Stem Cell Transplant in Treating Patients with High-Risk Acute Myeloid Leukemia or Myelodysplastic Syndrome; Thiotepa-Clofarabine-Busulfan with Allogeneic Stem Cell Transplant for High Risk Malignancies amongst the most recently listed trials: http://clinicaltrials.gov/ct2/results/rss.xml?term=stem+cells&rcv_d=14&count=1000 [Accessed 15 March 2009].

[95] International Society for Stem Cell Research. 2008. *Guidelines for the Clinical Translation of Stem Cells*. Available at: www.isscr.org [Accessed 12 May 2009].

[96] See website: http://www.isscr.org/about/index.htm [Accessed 12 May 2009].

cell research into safe and appropriate applications. These guidelines establish standards, by way of recommendations, to institutions, review committees and investigators on the proper standards to be observed in translational preclinical applications of stem cell technology. The *Guidelines* establish a comprehensive stand-alone set of guidelines for the conduct of stem cell research and clinical applications.

First, the ISSCR *Guidelines* restate the fundamental ethical requirements in human research of standard of care and patient/subject consent. The ISSCR *Guidelines* set out the minimal test requirement that the standard of care 'should compare new stem cell-based therapies against the best medical therapy currently available to the local population' (Recommendation 26); (following bracketed references refer to the *ISSCR Guidelines*) and equally importantly, ensuring the informed consent of those involved in highly innovative interventions (Recommendation 28).

Secondly, the *Guidelines* establish the institution's responsibility for the conduct of any stem cell-based intervention (Recommendation 1). Importantly, Recommendation 2 establishes that human subjects review committees must review the clinical research: '...involving (a) products from human embryonic or other pluripotent stem cells; (b) novel applications of fetal or somatic (adult) stem cells; and (c) haematopoietic or other stem cells used for applications outside established standards of care'. The review of stem cell-based clinical protocols should include advice from researchers with stem cell-specific scientific and ethical expertise. The ISSCR does not anticipate that stem cell research oversight committees will be required to conduct a separate review, although some members of stem cells research committees may be used as consultants to the human subjects review process.

Thirdly, the *Guidelines* provide helpful recommendations on cell processing, manufacture, sourcing of material (Recommendations 3–10). Importantly, the *Guidelines* are generally consistent with national codes of ethical conduct in human research in acquiring proper preclinical studies to be conducted on animal models (Recommendation 11) to assess the efficacy of any proposed stem cell-based intervention (Recommendations 13–15).

Fourthly, the ISSCR *Guidelines* recognise the likely toxicity of stem cells (Recommendations 16–17), and specifically recommend that: 'Risks for tumourigenicity must be assessed for any stem cell-based product, especially when extensively manipulated in culture or when genetically modified. A clear plan to assess the risks of tumourigenicity for any cell product must be implemented under the direction of an independent review body prior to approval for human clinical use' (Recommendation 18).[97]

Fifthly, and most importantly, these *Guidelines* set out, in detail, the required steps for stem cell-based clinical researchers developing any application. The required steps, that researchers should adopt, are as follows:

a. Cooperate with and share scientific expertise to assist other investigators and human subjects research review committees in assessing:
   i. the biological characteristics of the cells to be used in clinical trials;
   ii. whether these cells have been developed with appropriate manufacturing standards;
   iii. pre-clinical data on their use in animal and/or other models for evaluating their safety and efficacy; and
   iv. any early clinical data, if available, which address safety issues in the short- and medium-term and continued observations for long-term effects;
b. Address the risks of stem cell-based interventions including, for example, cell proliferation and/or tumour development, exposure to animal source materials, risks associated with viral vectors, and risks yet unknown;
c. Provide the utmost clarity regarding the potential benefits of participating in the trial with stem cells, since patients may have recourse to reasonable therapeutic alternatives; the informed consent process must emphasise the novel and experimental aspects of cell-based interventions — it is important to minimise misconceptions patients may have about the potential for therapeutic efficacy;
d. Disclose any financial and non-financial conflicts of interest among the investigators, sponsors, and institutions in which the stem cell research is being conducted;

[97] Ibid at 10.

e. Monitor research subjects for long-term health effects and protection of confidentiality of their health data;
f. Provide a clear, timely and effective plan for adverse event reporting;
g. Offer a clinical plan to provide treatment for toxicity, including treatment of tumours that might arise — this plan might include compensation for research-related injuries; and
h. Ensure that insurance coverage or other appropriate financial or medical resources are available to patients to cover potential complications arising from their research participation (Recommendation 20).

These recommended steps for stem cell research applications are supplemented by the requirement of independent regulatory oversight in Recommendation 21, which provides:

> 'All studies involving clinical applications of stem cells, whether publicly or privately sponsored, must be subject to independent review, approval and ongoing monitoring by human subjects research oversight bodies with supplemental appropriate expertise to evaluate the unique aspects of stem cell research and its application in a variety of clinical disciplines. This review and oversight process must be independent of the investigators regardless of whether it occurs at the institutional, regional or national level, and regardless of whether investigators employ the services of a contract research organisation'.[98]

Finally, the ISSCR *Guidelines* deal with peer review of any stem cell research application (Recommendations 23–25) and recommend patient/subjects should be monitored and adverse events reported (Recommendations 29–32).[99]

---

[98] Interestingly, the *Guidelines* recognise that some countries may not have an official national regulatory body and in these cases the ISSCR strongly urges governments to develop such regulatory competence before proceeding.

[99] There are also a number of recommendations about ensuring social justice (Recommendations 35–39).

The ISSCR *Guidelines* are a commendable set of guidelines for the future development of responsible stem cell therapies from research to clinic.[100]

Innovative Therapy

The introduction of any new procedure or therapy is generally treated as research and attracts the usual requirements of human research ethical review. In some countries, national codes of research governance include specific guidelines for innovative research and therapy. Stem cell research and applications are essentially experimental and subject to the usual human research review and prudential procedures.

For example, in Australia, the *National Statement on Ethical Conduct in Human Research* provides that innovations in clinical practice cover a wide spectrum from 'minor variations or extensions of existing methods, to new indications through to completely novel technologies'.[101] However, where a proposal is innovative and/or experimental, this should always be made *clear* to those who might be subject to it.[102] The *National Statement* also recognises the general requirements for innovative therapy to be assessed of a research mode by the institution's Science Review Committee and for an Ethics Committee to make a proper assessment of the risks and benefits involved and to ensure that there is proper monitoring of the procedure and the discontinuance of the therapy if there are any adverse reactions. The predominant requirement, in all these cases, is that the patient is provided with full information about the procedure and the risks and benefits involved and is able to provide a voluntary consent. In practice, this can be extremely difficult and there are often concerns that the patient is at risk and is invariably under pressure or has undue expectations for the procedure. The various national guidelines for ethical

---

[100] I. Hyun, *op. cit.* note 89.

[101] See: National Health and Medical Research Council. 2007. *National Statement on Ethical Conduct in Human Research.* Chapter 3.3: Interventions and Therapies, Including Clinical and Nonclinical Trials, and Invasions: at 33.

[102] Ibid.

conduct and research provide for additional considerations for vulnerable patients.[103]

Secondly, in addition to national research guidelines for innovative research and therapy, it is not uncommon for independent national advisory committees to be established as a reference point for those clinicians introducing innovative therapies. Again, using Australia as an example, the National Health and Medical Research Council (NHMRC) has established a Gene Therapy Research Advisory Panel that is available to provide independent advice to researchers and clinicians intending to undertake novel or innovative procedures or testing on volunteer patients. Stem cell applications are properly classified as innovative therapy.

Interestingly, the ISSCR *Guidelines* correctly assume that most stem cell applications are outside established standards of care and that any use of stem cells, involving a consenting patient, is properly described as innovative therapy. These guidelines accept that it may be permissible, in carefully managed circumstances, for clinicians to attempt a medically innovative application provided it is for the benefit of their patient outside the regulatory requirements for an official clinical trial.[104] Recommendation 34 focuses on stem cell-based medical innovation and recommends: 'Clinician-scientists may provide unproven stem cell-based interventions to at most a very small number of patients outside the context of a formal clinical trial, provided that:

a. There is a written plan for the procedure that includes:

    i. scientific rationale and justification explaining why the procedure has a reasonable chance of success, including any pre-clinical evidence of proof-of-principle for efficacy and safety;
    ii. explanation of why the proposed stem cell-based intervention should be attempted compared to existing treatments;
    iii. full characterisation of the types of cells being transplanted and their characteristics as discussed in Section 4, Cell Processing and Manufacture;

[103] See: for example, ibid. Chapter 4.4: *People Highly Dependent on Medical Care Who May Be Unable to Give Consent.*

[104] Hyun, *op. cit.* note 89.

   iv. description of how the cells will be administered, including adjuvant drugs, agents and surgical procedures; and
   v. plan for clinical follow-up data collection to assess the effectiveness and adverse effects of the cell therapy;

b. The written plan is approved through a peer review process by appropriate experts who have no vested interest in the proposed procedure;
c. The clinical and administrative leadership supports the decision to attempt the medical innovation and the institution is held accountable for the innovative procedure;
d. All personnel have appropriate qualifications and the institution where the procedure will be carried out has appropriate facilities and processes of peer review and clinical quality control monitoring;
e. Voluntary informed consent is provided by patients who appreciate that the intervention is unproven and who demonstrate their understanding of the risks and benefits of the procedure;
f. There is an action plan for adverse events that includes timely and adequate medical care and if necessary psychological support services;
g. Insurance coverage or other appropriate financial or medical resources are available to patients to cover any complications arising from the procedure; and
h. There is a commitment by clinician-scientists to use their experience with individual patients to contribute to generalisable knowledge. This includes:

   i. ascertaining outcomes in a systematic and objective manner;
   ii. a plan for communicating outcomes, including negative outcomes and adverse events, to the scientific community to enable critical review (for example, as abstracts to professional meetings or publications in peer-reviewed journals); and
   iii. moving to a formal clinical trial in a timely manner after experience with at most a few patients.

Despite its promise, the realisation of the potential of human stem cell technology in transplantation therapy or any other derivative therapy will require substantial research efforts. Clearly, the time from research result to clinical trial, much less any clinical application, are many years apart.

CONCLUSIONS

Stem cell technology provides a singular example of Professor Somerville's[105] staggered tripartite time scales of 1) fast-moving science time; 2) slower and deliberative public discussion in ethics time; and 3) the gradual move to social acceptance — with law time, limping along slowly behind these developments. The science of stem cells is not new, but the pace of the science has accelerated in the last decade. The international ethical debate has concentrated on the controversy of the embryonic stem cells,[106] while most of the stem cell applications and trials have involved autologous stem cells re-implanted in patients, sometimes in combinatorial therapy with other drugs. However, the science, ethics and law are not discrete considerations. The *European Life Sciences High Level Group* recognised this and stated 'that science alone is not sufficient for making decisions on stem cells, but that we cannot discuss the ethical issues raised by stem cells without clarifying the scientific facts'.[107]

Research science in relation to embryonic stem cells has been regulated at the national level in some countries either with outright bans or with the legislation or guidelines allowing research on surplus embryos but with considerable common 'restrictive-tilt' features. While research using adult stem cells is ethically less problematic, there may be less promise from adult cells, with reduced potentialities when compared with their embryonic counterparts.[108] These important scientific differences between adult and embryonic stem cell research have prompted most stem cell scientists to support the concurrent development of both strands of research. They argue that adult and embryonic (and now iPS) are complementary and may prove to be synergistic research pathways. It is recognised that there is a need for continuing research using embryonic as well as adult stem cells and now iPS cells.[109]

---

[105] M. Somerville. 2000. *The Ethical Canary: Science, Society and the Human Spirit.* Victoria: Viking.

[106] See: Chalmers and Nicol, *op. cit.* note 63.

[107] See: Chair Axel Kahn, 'Stem Cells: Therapies for the Future?' Statement from the *European Life Sciences High Level Group* at http://ec.europa.eu/research/quality-of-life/stemcells/pro_openad_en.html [Accessed 10 March 2009].

[108] See: National Academies Committee on the Biological and Biomedical Application of Stem Cell Research, *op. cit.* note 14, pp. 16–20.

[109] Nishikawa, *op. cit.* note 40.

The ISSCR *Guidelines* are an important contribution to the future development of responsible stem cell applications and therapies as stem cell research moves gradually into the clinic. The issue of the safety of stem cell applications for the patient is a prime consideration in the rapid move from laboratory to clinical application. Safety raises the tripartite considerations of independent scientific and ethical risk benefit assessment, risk communication in clear and unbiased terms to the patient and risk management during and after the stem cell application.

National research guidelines for innovative research and therapy, supplemented by the ISSCR *Guidelines* provide a sound foundation of core principles for the transitional phase from research to clinical trials. The ISSCR *Guidelines* also provide a foundation for the integrated harmonisation of international approaches to the translation of stem cell research to clinical applications. These *Guidelines* address major ethical issues in the translation of stem cell research to the clinic, especially issues of patient safety and risk communication, independent clinical assessment and ethical review and informed and voluntary patient consent to involvement in the trial. Apart from these ethical issues, the *Guidelines* address quality control, pre-clinical work and ethical clinical trials. Finally, these *Guidelines* should also use compliance standards in any assessments or criticisms of clinical applications of stem cell technology, particularly in countries with 'under legislation'[110] where clinics are offering dubious, stem cell 'treatments'[111] that have not undergone proper testing in approved clinical trials.

ACKNOWLEDGEMENTS

Professor Chalmers wishes to thank the Australian Research Council (Discovery Grant DP 0559760) for support; and Benjamin Capps for the assistance in preparing this chapter, especially for providing additional information on the science and international legal situation.

[110] An expression used by the Noelle Lenoir cited in Casado, *op. cit.* note 73.

[111] Kiatpongsan and Sipp, *op. cit.* note 6.

3

LEGAL IMPERIALISM IN THE REGULATION OF STEM CELL RESEARCH AND THERAPY: THE PROBLEM OF EXTRATERRITORIAL JURISDICTION

Daniela Cutas and Christian Munthe

INTRODUCTION

Since national regulations of embryonic stem cell (ES cell) research are very different around the world (where they exist at all), any effective global or multinational regulation of such research will imply some degree of imperialism in ethical and legal matters. That is, to achieve such regulation, involved parties will have to be willing to accommodate their respective positions regarding ES cell research to some extent, thus allowing national policy to be influenced by policies of other nations. This actualises familiar problems in research ethics, medical practice and international law. The Hinxton Group,[1] in a consensus statement from 2006, has pointed to a problem for researchers arising out of the fact that countries sometimes find reason to extend the applicability of their laws

---

[1] The group is a joint project between members of the Stem Cell Policy and Ethics Program (SCOPE) and The Johns Hopkins Berman Institute of Bioethics, undertaken for bringing 'together an esteemed, international and interdisciplinary group to explore the ethical and policy challenges of transnational scientific collaboration raised by variations in national regulations governing embryo research and stem cell science. ...Coordinated by a US/UK steering committee, the Hinxton Group is an informal collection of individuals interested in ethical and well-regulated science', on www.hinxtongroup.org [Accessed February 2009].

to regulate behaviour beyond their own borders.[2] In a recent paper, Heidi Mertes and Guido Pennings address this as a potential challenge to the feasibility of a process towards global regulation of the ES cell area in terms of so-called *extraterritorial jurisdiction* — the practice of a nation to apply its laws to, e.g. its citizens also when they are visiting a country where the law is different.[3] In this chapter, we will somewhat build on (but also criticise) this work, and add further dimensions that seem to affect the area of ES cell research with particular force: first, the strong case for the desirability of global substantial regulation; and second, the interests not only of researchers, but also those of clinicians and (potential) patients.

We will explore the implications of both a global regulation of ES cell research, and the extraterritoriality of national legislation, and their impact on researchers and research, clinicians and national health systems as well as private citizens. The premise of our analysis will be to tentatively accept the vision of an effective global or multinational regulatory framework for ES cell research. The phenomenon of extraterritorial jurisdiction will then be added as an ingredient that, through its effects on researchers, clinicians and patients, may affect the feasibility of the vision of global regulation.

We will not discuss the matter of research in Developing Countries — the reasons why some regulation is needed to prevent researchers from freely engaging in experimentation in areas which simply do not have the resources or authority to oversee or stop them, are of a particular kind. We do not contest the need for minimal international standards for performing research wherever — and in this regard we fully agree with the arguments presented by Mertes and Pennings.

---

[2] The Hinxton Group. 2006. *Transnational Cooperation in Stem Cell Research.* Available at: http://www.hinxtongroup.org/au_trans_cs.html [Accessed April 2009].

[3] H. Mertes & G. Pennings. Cross-Border Research on Human Embryonic Stem Cells: Legal and Ethical Considerations. *Stem Cell Review* 2008; 5: 10–17. The article offers a very clear presentation of the legal principles that may permit extraterritorial jurisdiction in some cases, and explains which of these, and in which ways, may be applied to stem cell research.

Neither will we, in this chapter, endorse any particular view on the moral status of the human embryo. We acknowledge the ethical disagreement as well as the entitlement of governments to protect whatever within those states is deemed to constitute a subject of protection, as well as the prioritisation of costs and benefits. However, in line with Mertes and Pennings' article, we also think that a legislature cannot legitimately disallow the public communication of dissenting opinions in ethical matters. Researchers, clinicians and patients can and do disagree about what is permissible and what is not, as well as about where their ethical duties, and those of others, lie.

At the same time, we believe the prospect of a globally harmonised regulatory framework to be considerably more vulnerable to the existence of very restrictive views and/or regulations of embryonic stem cell research than what is conceded by Mertes and Pennings. Their basically pragmatic/prudential reasons for why countries applying a restrictive legal stance should adopt a moderately relativistic and cautious attitude to extraterritorial jurisdiction as regards embryo research will not work when embryo destruction is viewed as on a par with murder. Since logic dictates that, on the basis of such a moral evaluation, ES cell research amounts to genocide, ES cell research would look like a classic example of the sort of act where — as mentioned by Mertes and Pennings — extraterritorial jurisdiction is often seen as acceptable within international law.

There are, basically, three categories of citizens that will be affected, in different ways, by the possible restrictions in respect to the regulation of stem cell science: the researchers in the first instance, then the clinicians and finally, the patients. In general, the result of our analysis is that, first, the idea of a globally harmonised regulatory scheme for ES cell research has much to say in its favour from the perspective of all of these parties. Second, however, the extreme range of actual ethical disagreement, combined with the room for extraterritorial jurisdiction, threatens to create a legal situation bound to effect substantial harm to central values in a number of areas besides research. Health care, the job market, basic freedom of movement and strategic international finance and politics may all be adversely affected. In effect, while extraterritorial jurisdiction may seem an attractive idea as regards a number of types of crime, it becomes a problematic feature in cases where deep and wide disagreement exists as to whether or not certain activities belong to one of these types.

Before coming to that, however, we need to say some things about what the vision of a global regulation of ES cell research may amount to and what reasons there are to view it as desirable.

THE VISION OF GLOBAL REGULATION OF ES CELL RESEARCH

Visions of global or far-reaching multinational regulation of any area of practice or policy share a similar set of ultimate objectives, all having to do with the evident benefits of cooperation between parties with (partly) conflicting interests. First, for individuals belonging to different countries, global or multinational rules make life easier in a number of important ways — in economic terms, they reduce the transaction costs of life in a globalised world. In concrete terms, this reduces the range of worries about, and necessary adaptations to, variations in national regulations as one moves about across national borders in the pursuit of health care, leisure, business, work or shelter from general hardships. On a population level, this creates a smoother situation for nations in their interaction with other nations, in spite of the many differences regarding morality, culture and institutionalised norms to be found around the world, as may be exemplified by EU directives facilitating citizens of member states to access various services in all member states. On a wider scale, both of these objectives make for the promotion of the general value of judicial security (for individuals and nations) and, perhaps most importantly, it reduces the room for serious international conflict.

When, as in the case of ES cell, vast and deep international disagreement exists on the subject of regulation, these objectives appear even more important. This was the main message of the above-mentioned consensus statement of the Hinxton Group from 2006, and the reason for why the phenomenon of extraterritorial jurisdiction was held out there as a particular problem. At the same time, as Mertes and Pennings observe,[4]

---

[4] Ibid.

the statement suffered the flaw of begging the question in its attack on extraterritorial jurisdictional ambitions in the ES cell area, since it assumed such ambitions to be directed at *ethically justified* ES cell research, while the nations harbouring them would, of course, do so on the basis of viewing this research as *un*ethical.

What this implies is that any practically workable global regulation of such an area will have to take into account this fact of fundamental disagreement. One aspect of this, obviously, is the general point made earlier about the right to publicly express dissenting opinions — any minimally decent regulatory scheme has to give room for that. A more important upshot, though, is that the vision of global regulation of ES cell research cannot be built on the idea that some parties to the disagreement have to completely abandon their basic outlook (and national laws based on that) in order to accommodate their rules to those of the other parties. Such ambitions of either ES cell restrictive or ES cell liberal countries would rather serve to undercut any willingness to discuss or create common rules, thus blocking completely the access to the objectives just mentioned. This will be a recurring theme in our analysis below, where we will pursue the idea that the problem with extraterritorial jurisdictional ambitions in the ES cell case, rather than being about clearly unjustified meddling in matters of an obviously morally innocent nature, is its tendency to block the access to the objectives of global regulation (and the widely recognised values attached to these).

One example of a multi-nationally legislative document in bioethics, which tries to comply with this condition, is the European so-called Bioethics Convention.[5] According to its Explanatory Report, the document 'lays down common standards with which States must comply, while allowing them to provide greater protection of the human being and of human rights with regard to applications of biology and medicine'.[6]

---

[5] The European Convention for the Protection of Human Rights and Dignity of the Human Being with regard to the Application of Biology and Medicine. Short title: Convention on Human Rights and Biomedicine, Oviedo, 1997, European Treaty Series — No. 164. Available at: http://conventions.coe.int/ [Accessed April 2009].

[6] Explanatory Report to the Convention at Article 27. Available at: http://conventions.coe.int/Treaty/EN/Reports/Html/164.htm [Accessed April 2009].

The definition of the Convention's purpose consisted of two elements: protecting every human being, which implied protection of the unborn human being; and guaranteeing the rights and freedoms of every person, only persons being regarded as having rights.[7] In the Convention, Article 27 reads:

> 'None of the provisions of this Convention shall be interpreted as limiting or otherwise affecting the possibility for a Party to grant a wider measure of protection with regard to the application of biology and medicine than is stipulated in this Convention'.[8]

Taken together, these formulations leave room for signing countries to implement national legislation before ratification that makes for a particular interpretative tendency as to central terms such as 'human being', 'human rights', 'person', etc. In effect, an ES cell restrictive country may have laws implying strong protection of embryos (in Europe at the moment, this is the case with, e.g. Germany, Ireland, Poland and Slovenia), while more liberal countries may create laws holding out the rights of born people who may want to use embryos for certain purposes, such as research, as central. For instance, in Sweden, a number of laws have been created that give ample room for embryo research in general, and ES cell research in particular (including the creation of embryos using somatic cell nuclear transfer SCNT) under the supervision of research ethical regulation and monitoring. The Netherlands, where a more restrictive view on SCNT has been adopted while otherwise permitting ES cell research on similar conditions as Sweden, chose to insure themselves against over-interpretations of this slightly less liberal stance by attaching a reservation to its signature/ratification, declaring that it interprets the term 'human being' as

[7] Preparatory Work to the Convention, Chapter I, Article 1, ii. Available at: www.coe.int/bioethics [Accessed April 2009].

[8] Convention on Human Rights and Biomedicine hereafter, the Bioethics.

referring exclusively to a human individual, i.e. a human being who has been born.[9]

One may ask what the point of a global regulatory framework of this sort is when it leaves room for preserving all substantial national differences. This question itself misses the point, however. The objectives of global or multinational regulation are (at least partly) reached by requiring of nations to create public, transparent and clear-cut rules within the (admittedly wide) frames set by the formulations of the Convention. In other words, one might say that a global regulation of ES cell research, if it is to be realistic and practically useful, will have to operate most specifically on a meta- and procedural level relative to the actual topic of the regulation (i.e. the actual ES cell research and related activities), while the regulative instruments applied directly to this topic will, as a matter of political necessity, be more open to interpretation of individual countries.

So, with a format similar to the European Convention in mind, let us ponder what happens if some countries find reasons to include, among their specified national standpoints, some portion of extraterritorial jurisdiction. This will be the baseline of our analysis in the sections to follow.

RESEARCH AND RESEARCHERS

It is usual that national legislation applies only within national borders. It can happen, though, that particular portions of a countries' legislation acquires extraterritorial jurisdiction. This can cover acts such as sex tourism, certain forms of weaponry, 'crimes against humanity' (whichever acts that are covered in those legislations under this name), etc. In some cases, national stem cell research regulations can have such extraterritorial jurisdiction. Until recently, this was the case in Germany: before August 2008, it was a common view among German researchers, as well as legal scholars, that a German researcher performing stem cell research in another country that is illegal in Germany, but legal in the other country,

---

[9] As indicated in the Chart of Signatures and Ratifications; Available at: www.coe.int/bioethics [Accessed April 2009].

could be prosecuted. The latest revisions of the German Stem Cell Act (Stammzellgesetz, StZG) make it explicit that the prohibitions therein only apply to the import of stem cells (which is subject to strict limitations), and not to German researchers' activities abroad.[10]

National extraterritorial regulations of the kind that was acted on in Germany (whether or not the strong interpretation of the restriction was in the intentions of the law-makers) create a very peculiar situation for researchers, whereby there is nowhere in the world where one can engage in work of a certain kind without being subjected to the legislation of the country one is a citizen of.

Alternatively, although being able to perform broad research that is illegal in their home-countries, researchers may not be allowed upon their return to use their research results. In other cases, the extraterritorial jurisdiction concerns the use of public funding for certain types of research (as is the case in the US and, according to some sources, was one interpretation of the German regulation until 2008); both of which may limit the opportunity to perform the research in question, and create a difference in this respect compared to research funded from other sources. Giuseppe Testa and Elena Cattaneo in their *Joint Statement on the Situation in Italy* (included in the ESTOOLS and EuroStemCell's statement on European legislation and stem cell research), identify another funding-related example[11]: although in Italy research on embryonic stem cells is permissible on already established cell lines, public funding for such research is not available — therefore, Italy-based researchers' collaboration with international teams, and their capacity to benefit from international research results in this field, are impaired.

---

[10] See: I. Herrmann, C. Woopen & O. Brüstle. 2008. *German Parliament Passes Amendment to Stem Cell Act*. Available at: http://www.eurostemcell.org/commentanalysis/german-parliament-passes-amendment-stem-cell-act [Accessed April 2009]; G. Vogel. Visiting German Profs Could Face Jail. *Science* 2003; 301: 577. We thank Bert Heinrichs for illuminating insights into the matter of German stem cell jurisdiction.

[11] Directors of ESTOOLS and EuroStemCell. 2007. *Joint Statement. The Impact of Legislation in Europe on Our Ability to Perform Research Using Stem Cells*. Available at: http://archive.eurostemcell.org [Accessed April 2009].

Yet another perspective[12] (regarding again the German pre-2008 case) is that researchers from countries with restrictive legislation can engage in international research based abroad, on the conditions that they are not employed and paid as researchers in their own countries. They can, however, participate if during the respective collaboration they take leave from their employment in the restrictive country.

Some international bodies involved in stem cell research may themselves acknowledge and accept the extraterritorial jurisdiction in the matter. For example, as noted by Mertes and Pennings,[13] the International Society for Stem Cell Research stipulates in its *Guidelines for the Conduct of Human Embryonic Stem Cell Research*, under the heading 'Responsibility for conduct', that

> 'International scientific collaboration and mutual trust among researchers are vital to the success and advancement of science and should be encouraged. Collaborations between scientists in different jurisdictions will raise issues due to the differences in the laws and regulations that govern stem cell research. An underlying principle of these guidelines is that any and all stem cell research shall be conducted in accordance with any applicable laws and regulations of the country or region where such research takes place, *recognising and respecting that certain laws and regulations may be applicable to individual researchers, regardless of where the research will take place*'.[14] (emphasis ours)

Each of the regulations referred to, as well as interpretations of rules made in particular contexts, have different implications. Whilst funding

[12] See Vogel, *op. cit.* note 10, and A. Abbott. German Stem-Cell Law Under Fire. *Nature* 2006; 444: 253. Available at: http://www.nature.com/nature/journal/v444/n7117/full/444253a.html [Accessed April 2009]. The original report by the German National Ethics Council presenting this perspective is available in German at http://www.ethikrat.org/stellungnahmen/stellungnahmen.html [Accessed April 2009].

[13] Mertes & Pennings, *op. cit.* note 3.

[14] International Society for Stem Cell Research. 2006. *Guidelines for the Conduct of Human Embryonic Stem Cell Research*: 4. Available at: http://www.isscr.org/guidelines/index.htm [Accessed April 2009].

restrictions or local regulations may leave room for 'research tourism' on the part of the researcher-citizen, a strong extraterritorial interpretation that connects the applicability of a national law to citizenship as such is (virtually) inescapable. Moreover, even if such a strict extraterritorial jurisdiction is not applied, as Mertes and Pennings note, many universities and national funding bodies will require of their employees or beneficiaries that they abide by laws and certain customs of their home country also when abroad. Moreover, adherence to certain 'ethics laws' is a condition for participation in the European Commission's Framework Programme for research.[15]

As we have seen, legislation not only may limit researchers' activities as regards embryos directly, but may forbid the derivation of stem cell lines in the country, while allowing their importation (as is the case, for example, in Germany and Italy). This is, however, inconsistent with the uncompromising view, which is the ground of the restriction, and according to which the destruction of unborn human life (i.e. of embryos) is unacceptable. The argument behind the compromise is that the setting up of cut-off dates coupled with the restriction to produce the stem cell lines will discourage the production of embryos for research (which may take the form of intentionally creating supernumerary embryos in IVF). The result is that research is allowed preferentially on 'foreign' unborn human life. Thus, their 'hands are clean' of the immorality of creating and destroying local embryos.

Mertes and Pennings use this actual stance, as adopted by several ES cell research restrictive countries, as an argument for why such countries should relax their view on what their citizens do abroad as regard ES cell research. After all, the argument goes, these countries have in fact not adopted rules that see the destruction of embryos as a form of murder. This, firstly, makes for too much of a conflation of the content of legislation and

[15] Hence, for example, Singapore is becoming increasingly 'ethical' according to international standards with respect to ES cell regulation — i.e. it basically takes on common regulations — such as those found in its endorsement of the *International Conference on Harmonisation Guidelines for Good Clinical Practice* — to 'fit in' with the 'Western' biotechnological powerhouses. See: K. Holden & D. Demeritt. Democratising Science — The Politics of Promoting Biomedicine in Singapore's Developmental State. *Environment and Planning D: Society and Space* 2008; 26: 68–86.

that of its underlying moral rationale. As hinted at above, what the rules of such countries imply is that the destruction of *domestic* embryos is indeed legally on a par with murder, while foreign embryos (and indeed embryos destroyed to create cell-lines before one or another cut-off date) are accorded less of a moral standing. But, we suggest, this is certainly not the underlying moral rationale for such regulations, but rather the outcome of a political compromise, where all sorts of strategic and tactical factors have been part of the story. Secondly, the argument ignores countries (such as Austria, Lithuania, Poland, Slovakia, Tunisia and several states/countries of the US and in Latin America) that do take a more uncompromising legal stance.[16] Both of these gaps in the argument serve to highlight the fact that a *consistent* legal application of the *moral* view underlying the restrictive legislations would imply that the ES cell research is, as a matter of fact, a case of genocide.

On such a basis, the pragmatic, prudential reasons offered by Mertes and Pennings lose their force, since their core rationale is the idea that a little compromise in morally important legal matters is not so bad if already the law itself expresses a compromise with basic moral standpoints. It is quite possible to argue against such an analysis that, while compromises in order to create laws are a political necessity, the *application* of law should be uncompromising from a moral point of view. Thus, supporters of the cut-off date solution as regards ES cell lines may find reasons to resist any *further* compromise with their underlying moral view of the destruction of embryos, and this conveys an understanding that embryo destruction in the course of research is an absolute moral wrong. In effect, a restrictive view that is either uncompromising in legal terms, or compromising only to the extent that is politically necessary to have the regulation adopted, would seem to imply that, morally speaking, ES cell research clearly falls into a category of legal violations for which, as Mertes and Pennings acknowledge, the room for very far-reaching extraterritorial jurisdiction is widely accepted.

Now, for sure, the adoption of such a stance by some country would be seen as absurd by countries with a more liberal stance towards ES cell

---

[16] See the information made available by the Hinxton Group at http://www.hinxton-group.org/wp.html [Accessed April 2009].

research (Belgium, Sweden and the UK, for instance). This, in turn, may imply that, by the same standards of international law just invoked, they have valid interests in protecting their citizens, settlers and institutions against being persecuted for alleged 'crimes against humanity' when this consists in the performance of ES cell research perfectly legal in those countries. A strong and principled *liberal* stance towards ES cell research may imply claims to valid reasons for extraterritorial jurisdiction — however, of course, in the direction opposite to that of a strong and principled restrictive view.

We conclude from all this that the case against the actual realisation of extraterritorial legislation and law enforcement regarding ES cell research is, in fact, much less robust than it is made out to be by Mertes and Pennings. Of course, from the point of view of the vision of constructing a substantial global regulation for ES cell research, we acknowledge the *desirability* of the sort of mutually moderately tolerant attitudes of countries with contrary views on ES cell research argued for by Mertes and Pennings. The sort of 'overlapping consensus' view of the matter, where pragmatically reasonable parties make mutual accommodations to avoid severe conflict is indeed an important tool for achieving global regulations of morally contested practices. However, as we have seen, strong forms of extraterritorial jurisdiction, impeding such mutual accommodations in the ES cell case, would indeed be the reasonable choice for parties not prepared to compromise with the values they assign (or do not assign) to the embryo, no matter the costs in other ethical 'currencies' (such as the risk of international conflict or the caring for people around the world). The mutual existence of such strong and principled (and consistently applied) outlooks thus seems to be what creates problems for the vision of a global and substantial ES cell research regulation.

CLINICIANS

During the work on this paper, the news was released of the forthcoming start of the first clinical trial of an ES cell-based therapy for disease.[17]

---

[17] A. Pollack. F.D.A. Approves a Stem Cell Trial. *The New York Times*. 23 February 2009. Available at: http://www.nytimes.com/2009/01/23/business/23stem.html [Accessed April 2009].

This event highlights the fact that not only researchers but also clinicians are affected parties to consider in the present context. Clinicians from reproductive medicine have been an essential party in ES cell research already at the preclinical stage, since it is through them that researchers gain access to sperm, ova, embryos and other cells. The initiation of bona fide clinical studies marks the starting point of a stage of ES cell research, where more and more clinical staff will gradually become more and more directly and visibly involved. Not least, it is the clinicians who will have direct contact with patients in the recruitment of research subjects.

Since the practice of medicine is a universally applicable skill, medical staffs — just like researchers — are a highly mobile part of the work force. Today, this mobility is an increasingly important factor for the functionality of the health care systems of many developed countries. Clinical specialists (doctors, nurses, technicians) may thus increasingly find themselves in situations equalling those of ES cell researchers subjected to extraterritorial jurisdiction. Besides the general problems described in the former section, the case of clinicians gives rise to particular issues, e.g. regarding whether or not they can participate — without fear of prosecution in their home country — in the assistance of a woman in a reproductive clinic that might end up donating embryos to research (or ova that might be used in SCNT procedures for the production of embryos for research).

Scenarios such as those discussed in respect to the extended jurisdiction of restrictive states, make the prospect of moving to countries with a more liberal regulation of ES cell research than one's own unattractive (or even impossible), in spite of the fact that such a move would benefit oneself (access to clinical resources) as well as the health care system of the host country (providing access to stem cell therapies). Of course, as the prevalence of clinical studies and trials of ES cell therapies increases, such consequences will increase proportionally.

The next step of development occurs, of course, once stem cell therapies become legally sanctioned within some countries. At that point, extraterritorial restrictions on this type of treatment could imply that an employee of the health system of such a country cannot offer the therapy to her patients, in virtue of her citizenship. Where a regulation that allows the treatment but does not fund it is in place (as would presumably be a continuation of the current status quo in Italy and the US), clinicians would be able to suggest the treatment to their patients, but access will be restricted by the patients' financial situation. A clinician specialised in stem cell therapy, for example, could in this scenario be constrained, against her own conscience, not to offer it to needy patients. She may not be allowed, as we will see in the next sub-section, to even mention it. Furthermore, if the holder of a national grant decides to pursue studies abroad in order to improve her clinical skill, she will not be able to choose the field which is illegal in her country. If she pursues it with independent funding, she may not be able to use this knowledge upon her return.[18]

To provide some context to these scenarios, it may be noted that in many legislatures, clinicians have a right to 'conscientiously object' to certain procedures — such as contraception, abortion or euthanasia — if such procedures are incompatible with their personal views. However, in the context of treatments that are illegal or not covered by medical insurance, they would presumably not be granted the same privilege, even while knowing that the failure to pursue the treatment in question is fatal for their patients. Therefore, in the case of abortion versus ES cell therapy, the clinicians' dissenting opinions would be accepted if she refuses to help the patient because of her own views, even if the patient is legally entitled to the procedure (which involves destruction of human life: the foetus, in the case of abortion), but not if she prefers to prioritise the needy patient above human embryos (in the case of ES cell therapy). All of this, of course, in a situation where the clinician is in fact practicing in a host country where ES cell therapy is legal, while it is restricted in the clinician's home country.

[18] There will also probably arise a number of very difficult legal line drawing issues. For instance, since ES cell research is a tool with wide applications, it is highly conceivable that ES cell research, just as genomic research, will contribute to the development of totally new and more efficient pharmaceuticals. Logic seems to dictate that if, due to the view that the destruction of embryos is very morally wrong, it is also wrong to use the cell-lines produced through ES cell research, then using drugs that have been developed due to such research (although they do not themselves contain any stem cells) is equally wrong. Perhaps, some of the ES cell restrictive countries will try to prevent such an outcome, in which case law scholars will have an interesting time studying the legal delicacies employed to achieve such a result.

From the perspective of the clinicians (a section on patients follows below), two things may thus be observed. Firstly, clinicians are already today involved in ES cell research and will be so even more in the future, thus exposing a much larger group to the problems produced by extraterritorial jurisdiction in the ES cell area. Secondly, as ES cell therapies are introduced in more liberal countries, similar problems will start to infect the health care sector on a broader basis. If as successful as their proponents hope for, such therapies will become very common and applied to all sorts of conditions. As a result, the problems created by extraterritorial jurisdiction will then attain huge proportions. Thirdly, and perhaps most important, such problems will not only affect those clinicians that might want to work in another country. Due to the need of many developed countries to 'import' health care staff from abroad, it may pose a serious threat to the ability of a country to provide a functioning health service. It is highly probable that the more liberal countries will respond to such effects with retaliations aimed at protecting visiting health care staff from prosecution. Given the size of the health care sector of such countries, extraterritorial jurisdiction regarding ES cell research and therapy may thus seriously upset the multinational reciprocity built into central concepts in international relations, such as mobility of the work force and the freedom of movement. The prerequisites for such outcomes are already in place in Europe, where high mobility of clinical staff is combined with very variable regulations of the handling of embryos in general and ES cell practices in particular.

The general outcome of the analysis regarding research thus is added to by another layer of difficulty when the case of clinicians is superimposed. From the perspective of the vision of a global regulation of ES cell research and (in this case) therapy, extraterritorial jurisdiction is a major impediment that threatens to deepen international conflict — in this case by producing risks of crippling the health systems of some countries and making political and financial retaliations probable.

PATIENTS

As indicated in the former section, once ES cell therapies are beginning to be introduced, extraterritorial jurisdiction in this area will affect (potential) patients. At first, this will relate to the possibility of and conditions for participating in clinical studies and trials — something which will be of importance primarily to patients suffering from severe conditions for which there is no effective treatment. It is highly conceivable, once attempts to make treatments evidence-based through controlled trials are initiated, that the research will be highly multinational. People whose home countries have adopted a restrictive legal stance will, of course, be legally impeded from entering any trials abroad by threat of being prosecuted at home (in some cases, where the cut-off date solution is applied, depending on when the cell lines used for the treatment where initially created). In the case of countries restricting mainly the public funding of ES cell research this may actually permit people to enter trials (at home or abroad) as long as these are funded in the right way.[19] Just as in the case with the US federal funding policy regarding embryo research in general, this has the peculiar effect that people from these countries are made more likely to enter trials where the exercise of proper research ethical control and monitoring is impeded due to commercial secrecy.[20]

After the clinical trial stage, there will probably be a number of treatments based on ES cell research (as noted, these treatments may but need not involve the use of actual stem cells) that, in liberal countries, will be adopted as new standard clinical responses to a number of conditions. This complicates the situation for patients even further.

Legal restrictions on (medically approved) ES cell-based *therapies* entail not only criminal, but also administrative law. First, there is the

---

[19] However, legal issues may arise if a research centre of such a country is involved in a multinational trial in which centres from more liberal countries also participate. Does the research in such a case involve the use of illegal materials (according to the law of the restrictive country)? Looking at the trial as a whole, the answer seems to be yes, while it appears to be negative if the outlook is restricted to a particular centre complying with the regulation of the restrictive country. Any patient from a restrictive country would thus need to have such matters cleared up, before being able to enter a trial without fear of prosecution.

[20] See C. Munthe. 1999. *Pure Selection: The Ethics of Preimplantation Genetic Diagnosis and Choosing Children without Abortion*. Gothenburg: Acta Universitatis Gothoburgensis: 246–249.

issue of medical insurance coverage. According to EU regulations,[21] if a life-saving treatment is not available (or if there is too long a waiting list) within a member state, patients can apply (using the form E 112) to have their treatment in another member state covered by their national health insurance. If, however, a treatment is not available in one's own country because it is illegal, the citizens' medical insurance would presumably not cover the expenses of that patient pursuing the treatment elsewhere. According to the said regulation, the treatment has to be deemed necessary by specialists in the needy patient's country of residence (and health insurance coverage). But if a treatment is not available because it is illegal, clinicians cannot prescribe it. Therefore, it cannot be covered.

Second, even when patients take it upon themselves to cover the costs of the treatment that is illegal in their countries, restrictive national legislation might still prevent them from seeking it. This may involve a number of impediments and troubles for patients. Obviously, there will be the threat of prosecution on arrival in one's home country after having had the therapy abroad. As in the case of clinicians this, in itself, may be seen as a threat to the principle of free movement. However, when it comes to patients, the situation may in fact become even more severe, since a restrictive country applying extraterritorial jurisdiction may want to not only punish their citizens for what they have done abroad, but actually apply concrete preventive measures in order to stop them from going abroad to commit the acts in the first place. This may include the steps mentioned in connection to clinicians above, restricting health care professionals' rights to actively seek information about what ES cell therapeutic possibilities exist abroad and/or to inform their patients about such things. In the name of legal coherence, therefore, applying similar restrictions to private citizens would seem to make perfect sense for a restrictive country that takes an extraterritorial stance to its bans. However, with regard to patients, there are further steps to be taken by such countries; all aimed at directly preventing these people from going abroad. Here, everything from invalidating or seizing passports to temporary freezing of

[21] Council regulation (EEC) no. 1408/71, art. 22.

private funds or outright detention of people suspected to be planning to seek ES cell therapies abroad may be applied. To be efficient, of course, such measures will have to be complemented by a system for monitoring those citizens in relation to whom such suspicions might arise (i.e. people suffering from severe diseases that may be treated by ES cell-based therapies banned in the country in question).[22]

Liberal minded people may undoubtedly find scenarios such as these so appalling that they might want to question if they are at all realistic. For this reason, we will flesh out these more speculative ideas with some hard facts regarding a very close analogy. Consider the case of Ireland's attempts to limit its citizens' access to (or even knowledge of) abortion, which (aside from when there is a direct threat to the pregnant woman's life) is a prohibited medical procedure in that country.[23] Two Ireland-based non-profit organisations (Open Door and Dublin Well Woman), which were providing information about abortion (more specifically, about how to access abortion services in the UK) were prohibited by the Supreme Court from further sharing it with patients. The organisations (along with a few patients) took the case to the European Court of Human

[22] We need to look no further than to pre-1989 Romania, presently a EU member state, to find a gripping example of how far the state's intrusion into its citizens' reproductive health and private lives can go: for many years, women of reproductive age in Romania, who were employed, had to submit themselves to regular gynaecological check-ups to establish whether they were or had recently been pregnant (the former discovery had to be reported so that the pregnancy was registered and monitored, and the latter would have suggested a performed abortion, which was illegal and thus was to be reported for investigation) (see G. Kligman. 1998. *The Politics of Duplicity: Controlling Reproduction in Ceausescu's Romania*. University of California Press: Berkeley and Los Angeles). We may comfort ourselves with the belief that such a political regime is no longer possible in Europe — however this does not prevent some EU member states from having very restrictive legislation on matters such as abortion and to show no mercy for those who do not respect it. And, indeed, such an optimistic belief becomes completely irrelevant when it comes to *global* regulation.

[23] According to article 40.3.3° of the Constitution of Ireland (the Eight Amendment), 'the State acknowledges the right to life of the unborn and, with due regard to the equal right to life of the mother, guarantees in its laws to respect, and, as far as practicable, by its laws to defend and vindicate that right'.

Rights (ECHR), on the grounds that the injunction violated article 10[24] of the European Convention of Human Rights, and won.[25] The consequence of this decision is that if women ask for counselling and information about abortion, the counsellor is now allowed to provide it. It may also be worth pointing out that *services* offered in the Well Woman Clinics are for a fee, except for, subject to funding, some special categories of needy patients.

This case of an attempt to apply the Constitution of Ireland so as to prevent citizens from seeking abortion services abroad is not unique. In 1992, the Irish High Court obtained an injunction whereby a 14-year-old girl who had been raped, and became pregnant, was to be prevented from travelling to the UK for the purpose of the termination of pregnancy.[26] The case was then taken to the Supreme Court, which withdrew the injunction, and ruled that the girl should be permitted to terminate her pregnancy in Ireland due to the risk in this particular case of suicide of the girl. However, two of the Supreme Court judges also held that the Constitution does allow preventing pregnant women from travelling abroad for the purposes of abortion. At any rate, it would seem that the decision leaves room for such prevention in the event that a clear risk of suicide cannot be established. Subsequent to this decision, however, two

---

[24] '1. Everyone has the right to freedom of expression. This right shall include freedom to hold opinions and to receive and impart information and ideas without interference by public authority and regardless of frontiers. This article shall not prevent States from requiring the licensing of broadcasting, television or cinema enterprises. 2. The exercise of these freedoms, since it carries with it duties and responsibilities, may be subject to such formalities, conditions, restrictions or penalties as are prescribed by law and are necessary in a democratic society, in the interests of national security, territorial integrity or public safety, for the prevention of disorder or crime, for the protection of health or morals, for the protection of the reputation or the rights of others, for preventing the disclosure of information received in confidence, or for maintaining the authority and impartiality of the judiciary'.

[25] *Open Door and Dublin Well Woman v. Ireland*. 64/1991/316/387-388. Council of Europe: European Court of Human Rights, 23 September 1992. Available at: http://www.unhcr.org/refworld/docid/3ae6b7020.html [Accessed April 2009].

[26] *The Attorney General v. X and Others* IESC 1; [1992] 1 IR 1, 5th March, 1992. Available at: http://www.bailii.org/ie/cases/IESC/1992/1.htm [Accessed April 2009]. The case is cited in the *Open Door and Dublin Well Woman v. Ireland* ECHR decision.

amendments were added to article 40.3.3° of the Constitution: it 'shall not limit freedom to travel between the State and another state' (amendment no. 13), and it 'shall not limit freedom to obtain or make available, in the State, subject to such conditions as may be laid down by law, information relating to services lawfully available in another state' (amendment no. 14).[27]

Outside Europe, in the US, the 1991 Rust vs. Sullivan[28] case is worth citing as an additional example. In this case, regulations according to which no public funds could be involved with family planning that mentions abortion, were challenged. The core of the matter thus regarded the refusal to fund the sharing of information regarding abortion in specified settings, and not whether or not to allow abortion at all (as in the Irish case). According to one of the Supreme Court judges on the case:

> '...the Title X programme regulations do not significantly impinge upon the doctor-patient relationship [...] Nor is the doctor-patient relationship established by the Title X programme sufficiently all-encompassing so as to justify an expectation on the part of the patient of comprehensive medical advice. The programme does not provide post-conception medical care, and therefore a doctor's silence with regard to abortion cannot reasonably be thought to mislead a client into thinking that the doctor does not consider abortion an appropriate option for her. The doctor is always free to make clear that advice regarding abortion is simply beyond the scope of the program. In these circumstances, the general rule that the Government may choose not to subsidise speech applies with full force.'[29]

The resemblances between the above examples and ES cell research or therapies developed through such research are more than technical. ES cell research and the continued production of stem cell lines available for

---

[27] Constitution of Ireland. Available at http://www.taoiseach.gov.ie [Accessed April 2009].

[28] Rust v Sullivan, III US 1759 (1991).

[29] Chief Justice Rehnquist, cited in T. Eastland, ed. 2000. *Freedom of Expression in the Supreme Court: The Defining Cases*. Washington: Rowman & Littlefield: 327. The regulation was withdrawn at the beginning of the Clinton presidency.

therapy involve the destruction of human embryos and, in many of these cases, also their creation for the purposes of destruction. The part of the Irish constitution motivating the abortion ban would seem to be equally applicable to such practices.[30] However, ES cell research that does not involve the destruction of embryos can be pursued in Ireland on condition that the cell lines are imported.[31] Similarly, it is common knowledge that the resistance to public funding of practices related to abortion in the US comes from the pro-life side of the underlying conflict. Hence, the underlying arguments in the abortion case are the same as in the Irish case and thus applicable to ES cell research as well.

Even if Ireland, in the case of abortion, finally ended up protecting the freedom of movement and right to information of their citizens at the expense of an extraterritorial take on the ban on abortion, the example goes to show that even when not explicitly formulated in such a way, national laws can be applied so as to prevent patients from getting access to medical services in other states (and even to prevent others from providing such information). All it takes, it would seem, is that the law is directed against acts perceived as fundamental moral wrongs — and in that respect, the analogy between abortion bans such as the case of Ireland and restrictions on ES cell activities appears to be almost perfect. Some consolation may be found in the endpoint of the Irish story regarding abortion. However, this case has important particularities (such as the closeness and sensitive relation to the UK) that may be suspected to have

[30] Accordingly, the Irish Medical Council's *Guide to Ethical Conduct and Behaviour* states that the creation of embryos for research purposes constitutes 'professional misconduct', and that spare embryos (obtained in the process of assisted reproduction) should not be destroyed. See: section F, Genetic Testing and Reproductive Medicine, 24.1 and 24.5. Available at: http://www.medicalcouncil.ie/professional/ethics.asp [Accessed April 2009].

[31] The current Irish development regarding ES cell research seems rather dynamic, though. In the fall of 2008, the governors of University College Cork allowed embryonic stem cell research to take place in their institution, subject to ethical review of the research proposal As reported in *Irish Times*: Barry Roche, *UCC gives go-ahead for embryonic stem-cell research*, 28 October 2008. Available at: http://www.irishtimes.com/newspaper/breaking/2008/1028/breaking67.htm [Accessed April 2009].

influenced the political outcome to land against an extraterritorial stance, but that are not present in the case of other countries that ban or restrict ES cell research. Thus, in other countries, attempts to apply extraterritorial enforcement measures with regard to ES cell activities also with regard to patients may very well occur and may also be sustained to a greater extent than the Irish attempts in the abortion case.

Now, in the face of such a possible reality, from the point of view of liberal countries, at some stage on the ladder of extraterritorial restrictions applied to patients, retaliation will start to look like a reasonable response. Again, therefore, we see how extraterritorial jurisdiction clouds the vision of a global substantial regulation of ES cell research and rather inspires international conflict. In this case, the reason for liberal countries to take this route will, of course, not be a perceived threat to the functionality of the health system, but rather humanitarian and general political concerns. A liberal country may very well apply the principle of live and let live *vis-à-vis* countries with less liberal policies in certain areas within their own borders. When restrictive countries claim the right to enforce their laws to events in other countries, and to severely restrict the freedom of movement of their citizens due to expected actions abroad that are perfectly legal in the host country, the line is approached when, for a liberal, the conclusion has to be drawn that restrictive countries fail to abide by basic regulations in international law, as these are interpreted in the liberal context. Ergo, extraterritorial application of the regulations of the liberal country becomes justifiable in the view of the liberal country. For instance, such a country may start to regard patients from restrictive countries that apply the extraterritorial outlook, as bona fide refugees from intolerable oppression, and may politically and financially retaliate against restrictions on people's abilities to visit and seek information about the liberal country as an illegitimate meddling in internal affairs. Of course, the restrictive country may take exactly the same attitude (and the extraterritorial stance to its restrictions would indeed suggest that route).

CONCLUDING DISCUSSION

The application of extraterritorial jurisdiction by ES cell restrictive countries is much less improbable than is conceded by Mertes and Pennings.

The ambition and strength of the moral basis of the legal restrictions of such countries is not made less strong by minor political compromises to achieve a national legislation. If taken seriously, this basis seems to imply that ES cell research and related activities are, in the eyes of such a moral view, crimes of a sort for which extraterritorial jurisdiction is particularly apt from both a legal and a moral standpoint. Since there is no reason to doubt the political or moral seriousness of countries that have adopted restrictive ES cell policies, we have concluded that extraterritorial jurisdiction has to be taken equally seriously as a possible ingredient in the international regulatory complex surrounding ES cell research and forthcoming therapies built on that.

Generally, we have identified a potential political process between states, where some of these extend very restrictive views on ES cell related activities beyond its borders. Such actions create severe troubles not only for researchers, clinicians and (potential) patients. They also adversely affect basic social institutions (such as health care) in more liberal countries, as well as finance, freedom of movement and freedom of expression at an international level. For this reason, extraterritorial ambitions of ES cell restrictive countries may be expected to create responses from liberal countries of an extraterritorial retaliating nature. As a result, the initial international moral and legal conflict will be sharpened, as well as transformed into a political strategic conflict. Such a development is the very opposite of what is required in international relations in order to facilitate global or multinational regulation in any area, and the ES cell case is no different in this respect.

Based on this general result, a peculiar side observation may be highlighted. Our argument implies that an ES cell restrictive country that does not endorse extraterritorial jurisdiction in this area may be rightly accused of not sticking up for the moral view held out as motivating its restrictive stance (i.e. the moral evaluation that the destruction of embryos amounts to murder). If embryo destruction really is morally on a par with murder, organised ES cell activities are either organised mass murder (genocide), or an organised scheme for exploiting on the occurrence of mass murder. And, if so, extraterritorial jurisdiction would seem to not only make sense and be allowed by international law. Morally, implementing such a stance would seem like an imperative.

However, if ES cell restrictive countries were to indeed go down such a path, they would risk undercutting any chance of global regulation of ES cell activities that they can use to protect their own right to apply their own national policies *within* their own borders (in line with the *Bioethics Convention*). Moreover, they would risk initiating a process bound to have themselves subjected to the extraterritorial legal measures of *liberal* countries. In effect, they would risk setting in motion a chain of events that would jeopardize international financial and political stability on a scale considerably larger than merely the ES cell area and, possibly, with vast effects in terms of life and health. In such a situation their (as all nations') abilities to uphold their own national legal and political integrity would, of course, suffer, and this would include ES cell policies as well. It remains to be seen how, in the light of such scenarios, ES cell restrictive countries choose to sum up the pros and cons.

The issue of extraterritorial jurisdiction raises a number of challenges for a global regulation of ES cell research and therapy. National legislation impacts on the three categories of potential stakeholders in many ways, and some provisions will have to be made in these regards in any future global regulation. The researchers, clinicians and patients stand to gain or lose from both their national and any global regulation. Will access to work (for the researchers and clinicians) and therapy (for the patients) be limited (or favoured) relative to one's state of origin? Will information be free to travel? Will people be punished in one country for research or medical intervention legally performed (by oneself or onto oneself) in another state in a manner that is legal in that state and protected by global regulation? Conversely, will citizens of a state with a liberal regulation of ES cell research and therapy be prevented from having their work internationally recognised and from collaborating with willing peers from other states, in virtue of not-so-liberal global regulation? Will conformation to not-so-liberal views be inescapable in the conditions of not-so-liberal global regulation? All of these questions will have to feature among those to be discussed in the making of global regulation on stem cell research and therapy.

POSTSCRIPT

The news of Obama's new policy on use of stem cell lines broke during proof reading of this chapter, but since the US ban of federal funding of embryo research still stands, the new policy has only a minor impact on our general arguments with regard to the US.

4

GOVERNING CLONING: UNITED NATIONS' DEBATES AND THE INSTITUTIONAL CONTEXT OF STANDARDS

W. Calvin Ho[1]

When an initiative was proposed calling on the United Nations (UN) to ban reproductive cloning, there was an expectation that little controversy would follow. This might have been premised on the assumption that a 'baseline' standard of human dignity was already present but required articulation. The danger perceived in the application of cloning technology for reproductive purposes, made credible by the successful cloning of Dolly the sheep, provided the occasion and the rationale for the initiative. Reproductive cloning was taken to be a threat to human dignity, which is essentially grounded in the notion that every individual person is unique and on this basis deserving of fundamental rights. In the course of the UN debates, the ambiguity of 'personhood' surfaced when the initiative was broadened to encompass not only reproductive cloning, but also therapeutic cloning (or somatic cell nuclear transfer). No agreement was reached on the issue of whether a human embryo could also qualify as a 'person' upon whom (or indeed, which) fundamental rights would attend. The lack of consensus ultimately resulted in the UN Declaration on Human Cloning ('Human Cloning Declaration'), regarded by many to be without moral

[1] The views and opinions expressed in this chapter are personal to the author.

or legal authority, aside from saying nothing about either cloning or human dignity.[2]

Ironically, the UN initiative had a catalytic effect on policy developments in a number of member states interested in therapeutic cloning. The threat of being subsumed into a disagreeable discourse motivated these states to articulate a national position that would be useful in at least two ways. First, it could serve as a discursive barrier against an allegation of condoning unethical scientific practices in exchange for some form of (often economic) benefit. Ethics is important as an intrinsic component to a member state's reputation of doing 'good science', which in turn influences the flow of, as well as its claim over, scarce resources and talent. Second, it enables solidarity in that a clear national position allows a member state to come into alliance with other member states that share in its position, and so amplify its political clout. For many of the member states not caught up in the fray however, the subject was of little relevance to them, even though they recognised, as a matter of principle, the danger of cloning technology if misapplied. As we shall see, these states had a strong influence over the outcome of the UN debates.

This chapter considers a possible reason for the failure of arriving at an effective international standard (or an exclusive global script) on cloning to be the difficulty of standards setting through resolving conflicts over meaning in the abstract. By further considering similar attempts that were made by domestic institutions, the significance of institutional context to standards creation is highlighted. To be sure, it is not the argument of this chapter that standards can only arise through the intermediation of domestic institutions. Rather, the domestic setting within which an institution subsists is a means by which the situatedness and historical specificity of standards are rendered more apparent. Key occurrences at the UN from the introduction of the initiative in 2001 to the promulgation of the Human Cloning Declaration are considered. However, the account of UN debates provided here differs from many other accounts in that they are presented from the standpoint of Singapore. When reproductive cloning was

[2] The Human Cloning Declaration is set out as A/Res/59/280, 23 March 2005. Available at: http://www.unescobkk.org/fileadmin/user_upload/shs/BEfiles/chapterE.eng/E8.2E.pdf [Accessed 30 June 2009].

presented as an issue at the UN, the absence of a sufficiently generic 'immutable mobile'[3] or 'boundary object'[4] that could be easily transplanted from one socio-political setting to another quickly became evident once the discussion was broadened to include the status of a human embryo. The notion of human dignity was itself too vague to inspire action, and also too ambiguous to enable consensus to be forged across a community with varied, and in some respects conflicting, interests and concerns.

Contrasting international with local developments, this chapter considers the role of domestic institutions in understanding and managing cloning in Singapore and in the UK. In Singapore, the work of the *Bioethics Advisory Committee* (BAC) in developing a national position on the subject is set out to explicate the rationale behind standards setting. Whereas the BAC's approach to cloning could be taken to be holistic, that of the UK was more incremental. The earlier institutional history of the UK's *Human Fertilisation and Embryology Authority* (HFEA) has been considered elsewhere.[5] This chapter is focused on the circumstances by which the supervisory authority of the HFEA was extended to include therapeutic cloning. The ethical premise that the BAC and the HFEA share, could arguably constitute an 'immutable mobile', even though the social and conceptual materials employed in the process differ. If such an argument could be made, the UN debate could well call into question the extent to which such an 'immutable mobile' or 'boundary object' could be transposed independent of a complementary social or conceptual context. One could go further to view the coalition that was opposed to therapeutic cloning to be advocating another 'boundary object', but neither succeeded in subsuming the other, perhaps owing in part to the failure of both coalitions in convincing a sizeable third group of member states that was largely disinterested in the technology. This chapter concludes with a discussion of the critical role that domestic institutions (and

---

[3] B. Latour. 1999. *Pandora's Hope: Essays on the Reality of Science Studies*. London, England: Harvard University Press: 102, 306–307.

[4] G.C. Bowker and S.L. Star. 2000. *Sorting Things Out: Classification and Its Consequences*. Cambridge, MA: MIT Press: 13–14.

[5] R.G. Lee and D. Morgan. 2001. *Human Fertilisation and Embryology: Regulating the Reproductive Revolution*. London, England: Blackstone Press Limited: Chaps. 1 and 4.

context) play in standards creation, dissemination and assimilation, and with a number of other observations.

CLONING AND THE UNITED NATIONS

In the 56th Session of the United Nations General Assembly (UNGA), France and Germany tabled a proposal for the promulgation of a legally binding treaty or convention to prohibit reproductive cloning of human beings. The original French-German proposal[6] was essentially directed at reproductive cloning and did not assume a firm position for or against therapeutic cloning. It merely cautioned:

> '[b]earing in mind that this purpose could lead to a step-by-step approach to addressing issues related to other forms of human cloning, including through the elaboration of a separate international instrument, as soon as negotiations on a convention against reproductive cloning of human beings have been concluded'.[7]

However, France and Germany subsequently amended their proposal to recommend that a moratorium be imposed on the conduct of therapeutic cloning immediately following the completion of negotiations on the reproductive cloning convention.[8] This amendment was made to reflect the growing number of delegations concerned with the practice of therapeutic cloning. With this amendment, France and Germany were able to retain a majority of countries supporting their proposal. These included countries that did not have a position on therapeutic cloning, but supported the proposal so that reproductive cloning could be prohibited at the international level.

Although the proposal was adopted by consensus at the 56th UNGA, contention arose a year later at the first meeting of the *Ad Hoc Committee*

---

[6] See A/C.6/57/WG.1/CRP.1.

[7] Ibid. See Paragraph 9. Paragraph 10 further indicates 'Bearing in mind that this purpose does not preclude the possibility of States Parties adopting stricter national regulations'.

[8] See A/C.6/57/L.8 (hereinafter, the 'French-German proposal'). The list of sponsors is set out in A/C.6/57/L.8/Corr.1.

of the Sixth (Legal) Committee in February 2002, brought about by the US, Spain, and Holy See-led coalition to seek a ban on therapeutic cloning along with reproductive cloning.[9] The basic premise for the position held by this coalition was that there could be no distinction made between therapeutic cloning and reproductive cloning, as both involved the use of a common technological process. Clarity in the simplicity of this formulation proved attractive to many countries (especially those with a predominantly large Catholic population) without having first arrived at a national position on the subject.

Various alternative proposals were put forward during the general debate within the Working Group to try and bridge the gap between the two camps in order to allow the broader agenda of prohibiting reproductive cloning to move ahead. The proposals included having a ban on reproductive cloning and a moratorium on therapeutic cloning, so as to allow the latter to be debated while resolving the former. This was suggested by Mexico, and supported by the Netherlands, Australia, and various Latin American and African countries.

Malaysia recommended a parallel track approach, whereby discussions on therapeutic cloning would be undertaken, at the same time as negotiations are ongoing on the reproductive cloning convention. The Republic of Korea suggested a variation of this when it proposed a 'two-tier' approach whereby the Convention could focus on reproductive cloning while proposing for therapeutic cloning to be regulated on an optional basis. These proposals were not greeted with much enthusiasm. Many considered the parallel approach to be onerous especially for small delegations. In addition, both the parallel and two-tier approaches were unacceptable to members of the US-Holy See faction because they were opposed to all forms of cloning.

Further complication arose when the US and Spain tabled a competing proposal in the Sixth Committee immediately after the close of the

[9] The *Ad Hoc* Committee on an International Convention against the Reproductive Cloning of Human Beings was formed through the UNGA's resolution 56/93 of 12 December 2001. It was tasked to 'consider the elaboration of a mandate for the negotiation of such an international convention, including a list of the existing international instruments to be taken into consideration and a list of legal issues to be address in the convention'. See http://www.un.org/law/cloning/ [Accessed 30 June 2009].

Working Group session without prior discussion in the Working Group itself.[10] The US-Spain proposal sought to commence negotiations on a convention which would ban both reproductive and therapeutic cloning, as well as to impose a moratorium on both immediately. Meanwhile, the French-German proposal was revised to a formulation that was more acceptable to countries which did not wish to preclude therapeutic cloning and was tabled with the Sixth Committee after the US-Spain proposal was tabled. Technically, the French-German proposal could be acted upon first since it was an amendment of the earlier proposal. Due to the intractable positions on the competing draft resolutions tabled by France and Germany on the one side, and the US-Spain-Holy See camp on the other side, a procedural decision was taken to defer action on the issue.[11]

When the UNGA reconvened for the 57th Ssession in the fall of 2002, the discussions were largely grounded in emotive rhetoric. Nevertheless delegates unfamiliar with science and who had no real national interest in the subject appeared to find the discussions persuasive. As Singapore has a national position on the subject by this time, one of the goals of the Singapore delegation was to deploy this as a basis for advancing the French-German proposal. Despite already having legislation that disallowed therapeutic cloning (and hence, having positions not inconsistent with the US), France and Germany were prepared to work with countries adhering to different views on therapeutic cloning in order to secure a legally binding treaty prohibiting reproductive cloning. They were motivated by a belief that human reproductive cloning was an imminent threat and prompt response on the part of the international community would be politically expedient. Hence, they took the pragmatic approach to focus only on reproductive cloning. In opposition, strong US support for a comprehensive ban on all forms of cloning could have been due in part to the need to play up to the domestic religious and pro-life lobby, and partly by the desire not to lose its scientific and commercial lead to other countries

[10] See A/C.6/57/L.3 (hereinafter, the 'US-Spain proposal'). The list of co-sponsors is set out in A/C.6/57/L.3/Rev.1/Corr.1.

[11] See A/C.6/57/L.24. See also Report of the Ad Hoc Committee on an International Convention Against the Reproductive Cloning of Human Beings, UN GAOR, 57th Session, Supp. No. 51, UN Doc. A/57/51 (2002).

that did not face similar political obstacles. Other countries that supported the US-Spain proposal were driven by ideological positions on the sanctity of life and the rights of the embryo. In addition, arguments advanced in support of a comprehensive ban on all forms of cloning included the following concerns:[12]

(1) If therapeutic cloning is not prohibited, it creates a loop-hole which prevents effectively enforcement of prohibition against the implantation of that cloned embryo into the uterus of a woman;
(2) 'Slippery slope' argument in that once scientists are allowed to carry out therapeutic cloning, there would be little to prevent them from going one step further and engage in reproductive cloning;
(3) Therapeutic cloning is against human dignity because it involves the killing of a life when stem cells are extracted from the cloned embryo thereby destroying it. The killing of this nascent life cannot be justified for any reason, even if it is to save other lives;
(4) Adult stem cell research, which is not ethically objectionable, will yield just as much benefit as embryonic stem cell research, including therapeutic cloning;
(5) Therapeutic cloning will lead to exploitation of women, especially in poor countries, as there will be illicit trade in eggs for profit;
(6) Chances are remote that developing countries can avail themselves of the potential benefits that might be derived from therapeutic cloning research; and
(7) There are more pressing concerns facing developing countries (such as malaria), and the resources that would be poured into therapeutic cloning research would be better utilised in these areas of pressing concern.

Aside from these, a stem cell science expert in the Singapore delegation observed that there were no serious discussions of the various multi-dimensional issues that reproductive cloning and therapeutic cloning

[12] These arguments are consolidated based on the author's interviews with some members of the Malaysia and Singapore delegations at the 57th UNGA.

entailed. Only a minority of countries that included Australia, Belgium, China, Israel, Singapore, South Africa, Sweden, Switzerland and the United Kingdom were fervent in keeping the door to therapeutic cloning open. When it eventually became clear that no agreement could be arrived at between the two factions, the Sixth Committee decided to continue discussions a year later.[13]

During this time, one of the most publicised controversy concerning stem cell research and cloning was the announcement of the implantations and births of two allegedly cloned babies by Clonaid, the US-based 'scientific' arm of a space alien-worshipping cult called Raelians. In July 2002, Clonaid's South Korean office also announced that a Korean woman had been successfully impregnated with a cloned embryo with the help of BioFusion Tech.[14] The South Korean government responded by commencing investigation and introduced legislation to ban human cloning, which was not then prohibited. In December 2003, the Korean Legislation and Judiciary Committee at the National Assembly passed a bill to ban all uses of cloning technology, as well as fertilising egg cells for the purpose of sex selection other than for use related to seeking cures of fatal diseases.[15] Apart from South Korea, political reactions were also triggered in India, Malaysia and the United States:

(1) The Indian government appointed a bioethics committee to consider the implications of stem cell research and cloning[16];
(2) In Malaysia, the National Fatwa Council, the country's highest religious authority, gave further consideration to its edict of March 2002 that prohibited the cloning of humans. It opined that research may be

[13] UN Doc. A/57/569 (2002) at page 7.

[14] *BBC News*. Clone Cult Firm Raided in South Korea. 30 Dec 2002. Available at http://news.bbc.co.uk/2/hi/health/2614341.stm [Accessed 30 June 2009].

[15] *Medical News Today*. Korea to Stop Cloning with Human Eggs, 19 Feb 2004. Available at: http://www.medicalnewstoday.com/index.php?newsid=6015 [Accessed 30 June 2009]. Legislation that explicitly prohibited reproductive cloning was passed in 2005: *Bioethics and Biosafety Act No. 7150*. 2005.

[16] R. Lakshmi. 2001. India Plans to Fill Void in Stem Cell Research. *The Washington Post*. 28 August: A07.

conducted on an embryo before 120 days from fertilisation. This is consistent with the Islamic belief that ensoulment only occurs four months from the time of fertilisation[17]; and

(3) In the US, a bill to ban both reproductive cloning and cloning for research purposes was introduced in the House of Representatives on 8 January 2003.[18] However, this bill did not succeed in its passage through the Democrat-controlled Senate.

At the 58th Session in 2003, countries remained divided along roughly similar lines. Costa Rica now led a group of 68 states with the most stringent proposal which recommended criminal sanctions and extradition of any person involved in any form of cloning.[19] The French-German position could not be sustained after strong domestic political pressure from the German legislature and public resulted in the withdrawal of Germany's support for its own proposal.[20] Belgium took over the initiative in the French-German proposal as it was consistent with its domestic policy of banning reproductive cloning as a matter of urgency. Following this development, the Belgian proposal gained the backing of the original supporters of the French-German proposal, in addition to a number of Nordic states.[21]

---

[17] See *LifeSiteNews*. Malaysia Muslims approve cloning, abortion up to 120 days. 9 January 2003. Available at http://www.lifesite.net/ldn/2003/jan/03010902.html [Accessed 30 June 2009].

[18] H.R. 234 Human Cloning Prohibition Act of 2003, introduced by Representative Dave Weldon (R-FL) to amend Title 18, United States Code, to prohibit human cloning. The Bill is reported to be similar to the cloning ban that passed the House of Representatives on 31 July 2001, which would have prohibited both reproductive and therapeutic cloning. See http://olpa.od.nih.gov/tracking/house_bills/session1/hr-234.asp [Accessed 30 Jun 2009].

[19] UN Doc. A/58/73 (2003). Available at http://www.un.org/law/cloning/#2003 [Accessed 30 Jun 2009].

[20] N.M. de S. Cameron and A.V. Henderson. Brave New World at the General Assembly: The United Nations Declaration on Human Cloning. *Minnesota Journal of Law Science and Technology* 2008; 9: 145–238, at 169, 189–191.

[21] UN Doc. A/C.6/58/L.8 (2003). Available at http://www.un.org/law/cloning/#2003 [Accessed 30 June 2009]. About a week before debate was resumed at the UNGA, the German government announced that it would no longer sponsor the French-German proposal, but would instead support the Belgian proposal: Ibid at 190.

In the course of the debates, both sides actively engaged with smaller states that did not have any immediate interest in cloning technology. When it seemed likely that the Costa Rican proposal would carry the day, the delegation of Iran, on behalf of the member states of the Organisation of the Islamic Conference (OIC), moved to adjourn the debate on the agenda item until the 60th Session of the UNGA in September 2005. The motion was passed by a narrow margin with 80 countries having voted in favour, 79 countries having voted against and 15 countries having abstained. The OIC regarded a treaty premised exclusively on the Judeo-Christian conception of 'personhood' to be wanting, and preferred to allow time for more discussion and deliberation. However, the UNGA was reported to have considered the report of the Sixth Committee on the agenda item at its 72nd plenary meeting held on 9 December 2003, and decided, without a vote, to include the item in the provisional agenda of its 59th Session in 2004.

The adjournment of the debate dealt a heavy blow to supporters of the Costa Rican proposal, as the push for a comprehensive ban of cloning by way of a legally binding treaty at the 59th Session of the UNGA did not proceed with the rigour that it did in earlier sessions. For some countries like Singapore, the near success of the Costa Rican proposal raised concern that international law instruments could be used in ways that could compromise its national interest. There was a progressive realisation that more active involvement in the negotiation and drafting of international law instruments was necessary, even if there were no critical interests or immediate benefit in doing so, in order to develop the member state's international standing and reputation. The adjournment did not strengthen the position of the Belgian faction however. Much to the contrary, the decision to resume the debate in 2004 instead of September 2005 might well have been reflective of a general skepticism among delegates that a consensus on therapeutic cloning could be reached.[22]

The 59th Session of the UNGA reconvened for general debate on 21 September 2004, with an address by US President George W. Bush that included a call on member states to ban all forms of cloning.[23]

---

[22] Ibid: 176.

[23] *President Bush addresses 59th U.N. General Assembly Opening*. 21 September 2004. Available at http://seoul.usembassy.gov/21-sep.04 [Accessed 30 June 2009].

Cloning remained an issue in US domestic politics as the nation prepared for its Presidential election in November that year. The position of the US federal government on embryonic stem cell research and therapeutic cloning was not shared by all of its constituents. In March 2004, 70 members of Congress wrote to President Bush to relax his ban of federal funding for research on embryonic stem cells created after 9 August 2001.[24] These legislators threatened to push for legislation to achieve this goal if the President failed to act. This followed from the confirmation by the National Institutes of Health that, of the 78 embryonic lines that qualify for federal funding, only 17 were actually ready for research. In addition, private institutions announced that they would push ahead in human embryonic stem cell research with private funds. Researchers at Harvard University have created 17 new embryonic stem cell lines with private funds.[25] The University has itself pledged US$100 million to finance a stem cell institute, putting it at that time ahead — in terms of funding — of Stanford University (US$12 million), the University of California San Francisco (US$11 million) and the University of Minnesota in Minneapolis (US$8 million). Later in the year, voters in the state of California approved of Proposition 71 on 2 November. This initiative established a US$3 billion bond measure to fund stem cell research in the state through the California Institute for Regenerative Medicine.[26]

Despite strong lobbying on both sides, no consensus was reached either by the UNGA or by the Sixth Committee when it met on 21 October 2004.[27] By that time, motivation in pushing for a legally binding treaty appeared to have significantly waned. Hence on 19 November 2004, the Sixth Committee decided to establish a Working Group to draft a

[24] B. Vastag. Private Efforts Pick Up Stem Cell Slack. *Journal of the American Medical Association* 2004; 291(17): 2059.

[25] C. A. Cowan *et al.* Derivation of Embryonic Stem Cell-Lines from Human Blastocysts. *New England Journal of Medicine* 2004; 350: 13.

[26] Information on Proposition 71 is available from the website of the California of Regenerative Medicine: http://www.cirm.ca.gov/?q=node/6 [Accessed 30 June 2009].

[27] Report of the Sixth Committee — Addendum, UN Doc. A/59/516 Add. I (2004). 71 states voted in favour, with 35 states voting against, and 43 states abstaining.

non-binding declaration instead of a convention on cloning.[28] The Working Group met in February 2005 to consider a draft non-binding declaration on human cloning that was submitted by the Italian delegation and another draft that was subsequently revised as a proposal by Honduras.[29] It was the amended proposal from Honduras that was subsequently adopted by the UNGA on 8 March 2005.[30]

Aside from the difficulty of reaching a consensus on a legally binding convention on cloning, active measures to regulate cloning introduced by key member states interested in the technology might have contributed to a change in the mindset of member states that had previously considered a treaty for a comprehensive ban on cloning to be the only effective safeguard against reproductive cloning. In this connection, this chapter will next consider some of the domestic — and essentially institutional — developments in Singapore and in the UK, before reflecting (comparatively) on the difficulties with standards setting at the supranational level of the United Nations.

STEM CELLS, CLONING AND THE BIOETHICS COMMITTEE OF SINGAPORE

The BAC took up the initiative to formulate ethical standards for embryonic stem cell research and cloning in early 2001 following its establishment in December of the preceding year. Already controversial in certain local quarters, this subject area became perhaps emblematic of the hopes and fears in biomedical technology with the widely publicised announcement by then US President George W. Bush on 9 August 2001,

[28] Press Release: Legal Committee Text Calls for Further Discussions on Human Cloning Aimed at 'Declaration'. U.N. Doc. GA/L/3270 (19 November 2004). Available at http://www.un.org/News/Press/docs/2004/gal3270.doc.htm [Accessed 30 June 2009].

[29] UNGA, Sixth Committee Working Group. 2005. Report of the Working Group Established Pursuant to General Assembly Decision 59/547 to Finalize the Text of a United Nations Declaration on Human Cloning. *U.N. Doc. A/C.6/59/L.27/Rev.1*. 23 February.

[30] UNGA Resolution 59/280 (2004) incorporates the United Nations Declaration on Human Cloning.

to deny federal funding for research on stem cells derived from embryos created after 10 August 2001.[31] In Singapore, public expression of concern over the practice of embryonic stem cell technology was received by the BAC as soon as its website was launched on 22 August 2001.[32]

During the time between the 56th UNGA and the first meeting of the Ad Hoc Committee, the BAC arrived at an interim ethical position on the subject, and public consultation commenced on 8 November 2001. While the BAC reasoned that reproductive cloning of human beings should be prohibited, embryonic stem cell research and therapeutic cloning was considered to be ethical provided that these proceeded on a strictly regulated basis and subject to particular ethical requirements. These aspects of the BAC's position were not altered by public feedback. Although particular groups expressed strong opposition to the research, their views could not be taken as representative of the society on the whole.

After the conclusion of BAC's public consultation, an article by Francis Fukuyama in the *Financial Times* referred to Singapore's stem cell initiative in implicitly negative terms; highlighting the eugenicist thinking of Minister Mentor (then Senior Minister) Lee Kwan Yew, and associating Singapore with China and South Korea as having fewer ethical constraints than the West in such research. Fukuyama appeared to be concerned as to whether non-industrialised, and especially non-Western, countries could be committed to ethical causes. Referring to the apparent lack of ethical constraints in Asian countries as 'The Asian advantage', Fukuyama argued:

> 'It is not just China, but also South Korea, Singapore and other countries in Asia that have expressed interest in moving ahead rapidly in stem cell research, cloning and other biotech fields, precisely because

---

[31] Office of the Press Secretary. 2001. *Remarks by the President on Stem Cell Research.* 9 August.

[32] A. Chang. 2001. Stem-Cell Research Draft Guidelines Out Next Month. *The Straits Times*, 13 September.

> they want to take advantage of the ethical constraints that western countries are imposing on themselves. Lee Kwan Yew, former prime minister of Singapore, was a strong believer in the hereditary basis of important qualities such as intelligence, and was a promoter of eugenics as a means of improving Singapore's global competitive position'.[33]

In rebuttal, Mr. Michael Eng, Singapore's High Commissioner in London published a reply the following weekend entitled 'Singapore's careful research' to highlight that 'Singapore places a priority on an ethical and legal framework to protect the rights and welfare of individuals, at the same time allowing the biomedical sciences to develop for the benefit of humanity'.[34] The BAC was referred to in the response as an expert body formed to consider concerns arising from biomedical research and development in Singapore.

In June 2002, the ethical recommendations for stem cell research and cloning were published by the BAC,[35] and these were accepted by the Singapore government in July that year. As it turned out, Singapore's position on the subject was similar to that of the UK, and did not differ in substance from the recommendations of the US *National Bioethics Advisory Commission* that was appointed under the Clinton administration.[36] However, the enunciation of ethical recommendations was not in itself sufficient to constitute Singapore as a

---

[33] F. Fukuyama. 2002. The Clone Traders. *The Financial Times Weekend Edition*. 18–19 May. A sub-heading appeared as: 'Advances in human biotechnology have highlighted the need for international regulation. But, as Fukuyama explains, religious and social differences between east and west could make this impossible'.

[34] M.C.T. Eng. 2002. Singapore's Careful Research. *The Financial Times Weekend Edition*. 25–26 May.

[35] BAC. 2002. *Ethical, Legal and Social Issues in Human Stem Cell Research, Reproductive and Therapeutic Cloning*. Singapore: BAC.

[36] US National Bioethics Advisory Commission. 1999. *Ethical Issues in Human Stem Cell Research*. A copy of this report is available at http://govinfo.library.unt.edu/nbac/pubs.html [Accessed 30 June 2009].

place for ethical research. Recognition had to be actively secured and defended.[37]

In August that year, an article in the *Far Eastern Economic Review* indicated that 'Singapore will have some of the most liberal stem-cell research guidelines in the world.'[38] A similar suggestion that a 'permissive climate for research' to draw top scientists to Singapore was proffered in *The Economist* that month.[39] This construction of 'permissive' as somehow 'ethically compromised' persisted for some time in the media, with hardly any discussion on why a community should be rendered less 'ethical' by permitting embryonic stem cell research, or *vice versa*.[40] But what this phenomenon seems to indicate is the associational and exclusionary effects of a particular viewpoint as a standard. When the Bush administration labelled human embryonic stem cell research and the related cloning technology as being ethically problematic, it provided or otherwise endorsed a standard by which the 'sacred' could be demarcated from the 'profane'. For a standard without clear parameters or goals, misappropriation and misrecognition would appear to be almost inevitable.

DOMESTIC AND INSTITUTIONAL RESPONSES IN THE UK

In the UK, the legislation that governed human embryonic stem cell research was construed by the judiciary as also covering therapeutic cloning. This development that has its origin in 2002 merits closer attention. The UK is one of a few countries that moved beyond the impasse of

[37] C. Taylor. 1994. The Politics of Recognition. In *Multiculturalism: Examining the Politics of Recognition*. A. Gutmann, ed. Princeton, NJ: Princeton University Press.

[38] T. Saywell. 2002. The New Frontier: Biomedics Could be the Next Big Thing. *Far Eastern Economic Review*. 11 July.

[39] *The Economist*. 2002. Send in the Clones: Will a Relaxed Attitude to Regulation make Singapore the Stem-Cell Research Capital of the World? 22 August.

[40] W. Arnold. 2003. Singapore Builds a Better Scientist Trap. *New York Times*. 27 August Arnold writes: 'For stem-cell researchers, Singapore offers one of the world's most liberal legal atmospheres. It allows stem cells to be taken from aborted fetuses, and human embryos to be cloned and kept for up to 14 days to produce stem cells'.

normative indeterminacy in relation to human embryological research. The *Human Fertilisation and Embryology Act* of 1990 ('HFE Act')[41] established a regulatory regime through the institution of a regulatory body — the HFEA — responsible for monitoring the creation and handling of human embryos. At the time the Act was passed, a genetic testing technique known as preimplantation genetic diagnosis ('PGD') was only a mere possibility. By the turn of the century, PGD has become an acceptable method employed to test for genetic disorder in an embryo created through IVF.[42] In 2002, controversy arose in relation to pre-implantation HLA typing,[43] a specific type of PGD that allowed the genetic composition of the embryo to be matched against the genetic composition of another person.[44] In 2002, the HFEA rejected the Whitakers' application for the use of this technique to produce a tissue-matching sibling for his brother, who was seriously ill with a rare disorder known as Diamond Blackfan anaemia. A person with

[41] The HFE Act has been amended by the British Parliament in November 2008 following a review that commenced in January 2004. The HFE Act of 2008 empowers the HFEA to regulate research involving human admixed embryos, namely (a) human cytoplasmic hybrid embryos, which are created by replacing the nuclei of animal eggs with that of human somatic cells, (b) true human-animal hybrid embryos, created by fusion of gametes from an animal and a human, (c) transgenic human embryos, which are human embryos that have animal DNA incorporated into their genome, (d) human-animal chimeric embryos, that are human embryos in which animal stem cells have been added, and (e) any other embryos that have human and animal nuclear or mitochondrial DNA but in which the animal DNA is not predominant.

[42] Y. Verlinsky *et al.* Preimplantation HLA Testing. *Journal of the American Medical Association* 2004; 291(17): 2079.

[43] HLA matching procedures have been used in 2002–2003 for nine couples with children affected by acute lymphoid leukemia, acute myeloid leukemia and Diamond-Blackfan anemia and so required HLA-matched stem cell transplantation. The procedure has been described as '[i]n 13 clinical cycles, DNA in single blastomeres removed from eight-cell embryos following *in vitro* fertilisation was analysed for HLA genes simultaneously with analysis for short tanderm repeats in the HLA region to select and transfer only those embryos that were HLA matched to affected siblings'. Of the 199 embryos tested, 45 HLA-matched embryos were selected, 'of which 28 were transferred in 12 clinical cycles, resulting in five singleton pregnancies and birth of five HLA-matched healthy children': see Ibid.

[44] S. Bhattacharya. 2003. Banned 'Designer Baby' is Born in the UK, *New Scientist*. 19 June.

this genetic disorder produces too few red blood cells and will not usually survive past 30 years old. The only known treatment is through the transplantation of perfectly matched stem cells. The HFEA rejected the application on the basis that tissue-typing of embryos would only be permitted in the UK if used in combination with screening for a serious genetic risk that poses a risk to the embryo.[45] Neither of the Whitakers possessed such a genetic pre-disposition. Undeterred, the Whitakers travelled to the United States, and Mrs. Whitaker successfully conceived a baby with the same genes for the immune system as his brother.

In 2003, another application was made to the HFEA for a similar treatment. This application was granted primarily because one parent was a carrier of the genetic disorder. The decision of the HFEA was successfully challenged by a pro-life group at the High Court but the High Court's ruling was overturned on appeal by the Court of Appeal.[46] The decision of the Court of Appeal merits evaluation as it provides a detailed analysis of the regime established by the Act.

Zain was born with a blood disorder known as beta thalassaemia major, and survived on a variety of drugs applied along with regular blood transfusion.[47] Mrs. Hashmi knew that she had a genetic disposition to producing children with this disorder and underwent a prenatal testing when she was pregnant with Zain. The test, however, failed to identify the disorder and Zain was carried to term. Zain's condition might be treated by a transplant of stem cells derived from the umbilical cord of a newborn child or from bone marrow of someone with matching tissue. Unfortunately, none of Zain's three older siblings has tissue that matched his. Determined to provide Zain with a matching tissue, Mrs. Hashmi conceived again. This child was tested to be with the same genetic disorder and was aborted. She

[45] See HFEA Press Release: HFEA confirms that HLA tissue typing may only take place when PGD is required to avoid a serious genetic disorder. 1 August 2002. Available at http://www.hfea.gov.uk/935.html [Accessed 30 June 2009].

[46] See HFEA Press Release: Court of Appeal Allows Tissue Typing for Human Embryos under Strict Conditions. 8 April 2003. Available at http://www.hfea.gov.uk/844.html [Accessed 30 June 2009].

[47] The factual description in this paragraph is essentially derived from the decision of the English Court of Appeal (Lord Phillips MR) in *R (Quintavalle) v. HFEA* [2003] 3 All ER 257 at 259–261.

was conceived with her fifth child and was carried to term as a healthy boy although he too did not provide a matching tissue sample for Zain. It was at this time that Mrs. Hashmi learnt from Dr. Fishel, the managing and scientific director of Centres for Assisted Reproduction Ltd ('CARE', the same centre that assisted the Whitakers in conceiving a child with tissue that matched that of his ill sibling), the largest provider of IVF services in the UK, that Reproductive Genetics Institute ('RGI') in Chicago has developed an advance medical procedure that may resolve her problem. The procedure was summarised as:[48]

> '(i) The fertilisation "*in vitro*" of a number of eggs taken from Mrs. Hashmi with sperm taken from her husband to form embryos. (ii) The removal from the developing embryo of a single cell by biopsy. (iii) The examination of that cell using molecular genetics to see whether the embryo carried the beta thalassaemia disease. The process is commonly described as "Pre-implantation Genetic Diagnosis" (PGD). (iv) Use simultaneously of the same process to identify whether the embryo had the same tissue type as Zain. Because this process involves examination of proteins known as human leukocyte antigens (HLA), this form of PGD is described as "HLA typing" [which is a specialised form of tissue typing]...(v) Jettison of embryos found by this analysis to be either disease bearing or of a different HLA type to Zain and implantation in the womb of Mrs. Hashmi of an embryo shown to be disease free and of the same HLA as Zain'.

As noted earlier, the creation, custody or use of a human embryo is prohibited in the UK under the HFE Act unless a license is first procured from the HFEA.[49] The HFE Act further empowers the HFEA to prescribe conditions relating to the creation, custody and use of the embryo.[50] In the present case, it was necessary for CARE to procure a license for treatment services before initiating such a procedure in the UK. The term 'treatment services' has been defined as 'medical, surgical or obstetric

[48] Ibid: 259–260.

[49] Section 3 of the HFE Act 1990.

[50] Sections 12 and 13 of the HFE Act.

services provided to the public or a section of the public for the purpose of assisting women to carry children…'[51] A license for treatment, including tissue typing, was granted by the HFEA but subject to certain conditions.[52] In particular, the HFEA indicated that tissue typing should only be permitted where PGD was already necessary to avoid the passing on a serious genetic disorder. Pursuant to the license, fifteen embryos were created through the first IVF treatment and biopsied cells were flown to RGI for analysis. Only one embryo produced a tissue match but it was not viable because it carried the beta thalassaemia disease. Mr. and Mrs. Hashmi then travelled to RGI for their second IVF treatment. Ten embryos were produced and of which two proved to be free of the genetic disorder and also provided a tissue match. One was implanted in Mrs. Hashmi but it did not result in a pregnancy.

Meanwhile, an action was filed at the High Court by Comment on Reproductive Ethics ('CORE').[53] It argued that the HFEA did not have the authority to issue a license that permitted the use of HLA typing to select between healthy embryos. Justice Maurice Kay found in favour of CORE

---

[51] Section 2(1) of the HFE Act. Paragraph 1(1) of Schedule 2 to the HFE Act further sets out the scope of authority of licenses for treatment as '(a) bringing about the creation of embryos *in vitro*, (b) keeping embryos, (c) using gametes, (d) practices designed to secure that embryos are in suitable condition to be placed in a woman or to determine whether embryos are suitable for that purpose, (e) placing any embryo in a woman, (f) mixing sperm with the egg of a hamster, or other animal specified in directions, for the purpose of testing the fertility or normality of the sperm, but only where anything which forms is destroyed when the test is complete and, in any event, not in, or determined in accordance with, regulations'.

[52] *op. cit.* note 47, p. 260. The HFEA indicated that license that couples tissue typing and PGD should be considered independently. The conditions attached were '(a) The condition of the affected child should be severe or life threatening, of a sufficient seriousness to justify the use of PGD. (b) The embryos should themselves be at risk of the condition affecting the child. (c) All other possibilities of treatment and sources of tissue for the affected child should have been explored. (d) The techniques should not be available where the intended recipient is a parent. (e) The intention should be to take only cord blood for the purposes of the treatment. (f) Appropriate counselling should be given to parent. (e) The intention should be to take only cord blood for the purposes of the treatment. (f) Appropriate counselling should be given to parents. (g) Families should be encouraged to take part in follow-up studies. (h) Embryos should not be genetically modified to provide a tissue match'.

[53] Ibid: 261. CORE is a group that argued for absolute respect for the human embryo.

and the continued treatment of Mr. and Mrs. Hashmi was suspended at that point.[54] However, leave to appeal was granted in view of the concern of the Secretary of State for Health over the breadth of the judgment which put into doubt the legitimacy of the beneficial practice of PGD screening for genetic diseases. The Secretary of State obtained permission to intervene to support the HFEA's appeal.

On appeal, the decision of the High Court was reversed. The Court of Appeal held that the legislative intent of the HFE Act was for the purpose of assisting women (who may not otherwise choose to conceive) to bear children free of hereditary diseases. The essential characteristic was accordingly in the avoidance of a particular genetic disorder rather than the power of the HFEA to license certain activities. In this case, HLA typing and PGD served the common purpose of selecting an embryo that was suitable for implantation into the woman and not solely for the purpose of selecting an embryo with the desired tissue match.

To assist in the interpretation of the expressions 'for the purpose of assisting women to carry children' and 'suitable for that purpose' in paragraph 1(1)(d) of Schedule 2 to the HFE Act, reference was made to the legislative history of the HFE Act. The first formal inquiry into the various challenges presented by developments in medicine and science related to human fertilisation and embryology in the UK was undertaken by the *Committee of Inquiry Into Human Fertilisation and Embryology*, whose report (generally known as the '*Warnock Report*') was published in July 1984.[55] Of relevance to the facts of the present case, the Committee of

---

[54] *R (on the application of Quintavalle) v. Human Fertilisation and Embryology Authority* [2003] 2 All ER 105. Justice Maurice Kay held that tissue typing — particularly in the genetic testing of the biopsied cells for the purposes of deriving a particular tissue match — involved the 'use' of an embryo that was not for the purpose of 'assisting women to carry children' and so fell outside the scope of the HFE Act.

[55] M. Warnock. 1984. *Report of the Committee of Enquiry Into Human Fertilisation and Embryology*. UK Committee on Human Fertilisation and Embryology. Great Britain, HMSO, Cmnd 9314. The Warnock Report addressed, in the main, the ethical, legal and social issues associated with the utilisation of technologically assisted reproductive techniques for the alleviation of infertility. Two of its recommendations were highlighted by the Master of Rolls in his judgment: (1) the proposal by the Committee of Inquiry for techniques relating to gender selection be allowed under license if justified by good medical reasons and (2) the establishment of a statutory licensing authority to regulate reproductive techniques and to monitor developments in this technology: *op. cit.* note 47, pp. 266–267.

Inquiry was in favour of gender selection to screen out gender linked diseases, 'which was the only form of PGD screening which seemed likely to prove feasible in the immediate future'.[56] Among the recommendations made by the *Warnock Report* is the establishment of a statutory licensing authority both to regulate infertility services determined as a matter of policy to be subject to regulatory control and to license research involving the use of embryos in circumstances where this is justified by the objectives of the research. This was necessary to allay public anxiety by keeping a number of specific technologically-assisted reproductive techniques and procedures, as well as other new techniques under constant review through the agency of this statutory authority. In addition, the statutory authority will also consider if further restrictions are required.[57] This recommendation to establish the statutory authority was taken up by the government [58] and Parliament further empowered it to license research — a matter which was left open in the White Paper.

Against this statutory backdrop, Lord Phillips was of the view that the provision 'for the purpose of assisting women to carry children' should be given a broad interpretation in order to prevent the legislative objective to be defeated. To this effect, his Lordship held that once it was established that an embryo is suitable for the purpose of being placed in a woman, PGD may be applied to determine the most suitable embryo that may be implanted for this purpose. The meaning of 'suitable' will have to depend on the context but is generally one that will lead to the birth of a child with the tissue typing in question:

> 'When concern as to the characteristics of any child that she may bear may inhibit a woman from bearing a child, IVF treatment coupled with

[56] Ibid: 269.

[57] Ibid: 266–267.

[58] The government followed-up on the recommendations presented in the Warnock Report with the White Paper (Human Fertilisation and Embryology: A Framework for Legislation (Cm 259)). The White Paper provided for the establishment of a statutory licensing authority to regulate 'infertility services' but left open the issue of embryonic research which Parliament could have either prohibited or permitted by way of licensing. In contextualising the provisions, the White Paper indicated that about 7000 babies a year are born in the UK with an obvious single gene inherited defect — a result that can be mitigated by PGD. In addition, it was indicated that IVF could alleviate male infertility, which was the sole cause in about 30% of cases of infertility: see Ibid: 267–268.

> PGD that will eliminate that concern can properly be said to be "for the purpose of assisting woman to carry children". When the Act was passed women who had reason to fear that they would give birth to children with genetic defects were probably the only section of the population for whom it was envisaged that IVF treatment could be justified on this basis. No evidence suggests that the wish of a woman to bear a child in order to provide a source of stem cells for a sick or dying sibling was anticipated at that time. Such a wish is now reality, and the case of Mr. and Mrs. Hashmi is not unique.'[59]

The decision of the Court of Appeal was upheld by the House of Lords, whose interpretation of the scope of the legislation by the courts is instructive. First, the legislative intent for the Act is for all activities involving the creation and handling of a human embryo to be subject to regulation. This was eloquently articulated by Lord Bingham in *R (on the application of Quintavalle) v. Secretary of State for Health*:

> 'There is no doubting the sensitivity of the issues. There were those who considered the creation of embryos, and thus life, *in vitro* to be either

[59] Ibid: 270–271. This broad reading was shared by Schiemann L.J. and Mance L.J. Schiemann L.J. noted that Parliament did not find objectionable the creation of embryos 'with the knowledge that some perfectly healthy embryos will deliberately be allowed to perish', nor did it consider to be unacceptable the use of an embryo by implantation after tests have revealed that it did not suffer from a genetic defect. Parliament did however expressly indicate the types of activities that would be considered unlawful, one of which would include the application of IVF for social selection purposes. The present use of PGD did not fall within the scope of prohibited activities articulated in the Act and further related to a purpose that was consistent with Parliamentary intent. For these reasons, the HFEA did not act outside the scope of its authority under the Act: see Ibid : 275–276. Mance L.J. added that the legislation itself contained a number of indications that the licensing authority of the HFEA extended beyond mere viability of an embryo: (1) Parliament was in favour of permitting research under license, (2) the Act permitted the mixing of sperm for the purpose of testing fertility or normality of the sperm, (3) Section 13(5) of the Act related to a wider concern of the well-being of both the future child and the sibling, and is not merely limited to the viability of an embryo for the purposes of 'being implanted, carried to term and born as a child', and (4) the term 'treatment services' should not be read as relating exclusively to woman but should also include the potential father who would have natural concern over the future health and welfare of his child: see Ibid: 283–284.

> sacrilegious or ethically repugnant and wished to ban such activities altogether. There were others who considered that these new techniques, by offering means of enabling the infertile to have children and increasing knowledge of congenital disease, had the potential to improve the human condition, and this view also did not lack religious and moral arguments to support it. Nor can one doubt the difficulty of legislating against a background of fast-moving medical and scientific development. It is not often that Parliament has to frame legislation apt to apply to developments at the advanced cutting edge of science. The solution recommended and embodied in the 1990 Act was not to ban all creation and subsequent use of live human embryos produced *in vitro* but instead, and subject to certain express prohibitions...to permit such creation and use subject to specified conditions, restrictions and time limits and subject to the regimes of control...The merits of this solution are not a matter for the House in its judicial capacity. It is, however, plain that while Parliament outlawed certain grotesque possibilities (such as placing a live animal embryo in a woman or a live human embryo in an animal), it otherwise opted for a strict regime of control. No activity within this field was left unregulated. There was to be no free for all'.[60]

A contextualised reading of the provisions of the Act was earlier proposed by Mance LJ so that PGD, as a health service, should not be limited to the assistance of women to carry children:[61]

> '...in relation to PGD screening to exclude abnormalities, the assistance to women to carry children which the Act contemplates is not limited to assistance in the narrow physical operation of becoming pregnant and giving birth. It extends to assistance in ensuring that any child born will so far as possible be free of genetic defects and not be a carrier of some hereditary problem which could affect a future generation. Considerations relating to the future well-being of yet-to-be-born children will weigh heavily with any prospective parents. So too will any

---

[60] *R v. Secretary for Health ex parte Quintavalle* (on behalf of Pro-Life Alliance) [2003] UKHL 13, paragraphs 12 and 13.

[61] *op. cit.* note 47, p. 286.

> effect that a new child would be likely to have on any existing sibling. Families cannot, for financial reasons or because of the needs of an existing sibling, accommodate another child, may take steps to avoid having one. Families may equally have another child with the idea in mind that he or she will be company for an existing child. Such considerations may no doubt also play a significant role in the clinical judgment, about the welfare of any child who may be born and of any other child who may be affected by the birth….'

Fost argues that PGD is less contentious and emotionally less stressful than prenatal diagnosis and abortion after pregnancy.[62] It may also be possibly employed as a means of saving the life of an existing child with an otherwise incurable disease. He observes[63] that conventional arguments against PGD, such as the utilitarian purpose in procreation and the use of a child as a means and then discarding the child are opinions not supported by evidence and parents who conceive a child to save a life, may be on higher moral ground than those who procreate as an unanticipated consequence of sexual pleasure or for some selfish purpose. Robertson and others criticised the position of the UK (and also that of Australia) on the basis that the policies of these countries interferes with the principle of procreative privacy and they argued for the use of cord blood donation from minors in order to avoid children being used as a means by their parents.[64] But as Fost observes, PGD for HLA typing is likely to already be an entrenched feature of medical technology. While some may continue to argue that such technology is immoral and should not be utilised, future debate is more likely to revolve around the safety and efficacy of this technique.

The reasoning of the English courts in extending the regulatory scope of the HFE Act finds an ethical equivalence in the BAC's

[62] N.C. Fost. Conception for Donation. *Journal of the American Medical Association* 2004; 291(17): 2125.

[63] Ibid: 2126.

[64] J.A. Robertson, J.P. Kahn and J.E. Wagner. Conception to Obtain Hematopoetic Stem Cells. *Hasting Center Report* 2002; 32: 34–40; and J.A. Robertson. Extending Preimplantation Genetic Diagnosis: The Ethical Debate. *Human Reproduction* 2003; 18: 465–471.

recommendations for cloning. In essence, the ethical reasoning of the BAC is that the 14-day limit that applies to human embryonic stem cell research provides an ethical premise within which therapeutic cloning could also be conducted.[65] A query was raised shortly after the publication of the BAC's recommendation in 2002 as to whether the Committee has adequately considered the ethical basis for therapeutic cloning.[66] It was argued that the Warnock Report, upon which the BAC has relied on in its ethical evaluation of the status of a human embryo, did not specifically consider therapeutic cloning. However, there was no mention of any additional ethical considerations that the BAC should have attended to. In 2004, Singapore joined an increasing number of states in passing national legislation that prohibit reproductive cloning.[67] The conduct of therapeutic cloning was specifically envisaged in the course of public consultation on the legislative bill, and also when it was debated in Parliament. A year later, the BAC considered the ethical, legal and social implications of PGD and HLA typing (referred to more generally as 'PTT' or Pre-implantation Tissue Typing), but they are construed as application of gene technology rather than cloning technology.[68] The reason for this could be that these techniques already have clinical relevance, whereas therapeutic cloning was still very much at the level of 'basic science'.

---

[65] See P. Lim. 2006. Bioethics: The Singaporean Approach. In *Life Sciences: Law and Ethics*. T. Kaan & E.T. Liu, eds. Singapore: Singapore Academy of Law and Bioethics Advisory Committee: 1–10; and J.M. Elliott. 2006. Ethical Considerations in Human Stem Cell Research. In *Life Sciences: Law and Ethics*. T. Kaan & E.T. Liu, eds. Singapore: Singapore Academy of Law and Bioethics Advisory Committee: 54–75.

[66] A. Ho. 2002. Bioethics Panel Should Revisit Therapeutic-Cloning Debate. *The Straits Times*. 29 June; and A. Ho. 2002. Cloning Can Wait Till Moral Issues Cleared Up. *The Straits Times*. 5 July. A response by the BAC was published: S. Lim. 2002. Stringent Research Behind Stem-Cell Recommendations. *The Straits Times*. 11 July.

[67] The Human Cloning and Other Prohibited Practices Act (Cap. 131B of Singapore) was enacted in Sep 2004 after the Ministry of Health conducted a public consultation on the legislative Bill in May 2004. The main features of this legislation include the prohibition of reproductive cloning: http://www.moh.gov.sg/mohcorp/legislations.aspx?id=7084 [Accessed 30 June 2009].

[68] BAC. 2005. *Genetic Testing and Genetic Research*. Singapore: BAC. See especially the discussion on Recommendations 9 to 11, pp. 31–37.

SOME OBSERVATIONS

The negotiations that led to the UN Human Cloning Declaration were described as a 'remarkable sort of culture war…[which give] the impression that the effort and resources are somewhat out of proportion compared to the output….[since] we are once again back to a situation where states are having to make their own decision — likely on a mixture of political, religious, and some scientific grounds — on when (individual?) '"human life" begins'.[69]

Arsanjani indicates that in attempting to achieve a balance between incompatible views on definition of human life, the Human Cloning Declaration neither defines 'human cloning' nor explicitly and unqualifiedly bans human cloning, including the reproductive cloning of human beings.[70] He notes in particular that 'cloning of human beings' is only referred to in the second preambular paragraph, and that the remaining paragraphs speak in general terms about the application of 'life sciences'. In addition, 'human dignity' is susceptible to various interpretations, and in respect of which Pronto has identified at least four sets of arguments that have emerged in the course of the UN debates.[71]

The two key operative paragraphs (a) and (b) of the Human Cloning Declaration are also problematic in that there is no mention of 'human cloning', and it is unclear what 'human life' could mean and how this would relates to a 'human being'. The UK voted against the Human Cloning Declaration due in part to the possibility of interpreting 'human life' as precluding therapeutic cloning, since this expression could refer to embryos.[72] While paragraph (b) is the only operative paragraph that appears to prohibit human cloning, the term 'inasmuch' could be a substantial limitation on its operation. In addition, paragraph (f) of the

---

[69] N. B. Andorno, 'It's Cloning Again!' *Journal of Medical Ethics* 2005; 31: 63.

[70] M.H. Arsanjani, Current Developments: Negotiating the UN Declaration on Human Cloning. *American Journal of International Law* 2006; 100: 164–179, at 177.

[71] A.N. Pronto. Consideration at the United Nations of an International Prohibition on the Cloning of Human Beings. *Leiden Journal of International Law* 2007; 20: 239–265, at 261.

[72] United Nations. 2005. *Press Release* GA/10333, 59th General Assembly Plenary, 82nd Meeting. March.

Human Cloning Declaration does not relate to human cloning at all, but rather to the financing of medical research to more pressing global health issues. Arsanjani observes that this would perhaps indicate the remoteness of the issues of human cloning in many developing countries where far more urgent medical and health concerns need to be prioritised.[73] In his view, it would be more realistic to let domestic law and industry take the initiative in regulating this field since attempting to 'universalise standards for application by 191 states marked by significant gaps in economic, scientific, and technological development, by way of an agreement on voluntary compliance or compulsory enforcement and monitoring is visionary'.[74]

When the French-German proposal was put forward in 2001, France and Germany proceeded under an expectation that a treaty specifically directed at prohibiting reproductive cloning would face little obstacle given that the European Union's *Additional Protocol to the Convention for the Protection of Human Rights and Dignity of the Human Beings with Regard to the Application of Biology and Medicine* and UNESCO's *Universal Declaration on the Human Genome and Human Rights* already signified a level of international consensus on the issue.[75] However, neither of these instruments provided a clear statement on therapeutic cloning. In the case of UNESCO's Declaration, Pronto argues that it could be construed as permissive or prohibitive of therapeutic cloning, depending on the normative stance of the interpreter.[76] In addition, cloning

[73] Arsanjani, *op. cit.* note 70, p. 178.

[74] Ibid: 179. Nikola Biller-Andorno similarly notes that 'if no meaningful universal agreement can be reached on reproductive cloning, at least not at the level of the United Nations, the prospect for reaching a global consensus on other issues in bioethics is rather bleak': Andorno *op. cit.* note 69.

[75] Arsanjani, *op. cit.* note 70, p. 166.

[76] Pronto, *op. cit.* note 71, pp. 259–262. These four sets of arguments advanced in the interpretation of 'human dignity' have been identified as: (a) the classical balancing of rights discourse, (b) attempts at construing the expression beyond a fundamentally Christian premise and hence on a more culturally-relativistic basis, (c) as a matter of domestic norms such as constitutional protection and judicial pronouncement, and (d) on different normative grounds.

technology is not a subject that all member states either have a real interest in or otherwise have a national position on — as paragraph 9 of the Human Cloning Declaration illustrates. On reflection, we can take away some useful lessons from the whole episode of negotiations on human cloning at the UN, and also from related developments in the UK and Singapore.

Minimum Common Denominator as Possibly a Prerequisite

First, if standards formation by a supranational body could be seen as an integrative operation, whereby a 'minimum common denominator' is sought from a community of practices,[77] the absence of any standard on the part of some of its constituents could impede efforts directed at establishing such a standard. As noted earlier, cloning is not a subject that is of immediate concern (or indeed, even in the foreseeable future) to many of the UN member states. While more countries including Singapore have responded by 2004 through the enactment of domestic legislation to prohibit some or all forms of cloning, many more countries remain undecided on the relevance of cloning technology. Furthermore, even in relation to reproductive cloning, the ethical premises that have been advanced for prohibiting such application of the technology are varied and by no means uncontestable. Roger Brownsword insightfully observes that:

> 'if anxieties about safety or reliability could be assuaged, those who presently cite such concerns in support of a prohibition on cloning might change their tune, arguing initially for a cautious and controlled permissive position and then, if and when doubts about safety and reliability have been largely laid to rest, for an even more permissive position. In other words, the consensus against human reproductive cloning is less deeply-rooted than it seems'.[78]

[77] A.A. Miralles. The Globalization of Bioethics: The Task of International Commissions. *Georgetown Journal of International Law* 2005; 37: 141–151, at 148–149.

[78] R. Brownsword. Stem Cells and Cloning: Where the Regulatory Consensus Fails. *New England Law Review* 2005; 39: 535–571, at 538.

Germany's dramatic change of stance from 2001 to 2005 suggests that the 'minimum common denominator' (or more generally concerns in a localised setting) matters, especially on issues that are of public concern in a liberal democracy. As noted earlier, Germany moved from being a co-sponsor of a limited ban on cloning in 2001, to assuming a more passive role as a supporter of the Belgian proposal in 2003, and to ultimately voting in line with the faction that called for a comprehensive ban on cloning in 2005.[79] This change may be attributed to the proximity of a particular construction of 'human dignity' entailed in cloning to the German identity.[80] This may further explain the ability of its co-sponsor, France, in consistently supporting a focused (rather than comprehensive) approach to cloning, even though this position contradicted its national policy.

Engagement and Representation as Legitimacy

Second, the absence of interest or national position on cloning for many of the member states might have rendered them susceptible to the influences of other member states or to forces and considerations that were unrelated to the subject matter.[81] If an effective and binding standard had been promulgated, some member states might have been deprived of an opportunity to give proper deliberation to the implications of the technology in the context of *their own* needs and circumstance. The Human Cloning Declaration is also problematic for the lack of recognition that could be accorded to a diversity of views on the subject. As it turned out, a particular discourse dominated the international forum on cloning and this ultimately undermined the legitimacy of the Human Cloning

---

[79] Cameron & Henderson. *op. cit.* note 20, pp. 189–191.

[80] Stefan Sperling observes: 'In a nation still haunted by memories of the Holocaust, the idea that scientists might once again conduct experiments on helpless human beings aroused special concern'. S. Sperling. Converting Ethics Into Reason: German Stem Cell Policy Between Science and the Law. *Science as Culture* 2008; 17(4): 363–375, at 364.

[81] It was suggested that the Organisation of the Islamic Conference acted 'as surrogate for those States most opposed to the comprehensive approach' even though it appeared to act in concert to undercut this approach by delaying the process in 2003: Cameron and Henderson. *op. cit.* note 20, p. 187. However, it could also be argued the OIC ultimately adopted a pragmatic approach as it did not consider the technology to be of immediate relevance or benefit.

Declaration. Mr. Vanu Gopal Menon, Singapore's permanent representative to the UN said he had voted against the resolution (that incorporated the Human Cloning Declaration) because it did not capture the diversity of views on the issue. He noted that four years ago, the Assembly endorsed an initiative to begin work on an international convention on human cloning. Although there was unanimity that reproductive cloning should be banned, he felt it was unfortunate that that initiative was hijacked, and culminated in the adoption of a text which sought to impose a single set of regulations on member states regarding all forms of human cloning.[82] Isasi and Annas provide an interesting observation that 'if the population of each voting country is considered, the results would be as follows: 1.5 billion people voting in favour of the declaration, 3.1 billion people voting against it, and 1.6 billion people not voting at all'.[83] With support by countries representing less than one-fourth of the world's population and opposed by many countries now engaged in cloning research, it would be difficult to argue that the Human Cloning Declaration carries any moral force.[84]

Heterogeneity in Standards

Third, standards generate knowledge about products, processes and people by specifying particular practices and in defining who the risk-bearers are and what sort of activities are risky. Elizabeth Dunn argues that '[s]tandardisation thus implied *legibility*, *commensuration, and hierarchy*', as a 'normative governmentality' is entailed in 'harmonisation' and 'integration'.[85] Her argument is well illustrated in her study of the adoption of European Union standards for food processing by Poland. These standards were designed to reduce risk of food-borne illnesses such as

[82] United Nations. *op. cit.* note 72.

[83] R.M. Isasi and G.J. Annas. To Clone Alone: The United Nations Human Cloning Declaration. *Development* 2006; 49(4): 60–67, at 63.

[84] Ibid.

[85] E. Dunn. 2005. Standards and Person Making in East Central Europe. In *Global Anthropologies: Governmentality, Technology, Ethics*. A. Ong & S. Collier, eds. London: Blackwell: 173–193, at 183.

trichinosis and Creuzfeld-Jakobs ('mad cow') disease, and also to reduce spread of livestock epidemics like foot-and-mouth disease. Regulations that came into effect for every meatpacker in Poland in late 2003, and enforced via regular inspections both by the Polish Head Veterinarian's Office and EU inspectors, included detailed specifications for the physical plant of abattoirs and meat processing plants, as well as specifications on documentation and tracking.

Compliance with the more rigorous standards of the European Union elicited trust on the part of foreign investors and opened the flow of capital into Poland. The arrival of American corporation Smithfield Meats and other multinational corporations had at least two effects: standardisation of meat products as very lean hogs are preferred to genetically irregular and often fatty hogs produced by smallholder farmers, and small and medium meatpackers in the countryside were forced out of business.[86] Consequently, an informal 'gray zone' market in agricultural products emerged as a direct result of increased standardisation since standards could not account for every situation, especially given its failure to take into account distinct local conditions. The re-emergence of midnight meat companies and post-socialist black markets in Eastern Europe was seen as an attempt by some local firms to 'try to create commodity chains other than the industrialised ones controlled by the multinationals'.[87] Dunn highlights the need to be mindful that standardisation does not homogenise persons, but it creates significant inequalities and gives people strong incentives to find ways around the standards.[88]

The divisiveness of the negotiations on cloning at the various sessions of the UNGA arises in part from the label of 'profanity' that a promulgated standard would imprint on supporters of some forms of cloning. The dominance of a particular discourse on the subject has also been shown to be problematic in that member states that did not subscribe to that discourse either felt excluded or otherwise subjugated within a process that embodied (or at least sought to embody) communal effort and consensus.

[86] Ibid: 178–179.
[87] Ibid: 188.
[88] Ibid: 189.

In October 2008, the International Bioethics Committee of UNESCO has announced that it has appointed a working group to explore whether the scientific, ethical, social, political and legal developments on human cloning in recent years justify a new initiative at the international level.[89] Perhaps the implications of establishment of a regulatory standard on cloning should be given further deliberation before embarking on such a course.

CONCLUSION

There may be a need for international organisations to give greater recognition to domestic institutions and context in standards setting.[90] There are often large gaps that can persist between formal rules and institutions, and between expected behaviour and actual behaviour. Even where international standards are available, complex adaptation rather than simple adoption is entailed. In reviewing policy developments from 2001 to 2005 on cloning in Singapore and in the UK, domestic institutions have been instrumental in developing and adapting standards for the development and application of cloning technology. These standards were developed in ways that have meaning within their local context, and it is also within this context that the political and socio-cultural impetus and resources in resolving conflicts over meaning are found. Often, imagined possibilities — both positive and negative — can only be properly addressed within a more limited, situated setting. In their ethnographic study of PGD, Sarah Franklin and Celia Roberts proposed a form of social contract for understanding the uptake of embryo research and new reproductive technologies in Britain.

Their approach returns to the social contract that grounds the Warnock Committee's recommendations and to the key principle guiding the

[89] See announcement of UNESCO entitled 'Human Cloning and International Governance'. Available at: http://portal.unesco.org/shs/en/ev.php-URL_ID=12279&URL_DO=DO_TOPIC&URL_SECTION=201.html [Accessed 30 June 2009].

[90] The notion of boundary infrastructure (Bowker & Star. *op. cit.* note 4, p. 290) could perhaps be a more abstract way of thinking about domestic institutions and context, although the 'scaling up' process is problematised here differently.

'Warnock strategy'. They argue that in exchange for permitting a limited amount of embryo research, the state would assure the public of strict regulation that is subject to the very highest standards of public accountability. It was in this context that Mary Warnock posed a question about feeling, judgement and belonging to which she offered a solution of tolerance, compromise and regulation.[91] In creating a sense of a whole that is greater than the sum of its parts, a kind of 'social contract' emerges that marks the 'British way forward' with techniques such as PGD and IVF, as well as with human cloning, stem cell technology and biobanking. Franklin and Roberts allegorise this as a firm hand that disciplines the troops, so that if discipline and order can be maintained, much faster progress will be made — to everyone's benefit.[92] Also of pertinence is their ethnographic finding that, contrary to the view of PGD as careering forward out of control, by offering 'too much choice', their study suggests a much more careful and thoughtful engagement with the difficulties presented by PGD, evidenced in the range of ways couples plan ahead on how they will move on if treatment is unsuccessful, the difficulties they acknowledge in knowing where to 'draw the line', and the ambivalence expressed by professionals about the decision to encourage or dissuade borderline PGD candidates. It is the *ambivalence* of PGD that enables would-be parents to move simultaneously forward, and back and forth, between different alternatives to PGD.[93] Franklin and Roberts further observe that PGD is in many ways the opposite of the dangerous and dystopian 'designer baby' characterisation, which so unhelpfully continues to dominate much public and media discussion of the increasingly difficult choices and challenges PGD presents to individuals, couples, professional, and wider society of which they are a part.[94] It may be further argued that this approach in social contract would not be possible without the presence of supporting institutions as contracts are always informationally incomplete. As Annelise Riles notes, policy documents

---

[91] S. Franklin and C. Roberts. 2006. *Born and Made: An Ethnography of Pre-implantation Genetic Diagnosis*. Princeton, NJ: Princeton University Press: 197.
[92] Ibid: 198.
[93] Ibid: 217.
[94] Ibid.

(arguably similar to social contracts) are often less interested in specificities like expounding concepts or terminologies (such as 'women') than they are in ensuring institutional continuity within which the document (or contract) derives value and meaning.[95]

This is not to say that the international community has no role to play in the governance of technology such as cloning, but for standards to make sense, it is often necessary for them to be linked or referenced to the history and identity of shared (and typically domestic) institutions and circumstance. Otherwise, imagined possibilities that span from prospect of a new salvation to a world populated by single-profiled clones are bountiful and often an obstacle to meaningful engagement.

[95] A. Riles. 2001. *The Network Inside Out*. USA: University of Michigan Press: 80–81. At page 80, she observes: 'For example, if one takes the general subject of this conference 'women', certainly the word *women* appeared frequently enough in the thousands of documents that circulated through the meeting. Yet in practice, it was hardly clear what this word 'meant' at all and how it might be delineated by the scope of other UN conferences on subjects such as development, human rights, population, children, or environment'.

(b) The Enduring Ethical Debate

5

SOCIOLOGICAL REFLECTIONS ON ETHICS, EMBRYONIC STEM CELLS AND TRANSLATIONAL RESEARCH

Claire Williams and Steven Wainwright

SOCIOLOGY AND BIOETHICS

Sociology and bioethics is a growing area within the expanding research fields of bioethics and the social sciences.[1] *Sociology* ***in*** *bioethics* explores the links between bioethics, medicine, science and society and aims to ground more abstract philosophical ethical debates in empirical case studies which explore and describe the embodied ethics of 'real actors' in particular social worlds.[2] Sociological approaches to ethics explores 'the social processes, meanings and institutions that frame and produce 'ethics' and 'ethical problems',[3] and the way in which 'ethical material' informs what we take to be empirical'.[4] Hence, from this

---

[1] B.K. Rothman, E.M. Armstrong & R. Tiger. 2008. *Bioethical Issues, Sociological Perspectives*. Amsterdam: Elsevier.

[2] A. Hedgecoe. Critical Bioethics: Beyond the Social Science Critique of Applied Ethics. *Bioethics* 2004; 18: 120–143; R. de Vries *et al.* 2007. *The View From Here: Bioethics and the Social Sciences (Sociology of Health and Illness Monographs).* Oxford: Blackwell; and C.L. Bosk. 2008. *What Would You Do? Juggling Bioethics and Ethnography.* Chicago: University of Chicago Press.

[3] E. Haimes. What Can the Social Sciences Contribute to the Study of Ethics? Theoretical, Empirical and Substantive Considerations. *Bioethics* 2002; 16: 110.

[4] R. Ashcroft. Constructing Empirical Ethics: Foucauldian Reflections on the Empirical Turn in Bioethics Research. *Health Care Analysis* 2003; 11: 11.

perspective, sociologists analyse the ways in which ethical problems are 'identified, classified, debated, managed, resolved or stalemated in clinical [and scientific] situations'.[5]

In contrast, *sociology **of** bioethics* charts the social forces that help shape particular (dominant) varieties of philosophical bioethics (e.g. principlism, utilitarianism, etc.) and so examines the ways in which certain kinds of ethical questions are privileged, promoted and funded within bioethics, whilst other approaches tend to be marginalised.[6] Moreover, from this perspective, bioethics as a field is seen as limiting the types of questions that can be asked and researched. It has been argued that there has been a 'leaching out of the social', particularly in mainstream US bioethics, which has limited ethical debates to questions around means rather than questions about ends.[7] Consequently, the discipline of bioethics tends to bracket out the social and so largely ignores discussion of what many see as the central question of ethics, namely, 'what counts as a good life'.[8]

In this chapter we will summarise some of our recent work on empirical ethics, particularly in the fields of embryonic stem cells and translational research, in order to illustrate the nature of empirical ethics, i.e. sociology *in* bioethics. We will then move on to a discussion of the ethical implications of hybrid embryo research and translational research in neuroscience as examples of two areas that have developed from our work on the empirical ethics of stem cell translational research.

---

[5] C.L. Bosk. 2000. The Sociological Imagination and Bioethics. In *Handbook of Medical Sociology.* C. Bird *et al.*, eds. New Jersey: Prentice Hall: 406.

[6] J.H. Evans. 2002. *Playing God? Human Genetic Engineering and the Rationalisation of Public Bioethical Debate.* Chicago: University of Chicago Press; D.J. Rothman. 2003. *Strangers At the Bedside: A History of How Law and Ethics Transformed Medical Decision Making: Second Edition.* New York: Aldine de Gruyter; and R.C. Fox & J.P. Swazey. 2008. *Observing Bioethics.* New York: Oxford University Press.

[7] J.H. Evans. 2002. *Playing God? Human Genetic Engineering and the Rationalisation of Public Bioethical Debate.* Chicago: University of Chicago Press; and R.C. Fox. The Bioethics That I Would Like to See. *Clinical Ethics* 2008; 3(1): 25–26.

[8] For a more embodied and social vision of bioethics, see A. Cribb. 2005. *Health and the Good Society.* Oxford: Oxford University Press; and A.V. Campbell. 2009. *The Body in Bioethics.* London: Routledge-Cavendish.

The chapter ends with some final thoughts on making bioethics more multidisciplinary.

EMPIRICAL ETHICS: EMBRYONIC STEM CELLS AND TRANSLATIONAL RESEARCH

Although innovative technologies may have the potential to diagnose, treat and possibly even prevent illness and disease, they concurrently raise new risks that highlight a set of important questions linking social studies of medical and scientific technologies with debates around the ethical, legal, and policy dimensions of innovative but controversial biomedical practices.[9] These technologies are redefining the scale, scope and the boundaries of science and medicine, and the relationship between biomedical technologies, science and the social.[10] Within this emerging context, scientists must nevertheless demonstrate their commitment to 'ethics' as the audiences of science include various public and regulatory constituencies who, in one way or another, lend the whole bio-scientific enterprise legitimacy.[11]

---

[9] C. Williams, P. Alderson & B. Farsides. Dilemmas Encountered by Health Practitioners Offering Nuchal Translucency Screening: A Qualitative Case Study. *Prenatal Diagnosis* 2002a; 22: 216–220; C. Williams, P. Alderson & B. Farsides. Too Many Choices? Hospital and Community Staff Reflect on the Future of Prenatal Screening. *Social Science and Medicine* 2002b; 55: 743–753; C. Williams, P. Alderson & B. Farsides. Is Non-Directiveness Possible Within the Context of Antenatal Screening and Testing? *Social Science and Medicine* 2002c; 54: 17–25; and C. Williams, P. Alderson & B. Farsides. 'Drawing the Line' in Prenatal Screening and Testing: Health Practitioners' Discussions. *Health, Risk and Society* 2002d; 4: 61–75.

[10] N. Brown & A. Webster. 2004. *New Medical Technologies and Society.* Cambridge: Polity; and A. Webster. 2007. *Health Technology and Society: A Sociological Critique.*

[11] B. Salter. Bioethics, Politics and the Moral Economy of Human Embryonic Stem Cell Science: The Case of the European Union's Sixth Framework Programme. *New Genetics and Society* 2007a; 26: 260–288; and B. Salter. Bioethics and the Global Moral Economy: The Cultural Politics of Human Embryonic Stem Cell Science. *Science, Technology and Human Values* 2007b; 32(5): 1–28.

The interaction between bench and bedside, or translational research, is an increasingly important topic in biomedicine that is strongly shaping the biomedical research agenda of both the Medical Research Council (MRC) in the UK;[12] and of the National Institutes of Health (NIH) in the USA.[13] The key thrust of translational research is that work in the laboratory is translated as quickly as possible into effective treatments in the clinic, thereby bringing benefits to patients and to society. Translational research entails encouraging the translation of basic science methods and findings into research designed to reduce the burden of disease, together with the development of novel therapeutic and diagnostic approaches.[14] Translational research is often seen as bi-directional, working from the bench to the bedside and from the bedside to the bench.[15] The scope of translational research is now seen as incorporating Type 1 and Type 2 translation.[16] *Type 1 translation* entails the transfer of new understandings of disease mechanisms gained in the laboratory into the development of new methods for diagnosis, therapy, and prevention, and their first testing in humans (and this has been the object of our sociological research); whilst *Type 2 translation* encompasses the translation of results from clinical studies into everyday clinical practice.

Social scientists have conducted a number of seminal ethnographic studies of laboratory life that are central to the overlapping disciplines of sociology, anthropology, and science and technology studies (STS).[17] There is also a strong tradition of qualitative social research on the nature

---

[12] MRC. 2004. *Translating Research: Annual Review 2003/04*. London: MRC.

[13] E. Zerhouni. The NIH Roadmap. *Science* 2003; 302: 63–72.

[14] R.B. Sartor. Translational Research: Bridging the Widening Gap Between Basic and Clinical Research. *Gastroenterology* 2003; 124: 1178.

[15] F.M. Marincola. Translational Medicine: A Two-Way Road. *Journal of Translational Medicine* 2003; 1: 1; and P. Martin, N. Brown & A. Kraft. From Bedside to Bench? Communities of Promise, Translational Research and the Making of Blood Stem Cells. *Science as Culture* 2008; 17: 1–13.

[16] S.H. Woolf. The Meaning of Translational Research and Why It Matters. *The Journal of the American Medical Association* 2008; 299(2): 211–213.

[17] e.g., see B. Latour & S. Woolgar. 1986. *Laboratory Life: The Construction of Scientific Facts (Second Edition)*. Princeton: Princeton University Press; and P. Rabinow. 1996. *Making PCR: A Story of Biotechnology*. Chicago: Chicago University Press.

of clinical medicine.[18] Whilst there is a plethora of ethnographies that focus on either the laboratory or the clinic, few social research studies have examined both the bench and the bedside. Examples of this approach have explored the culture of clinical experimentation in oncology[19] and the relationships between immunology and oncology.[20] These studies do not, however, focus specifically on the *interactions* between bench and bedside. In contrast, much of our recent research has explored these interactions, specifically in relation to the use of stem cells as a potential cure for diabetes and for neurodegenerative diseases.[21] This set of papers uses

---

[18] e.g., see P. Atkinson. 1995. *Medical Talk and Medical Work: The Liturgy of the Clinic.* London: Sage; F. Baylis. Animal Eggs for Stem Cell Research: A Path Not Worth Taking. *The American Journal of Bioethics* 2008; 12: 18–32; and M. Lock. 2001. *Twice Dead: Organ Transplants and the Reinvention of Death.* Berkeley: University of California Press.

[19] I. Lowy. 1997. *Between Bench and Bedside: Science, Healing and Interleukin-2 in Cancer.* Cambridge: Harvard University Press.

[20] P. Keating & A. Cambrosio. 2003. *Biomedical Platforms: Realigning the Normal and the Pathological in Late-Twentieth Century Medicine.* Cambridge: MIT Press.

[21] S.P. Wainwright *et al.* From Bench to Bedside? Biomedical Scientists' Expectations of Stem Cell Science as a Future Therapy for Diabetes. *Social Science and Medicine* 2006a; 63: 2052–2064; S.P. Wainwright *et al.* Ethical Boundary Work in the Embryonic Stem Cell Laboratory. *Sociology of Health and Illness* 2006b; 28: 732–748; S.P. Wainwright *et al.* Remaking the Body? Scientists' Genetic Discourses and Practices as Examples of Changing Expectations on Embryonic Stem Cell Therapy for Diabetes. *New Genetics and Society* 2007; 26: 251–268; S.P. Wainwright, M. Michael & C. Williams. Shifting Paradigms? Reflections on Regenerative Medicine, Embryonic Stem Cells and Pharmaceuticals. *Sociology of Health and Illness* 2008; 30: 959–974; S.P. Wainwright *et al.* 2009. Stem Cells, Translational Research and the Sociology of Science. In *Handbook of Genetics and Society: Mapping the New Genomic Era.* P. Atkinson, P. Glasner & M. Lock, eds. London: Routledge; S.P. Wainwright & C. Williams. Spaces of Speech and Places of Performance: An Outline of a Geography of Science Approach to Embryonic Stem Cell Research and Diabetes. *New Genetics and Society* 2008a; 27: 161–173; C. Williams *et al.* Facilitating Choice, Framing Choice: Staff Views on Widening the Scope of PGD in the UK. *Social Science and Medicine* 2007; 65: 1094–1105; M. Michael *et al.* From Core Set to Assemblage: On the Dynamics of Exclusion and Inclusion in the Failure to Derive Beta Cells from Embryonic Stem Cells. *Science Studies* 2007a; 20(1): 5–25; M. Michael, S.P. Wainwright & C. Williams. Temporality and Prudence: On Stem Cells as 'Phronesic Things'. *Configurations* 2007b; 13: 373–394; and A. Cribb *et al.* Towards the Applied: The Construction of Ethical Positions in Stem Cell Translational Research. *Medicine, Health Care and Philosophy* 2008; 11: 351–361.

data from two ESRC funded projects (2005–2009) on the prospects and problems of translational research in the field of stem cell research. This empirical research programme drew on over 70 in-depth interviews with scientists and clinicians in some of the leading labs and clinics in the UK and the USA, exploring their views on the bench-bedside interface in the fields of neuroscience and diabetes.

Many of the social science papers that touch on stem cell ethics draw upon analysis of documentary sources.[22] In contrast, our own research examined the views of laboratory scientists and transplant clinicians on the ethics of biomedical science research using embryonic stem cells,[23] and on the ethics of translational research.[24] In these papers we add to the relatively few sociological and anthropological studies which explore the ways in which ethical dilemmas and reasoning occur in the clinical setting;[25] and to an even smaller body of work, exploring scientists' views on the ethical issues relating to their research.[26] Such studies contrast with

[22] e.g., see S. Franklin. Culturing Biology: Cell Lines for the Second Millennium. *Health* 2001; 5: 335–354; C. Waldby. Stem Cells, Tissue Cultures and the Production of Biovalue. *Health* 2002; 6: 305–323; S. Parry. The Politics of Cloning: Mapping the Rhetorical Convergence of Embryos and Stem Cells in Parliamentary Debates. *New Genetics and Society* 2003; 22: 145–168; S. Franklin. 2005. Stem Cells R Us: Emergent Life Forms and the Global Biological. In *Global Assemblages: Technology, Politics and Ethics as Anthropological Problems.* A. Ong & S.J. Collier, eds. New York: Blackwell; and S. Jasanoff. 2005. *Designs on Nature: Science and Democracy in Europe and the United States.* Princeton: Princeton University Press. For a recent interview study see E. Haimes *et al.* 'So, What is an Embryo?' A Comparative Study of the Views of Those Asked to Donate Embryos for hESC Research in the UK and Switzerland. *New Genetics and Society* 2008; 27: 113–126.

[23] S.P. Wainwright *et al.* From Bench to Bedside? Biomedical Scientists' Expectations of Stem Cell Science as a Future Therapy for Diabetes. *Social Science and Medicine* 2006a; 63: 2052–2064.

[24] A. Cribb *et al.* Towards the Applied: The Construction of Ethical Positions in Stem Cell Translational Research. *Medicine, Health Care and Philosophy* 2008; 11: 351–361.

[25] e.g., see R. Anspach. 1993. *Deciding Who Lives: Fateful Choices in the Intensive Care Nursery*. Berkeley: University of California Press; and C. Williams. Framing the Fetus in Medical Work: Representations and Practices. *Social Science and Medicine* 2005; 60: 2085–2095.

[26] e.g., M. Michael & L. Birke. Animal Experimentation: Enrolling the Core Set. *Social Studies of Science* 1994; 24, 81–95.

the dominant, disembodied ways in which ethical reasoning is traditionally presented in philosophical bioethics[27] and in philosophical science ethics.[28] In the next two sections of the chapter we summarise a small part of our stem cell research findings. First, we illustrate how embryonic stem cell scientists' practice ethical boundary work. Second, we briefly examine one aspect of how stem cell scientists' and transplant clinicians' ethical positions shape their perspectives on translational research.

Embryonic Stem Cells and Ethical Boundary Work

Building on the concept of boundary-work[29] we introduced the notion of 'ethical boundary-work' to analyse how scientists involved in hES cell science practice ethics in the lab.[30] Gieryn[31] outlines the ways in which scientists defend their intellectual territory and how the demarcation of science from non-science works to maintain an image of expertise, authority and credibility. We extended Gieryn's work, exploring how scientists also present themselves as ethical, as well as expert, actors by drawing the boundaries of ethical scientific activity. We discussed three key issues: what individual scientists themselves view as ethical sources of human embryos and stem cells; their definitions of human embryos and stem cells; and how scientists perceive regulatory frameworks in stem cell research. These dimensions of laboratory practice are all examples of what we describe as 'ethical boundary-work'. Practical ethics here took

---

[27] E. Haimes. What can the Social Sciences Contribute to the Study of Ethics? Theoretical, Empirical and Substantive Considerations. *Bioethics* 2002; 16: 90–113; and A. Hedgecoe. Critical Bioethics: Beyond the Social Science Critique of Applied Ethics. *Bioethics* 2004; 18: 120–143.

[28] D.B. Resnik. 1998. *The Ethics of Science: An Introduction.* Routledge: London; and B.E. Rollin. 2006. *Science and Ethics.* Cambridge: Cambridge University Press.

[29] T.F. Gieryn. Boundary-Work and the Demarcation of Science from Non-Science: Strains and Interests in Professional Ideologies of Scientists. *American Sociological Review* 1983; 48, 781–795.

[30] S.P. Wainwright et al. From Bench to Bedside? Biomedical Scientists' Expectations of Stem Cell Science as a Future Therapy for Diabetes. *Social Science and Medicine* 2006a; 63: 2052–2064.

[31] T.F. Gieryn. 1999. *Cultural Boundaries of Science: Credibility on the Line.* Chicago: Chicago University Press.

the form of a number of choices over how to conduct oneself in a complicated political, moral and scientific context. In this section we illustrate how scientists acted in ethically nuanced ways by focussing on scientists' ethical reasoning around what source of embryos to use (or not use).

In brief, scientists discussed the ethical issues surrounding four sources of embryos for laboratory work with hES cells. For example, much was made of the fact that if 'spare embryos' were not used for scientific research they would be discarded:

> '*With rare exceptions, the embryos that are used in stem cell research are embryos that have no future, either because they are not implantable…or they've been screened by PGD* [pre-implantation genetic diagnosis] *and been shown to have, or be at high risk of having, a genetic disorder…If all we're doing is using something left over and destined to be discarded, then if some good can come out of it, it's worth doing*'. (Scientist 8)

In their analysis of media coverage of the stem cell debate in the UK in 2000, this was one of the rhetorical strategies Williams *et al.*[32] identified as used by proponents of stem cell research to assert an ethical position, that embryos would otherwise be 'discarded' or 'left to perish'. This meant that not only could stem cell research be presented as 'less wasteful' of spare embryos, but also that stem cell research could be presented as a form of rescue. Similarly, Waldby states:

> 'Advocates of stem cell research generally portray the spare embryo as a precious substance. If it is not freely donated it will be simply wasted, a recklessly squandered resource…Stem cell technologies are, in these terms, particularly productive sources of bio-value precisely because they can rehabilitate what would otherwise be needless waste and transform it into a spectacularly active, flexible and manageable tissue resource'.[33]

[32] C. Williams, J. Kitzinger & L. Henderson. Envisaging the Embryo in Stem Cell Research: Discursive Strategies and Media Reporting of the Ethical Debates. *Sociology of Health and Illness* 2003; 25: 793–814.

[33] C. Waldby. Stem Cells, Tissue Cultures and the Production of Biovalue. *Health* 2002; 6: 314.

A few scientists stated that they would only work on embryos donated from PGD and were not prepared to work with embryos from IVF programmes:

> '*I've got large ethical problems with using spare embryos from routine IVF cycles for stem cell research. I believe if an embryo is rejected as too poor quality to freeze on day 3 for potential future implantation, and then it turns into a blastocyst suitable for stem cell derivation, it may have some clinical potential and should probably be frozen. PGD doesn't have the same ethical baggage — those embryos can't be replaced*'. (Scientist 10)

Here Scientist 10 is arguing that some 'spare' IVF embryos may turn out to have the clinical potential to be used in treatment by the couple, and should therefore be frozen. This situation cannot arise if only genetically affected PGD embryos are used as a source of stem cells as, by definition, such embryos would be deemed unsuitable for replacement. Scientist 10 supports the work of Throsby, who draws attention to the way in which PGD embryos are constructed as 'pre-discursively *spare*, and therefore unproblematically available, obscuring the [social] process of their production and acquisition'.[34]

All of the scientists interviewed were prepared to use 'spare' embryos for research, although their definitions of 'spare' varied. In contrast, many of the scientists we interviewed were opposed to creating embryos solely for research:

> '*At the moment the way you grow human stem cells is you get embryos that will be thrown away if you don't use them, and the parents have given informed consent for them to be used by researchers. I don't think that's unethical. I think it would be unethical to let those embryos be thrown away when there's a choice. But I wouldn't agree with working with embryos that have been created solely for the purpose of harvesting stem cells — I would definitely refuse to work on those cells*'. (Scientist 1)

---

[34] K. Throsby. 2004. *When IVF Fails: Feminism, Infertility and the Negotiation of Normality*. London: Palgrave: 22.

> *'We get embryos from IVF and PGD and those embryos would be thrown away so it's not as if we're making them specifically for cell work. I wouldn't do that, I wouldn't be happy to produce just a continuous supply of fertilised embryos for lab work'*. (Scientist 2)

This stance is interesting in view of the fact that the UK *House of Commons Science and Technology Committee* has recommended that, 'where necessary, embryos can be created specifically for research purposes'.[35] Scientists are often portrayed as pushing the ethical limits of biomedical work,[36] but here we see examples of scientists resisting a more permissive public policy on stem cell research. We argue that this is a further example of our respondents distinguishing between two forms of waste: material that has been created unnecessarily; and existing material that risks not being used. The agency and responsibility of these scientists is deeply embedded in this distinction and, in particular, in not crossing the boundary into the former zone. From their accounts, it seems that they view the source of embryos along an ethical continuum. At one end scientists are simply redeeming the situation, whilst at the end, embryos are being created for their 'own' purposes alone. The ideal for many of our respondents appears to be redeeming and transforming material created for other purposes — in other words, the agency of the scientists enters after the 'waste' appears, and not before.

The scientists' views also echo the global politics of hES cell science, in that whilst the formal government policy of 18 countries (at the time of our research) allowed the procurement of hES cells from supernumerary embryos, only six, including the UK, also allowed the creation of human embryos for research purposes. As Salter argues 'the IVF "supernumerary" embryo is the morally superior option (ironically, because it is "spare" to the needs of reproduction it is then seen as having less intrinsic value) over… cloned embryos'.[37] So rather than supporting the UK's more liberal

[35] Science and Technology Committee. 2005. *Human Reproductive Technologies and the Law, Fifth Report, Volume 1*. London: House of Commons: 24.

[36] e.g., see J. Turney. 1998. *Frankenstein's Footsteps: Science, Genetics, and Popular Culture*. New Haven: Yale University Press.

[37] B. Salter. 2005. *Working Paper 2, Project: 'The Global Politics of Human Embryonic Stem Cell Science', ESRC Stem Cell Programme*. University of East Anglia: 20.

regulations, many of our respondents supported the majority global view of the time. Indeed, we might tentatively suggest that, in the context of the ethical contrast between PGD and IVF, our scientists present themselves as *predisposed* to taking a more ethically stringent position. By performing such ethical boundary-work around the sources of human embryos used in their work, our respondents were thus able to articulate and enact an ethical position that aligned them with the more ethically cautious countries amongst those who permitted hES cell research.

When we document aspects of the ethical boundary-work scientists undertake, what precisely are we witnessing? Most obviously, we argue that we are observing the delineation of a positive 'ethical space' which scientists can occupy — a space which signals both ethical reflection and rectitude. The rectitude is largely underpinned by reference to the formal legal and ethical framework that defines and allows 'ethical science', but it is also signalled by the reflection itself and a preparedness to venture into ethical argumentation and thereby enter the foothills of normative as opposed to merely conventional ethics.[38] Our scientists' refusal to create embryos for research, even though this is legal in the UK and is something that is promoted by many bioethicists,[39] is one striking example of this. It also, we argue, illustrates the value of empirical ethics in challenging 'normative bioethics'. Ethical boundary-work of scientists involves working across a dichotomous and even contradictory terrain. It means maintaining the distinction between 'real science' and 'associated ethics', whilst at the same time incorporating ethical acceptability into the heart of the scientific work.

Translational Research and Ethical Positions

As an approach to the sociology of translational ethics we have also explored these implicit themes of 'embodied ethics' through the notion of

---

[38] A. Cribb *et al.* Towards the Applied: the Construction of Ethical Positions in Stem Cell Translational Research. *Medicine, Health Care and Philosophy* 2008; 11: 351–361.

[39] S. Holm. Going to the Roots of the Stem Cell Controversy. *Bioethics* 2002; 16: 493–507; and L. Gruen, L. Grabel & P. Singer. 2007. *Stem Cell Research: The Ethical Issues.* Oxford: Blackwell.

'ethical positions' to illustrate some of the medical, scientific and ethical dilemmas involved in experimental translational research/treatment.[40] Using the example of stem cell science to illuminate the uneven ethical terrain of translational research, we examined how roles shape ethics. Our core argument — which emerged from, and was suggested by our data — is that the normative structures produced by the 'institutions and organisations' of the scientific and the clinical construct different ethical spaces and role positions, and that translational research has to be understood as a process of movement and negotiation across ethical spaces and not simply across physical and social places and spaces.

A number of (philosophical) bioethicists have developed lists of stem cell related ethical issues that encompass issues such as: the use and destruction of embryos; informed consent; commercialisation and the commodification of bodies; the 'threat' of reproductive cloning; animal rights and species integrity; resource allocation.[41] As a partial corrective to this 'view from nowhere' we argue that translational research entails a 'view from somewhere' which produces a 'normative analysis of lived moral experience'.[42] As part of this stream of work, we examined how role positions are constructed within, and defined by the differentiated ethical spaces of the scientific and the clinical; that is, the ethical positions and ethical burdens of doctors and scientists are institutionally produced.[43] Translational research, by its very nature, depends upon processes that transcend the ethical spaces of science and medicine and the case of translational

---

[40] A. Cribb *et. al.* Towards the Applied: the Construction of Ethical Positions in Stem Cell Translational Research. *Medicine, Health Care and Philosophy* 2008; 11: 351–361.

[41] e.g., see: S. Holm. Going to the Roots of the Stem Cell Controversy. *Bioethics* 2002; 16: 493–507; G. Outka. The Ethics of Human Stem Cell Research. *Kennedy Institute of Ethics Journal* 2002; 12: 175–213; L. Bortolotti & J. Harris. Stem Cell Research, Personhood and Sentience. *Reproductive Biomedicine Online* 2005; 10 Suppl: 76–79; M. Giacomini, F. Baylis & J.S. Robert. Banking On It: Public Policy and the Ethics of Stem Cell Research and Development. *Social Science and Medicine* 2007; 65: 1490–1508; and L. Gruen, L. Grabel & P. Singer. 2007. *Stem Cell Research: The Ethical Issues.* Oxford: Blackwell.

[42] A. Hedgecoe. Critical Bioethics: Beyond the Social Science Critique of Applied Ethics. *Bioethics* 2004; 18: 121.

[43] A. Cribb *et al.* Towards the Applied: The Construction of Ethical Positions in Stem Cell Translational Research. *Medicine, Health Care and Philosophy* 2008; 11: 351–361.

research enabled us to investigate the ways in which stem cell researchers and transplant clinicians 'assume', 'share' and 'refer' ethical responsibility. Applying science is not, as it is sometimes conceived, a move from 'theory' to the 'thorny ethics of practice'. Rather it is series of negotiations and collisions between value fields in which 'thorns' are everywhere present. In what follows we illustrate some of these ethical issues by drawing on one of the themes of our ethical positions paper — experimental treatments.[44]

The distance between the scientific and the clinical are reflected and refracted in the distance between the bench and the bedside. This distance is constructed in our interview data simultaneously as 'a huge gulf' and as 'tremendous potential'. Applying stem cell research, or thinking about 'what works', means recognising the multiple senses and layers of what counts as 'working':

> '*No doubt there's tremendous potential, but it's still a huge gulf between what is observational experimental stuff and something that's going to be clinically applicable*'. (Scientist 41)

> '*My concern is, however, we are not cells. We are a body made up of cells. And to, just to try to study something in a petri dish, does not equate to the human state. There's something in it, but don't extrapolate that just because it works in a dish, it will work in a human...The general population doesn't understand the difference between clinical and research. I don't think we explain it very well as scientists. And I think we're all too happy to allow people to think that research is something in a nasty dark laboratory with people doing scary things, where anything clinical is safe. And neither are correct. It's somewhere in between the two*'. (Physician 37)

Although both the scientists and the doctors that we interviewed were clear about the challenges of making stem cell research clinically relevant and effective, there was a rather different emphasis to their concerns about this

[44] Ibid.

process. We argued that the role positions of scientists are oriented towards the horizon of scientific knowledge whereas the role positions of doctors are sharply defined by the immediate presence of patients and the demands of clinical relationships.[45] Given these role positions it would not be surprising if doctors were inclined to look for what might be experimentally applicable today to improve treatment, whilst scientists were more inclined to be sceptical about the knowledge base underlying experimental treatments. In fields like organ and cell transplants, it is clinicians who have embarked on 'experiments perilous'[46] as they have had 'the courage to fail'.[47] This ethos, of making bold decisions about potentially lifesaving treatments can become part of the disposition of transplant surgeons:

> '*Who took it* [transplantation] *forward? It was the clinicians. People had to bold about it*'. (Surgeon 46)

> '*In some respects it's easier when you're dealing with patients than when we started out. But your decisions technically are often black or white in that, if you're going to die and you have an experimental treatment, most patients will take it and ethically one feels comfortable offering it, providing that one explains clearly what the risks are and the background leading up to making that decision*'. (Surgeon 32)

Amongst the scientists we spoke to there was a high level of scepticism, and some consternation, about the clinical imperative which is used to justify the 'rush' to experimental treatment in some areas of stem cell research (and elsewhere):

> '*I know a surgeon in x, who has a small trial, a phase 1 trial. He comes over as a cutting edge "stem cell researcher" and he wouldn't actually know one if it jumped up and bit him on the backside!... And he's*

---

[45] Ibid.

[46] R.C. Fox. 1998. *Experiment Perilous Physicians and Patients Facing the Unknown.* New Brunswick: Transaction.

[47] R.C. Fox & J.P. Swazey. 2002. *The Courage to Fail: A Social View of Organ Transplants and Dialysis. Third Edition.* New Brunswick: Transaction.

> *injecting in a rather cavalier fashion..., but it's based upon NO good animal models. And he may be exacerbating the situation, he may be causing more [complications]. I don't know. He's now going back and doing some animal model work, but the clinical trials have gone ahead! Okay, he hasn't killed anyone! He's cavalier...The way forward in research is normally you've got something you do in vitro, then you maybe have some pre-clinical models whether you're doing fish, flies or rats and mice. And then go on to maybe a human trial. It seems to me that often now, such is the anxiety of people to become known in this field, and get on, that the clinical trials are coming before any decent animal experiments. Maybe to their detriment...*[A scientific colleague], *who's from* [another university] *actually said '"These guys are an embarrassment to the stem cell community"'*. (Scientist 40)

> *'They basically said, '"Oh we've got some sick patients, got some cells, chuck one into the other and see what happens"'. With absolutely no biology behind it at all! And, of course, it didn't work. It's not surprising. So a lot of trials were done, in a completely sub-optimal fashion, and nobody tried to do the biology first'*. (Scientist 47)

These sceptical remarks highlight the differences reviewed above between the 'internal' imperatives of science and medicine — the imperative of finding treatments versus the imperative of validating truth claims.[48]

Applying stem cell research, or thinking about 'what works', means recognising the multiple senses and layers of what counts as 'working'. Although both the scientists and the doctors we interviewed were clear about the challenges of making stem cell research clinically relevant and effective, there was a rather different emphasis to their concerns about this process. The role position of scientists was oriented towards the horizon of scientific knowledge, whereas the role position of doctors was sharply defined by the immediate presence of patients and the demands of clinical relationships. Doctors and scientists recognised that cure, especially with novel treatments like cell transplants, was often not currently possible.

---

[48] S.P. Wainwright *et al.* Ethical Boundary Work in the Embryonic Stem Cell Laboratory. *Sociology of Health and Illness* 2006b; 28: 732–748.

Experimental treatments were seen as much more ethically complex than simply contending that medicine is about exhibiting 'the courage to fail'. For example, one eminent ES cell biologist we interviewed in the US described the clinicians engaged in 'stem cell trials for heart disease' as 'third rate scientists, misled by bad data' (Scientist 27), which captures the difference between 'the two cultures' of science and medicine in a particularly vivid aphorism.[49]

We hope that the two examples we have drawn upon above illustrate that developments in embryonic cell science and translational research provide a fertile ground for developing empirical ethics, as they require grounding in the evolving contexts of the perspectives of scientists, health professionals, policy makers and publics, in addition to the arguments of philosophers and social scientists.

TRANSLATIONAL RESEARCH, HYBRID EMBRYOS AND EXPERIMENTAL NEUROSCIENCE

In this next section of the chapter we focus on recent key developments in stem cell science and neuroscience as critical instances of the interface between research and treatment, and between science and medicine. We are beginning a Wellcome Trust-funded five-year research programme (2009–2014) that will provide a series of multidisciplinary perspectives on these issues, but in what follows we outline the background to this ongoing research to illustrate the potential for multidisciplinary research on translational ethics.[50] Our multidisciplinary team includes five social scientists (from the fields of medical sociology, science studies and political science), three clinician/scientists (from the fields of stem cell biology,

---

[49] S.P. Wainwright *et al.* 2009. Stem Cells, Translational Research and the Sociology of Science. In *Handbook of Genetics and Society: Mapping the New Genomic Era.* P. Atkinson, P. Glasner & M. Lock, eds. London: Routledge.

[50] C. Williams. Reflections on the Ethics of Translational Research. *Clinical Ethics* 2009; 4(2): 55–56. C. Williams, P. Alderson & B. Farsides. Dilemmas Encountered by Health Practitioners Offering Nuchal Translucency Screening: A Qualitative Case Study. *Prenatal Diagnosis* 2002a; 22: 216–220. For further details on this work see our webpage: http://www.kcl.ac.uk/schools/sspp/interdisciplinary/cbas/research/projects/labtec [Accessed 11 May 2009].

reproductive medicine, and neuroscience), and three philosopher/ethicists (from the fields of law, bioethics and clinical ethics).

Since the late 1990s, the government has strongly promoted the UK as a global centre for hESC research and translational research. For this investment to fulfil its potential it is important that progress is seen to occur, particularly in terms of translation to patient treatment, and that hope rather than hype is used to assess progress.[51] However, the variety of sources of stem cells and the patient-driven urgency for stem cell treatments have created numerous ethical issues for clinicians, scientists, patients and society which show no signs of abating.[52] We argue that two discrete but inter related areas selected pose profound and ongoing ethical, social, clinical, scientific, legal and regulatory issues. They are:

- The use of inter-species embryos, recently described in the UK Human Tissue and Embryos (Draft) Bill (2008)[53] as 'one of the most contentious issues in our inquiry and one in which many witnesses had opposing, deeply held views';
- The interface between experimental research and treatments for Motor Neuron Disease (MND) and Parkinson's Disease (PD). These are examples of serious neurological diseases where there is particular concern that experimental treatments could be introduced prior to adequate scientific testing, including controversial animal research on non human primates.

The central ethical question raised by both these areas is the ethical acceptability of changing what it means to be human and/or a person,

---

[51] P. Braude, S.L. Minger & R.M. Warwick. Stem Cell Therapy: Hope or Hype? *British Medical Journal* 2005; 330: 1159–1160.

[52] F. Baylis. Animal Eggs for Stem Cell Research: A Path Not Worth Taking. *The American Journal of Bioethics* 2008; 12: 18–32; B. Capps. Authoritative Regulation and the Stem Cell Debate. *Bioethics* 2008; 22: 44–55; and J. Maienschein, R.A. Ankeny & J.S. Robert. The Ethos and Ethics of Translational Research. *The American Journal of Bioethics* 2008; 8: 43–51.

[53] Department of Health. 2007. *Human Tissue and Embryos (Draft) Bill (2007). Cm 7087.* London: The Stationery Office.

but other related issues include the impact on human/animal rights and human/animal dignity; the interests of future generations; the interpretation of safety and risk; boundaries/overlaps between experimental research/treatment; the ethical evaluation of research; the relationship between personal beliefs and professional demands/responsibilities; the challenges for practitioners of fulfilling the overlapping roles of clinician, scientist, carer and investigator; the place of values in patient choice; and the shifts in moral landscapes as research progresses. The fact that the UK Prime Minister took the unusual step (on 25 March 2008) of allowing Labour MPs a free vote on three sections of the embryology bill before parliament, including the creation of inter-species embryos, indicates the level of ethical concern surrounding our chosen research area.

Experimental Science: Stem Cells and Hybrid Embryos

One of the long-term goals of stem cell research is to develop cell based treatments, using hES cells to replace damaged cells and tissues. The availability of human oocytes for research purposes is limited by both the prior needs of patients undergoing fertility treatment and the invasiveness of the donation procedure, which raises ethical concerns, particularly about acquiring embryos outside a therapeutic context. In this dynamic area there are frequent developments in medical and scientific technologies. Induced pluripotent stem cells (iPS), the reprogramming of adult cells back to embryonic-like stem cells, thus avoiding the need for eggs or the creation of embryos, is one such recent development which will be explored in this programme.[54] It is argued that if successful, this has the potential to circumvent many of the ethical issues associated with hESC research, although researchers caution that because of the use of retroviruses and cancer genes in their production, iPS cells are currently unsafe for human therapy.

[54] S. Holm. Time to Reconsider Stem Cell Ethics — The Importance of Induced Pluripotent Cells. *Journal of Medical Ethics* 2008; 34: 63–64; and K. Takahashi. Induction of Pluripotent Stem Cells from Adult Fibroblasts by Defined Factors. *Cell* 2007; 131: 861–872.

UK scientists have also recently argued that SCNT techniques, in which the nucleus of an adult somatic cell is transferred into an animal oocyte from which the nucleus has been removed (a type of inter-species embryo known as a cytoplasmic hybrid embryo or admixed embryo), offers a promising way forward which will provide them with increased knowledge about, for example, the factors required for reprogramming somatic cells.[55] Human made chimeras have long been a part of medical and scientific research, and the chimeric notion includes, for example, many people who have received pig heart valves.[56] However, what is novel here is combining stem cells with increasing knowledge of animal development and improved scientific techniques to create new chimeric entities at the level of the embryo. The earlier in development that the embryo is manipulated, the more profound the result is likely to be.[57]

The Academy of Medical Sciences report[58] on inter-species embryos states that, 'regulatory questions will increasingly arise from research involving non-human embryos and animals incorporating human material'. It goes on to argue that 'the interface between regulatory regimes involving human embryos, hES cells and animal research will become increasingly important'. In addition to focusing specifically on this interface, our research programme will also document the area of transgenic research. The report points out that as the science of transgenics has progressed, ever more 'ambitious' transgenic animals have been 'constructed', and that ever increasing amounts of human DNA will be engineered into animals. Although it considers that current UK activity is covered by existing regulatory regimes, it argues that the presence of significant amounts of human material in non-human animals will raise further ethical and social issues not covered under existing regimes. There is particular concern about the transplantation of

---

[55] Academy of Medical Sciences. 2007. *Inter-Species Embryos: A Report by the Academy of Medical Sciences*. London.

[56] I. Hyun *et al*. ISSCR Committee Forum: Ethical Issues in Human-to-Animal Chimera Experiments in Stem Cell Research. *Cell Stem Cell* 2007; 1: 59–63.

[57] C.T. Scott. Chimeras in the Crosshairs. *Nature Biotechnology* 2006; 24: 487–490.

[58] Academy of Medical Sciences. 2007. *Inter-Species Embryos: A Report by the Academy of Medical Sciences*. London: 39.

human neural stem cells into non-human primates, as advocated by some stem cell biologists.[59]

The problematic interface between experimental research and treatments, particularly in serious diseases, is not a new phenomenon. As Holm[60] argues, it is ethically problematic to raise false expectations in seriously ill people, particularly if this is done from self-interest or promotion, or to gain public and political acceptance of particular forms of treatment. However, there are a number of shifts which are potentially reshaping this interface. These include the rise of Internet use, meaning patients can access information about experimental treatments available globally; the increasing emphasis placed on patient autonomy and informed choice, as exemplified by Department of Health 'Expert Patient' Initiatives; and the changing nature of the clinician/patient relationship in uncertain research fields such as Parkinson's Disease (PD) and Motor Neuron Disease (MND), where high expectations serve in the 'mutual motivation' of scientists, clinicians and patients. With serious neurological diseases and treatments, it is also argued that some of these might be seen as fundamentally different from other medical interventions, because of their potential to alter our understanding of the species and/or modify our sense of self.[61] This is a key reason that some stem cell biologists believe testing should be carried out on non-human primate models. Conversely, others[62] argue that knowledge gained from animal models is not sufficiently transferable to humans, and that experimental therapies should instead be tested on terminally ill patients.

We argue that interspecies embryos raise a series of ethical, clinical, scientific, legal and regulatory issues that will help shape current and

---

[59] C.T. Scott. Chimeras in the Crosshairs. *Nature Biotechnology* 2006; 24: 487–490; and I. Hyun *et al.* ISSCR Committee Forum: Ethical Issues in Human-to-Animal Chimera Experiments in Stem Cell Research. *Cell Stem Cell* 2007; 1: 59–63.

[60] S. Holm. Going to the Roots of the Stem Cell Controversy. *Bioethics* 2002; 16: 493–507.

[61] F. Baylis & J.S. Robert. 2006. *Primer on Ethics and Crossing Species Boundaries.* American Institute of Biological Sciences. Available at: http://www.actionbioscience.org/biotech/baylis_robert.html [Accessed 11 May 2009].

[62] e.g., see I. Wilmut. 2006. *After Dolly: The Uses and Misuses of Human Cloning.* New York. Norton.

future landscapes of experimental science.[63] For example, what are the key ethical, clinical, social and legal issues stem cell laboratory staff consider when deciding which entities they will work with? What are the main approaches employed in the philosophical debate concerning the use of inter-species embryos? How have the legal, policy and regulatory debates been conducted differently in different settings? How has the media portrayed ethical debates around inter-species embryos? These are all questions that we will address from the multidisciplinary bioethical perspectives of sociology, science studies, political science, medicine, bioscience, philosophy and law — drawing on the expertise of our 11 co-applicants.

The proposed use of inter-species embryos in research has generated significant media coverage in the UK, stemming from applications for licenses made by two teams to create cytoplasmic hybrid embryos through the process of SCNT.[64] This involves human non-gametal cells such as skin cells being inserted into enucleated animal oocytes, enabling the study of human genetic diseases including Alzheimer's Disease, Huntington's Disease, PD and MND, using disease-specific embryonic stem cells cloned from patients. It is argued that this will reduce researchers' reliance on scarce human oocytes, in part avoiding the medical and ethical concerns associated with obtaining oocytes from women,[65] and that it will reduce the numbers of animal experiments.[66]

Responding to the license applications, the Human Fertilisation and Embryology Authority (HFEA) initiated a public consultation on the

---

[63] N. Brown & M. Michael. Risky Creatures: Institutional Species Boundary Change in Biotechnology Regulation. *Health, Risk and Society* 2004; 6(3): 207–222.

[64] S.L. Minger. Interspecies SCNT-Derived Human Embryos — A New Way Forward for Regenerative Medicine. *Regenerative Medicine* 2007; 2: 103–106; H. Gottweiss & S.L. Minger. iPS Cells and the Politics of Promise. *Nature Biotechnology* 2008; 26: 271–272; and F. Baylis. Animal Eggs for Stem Cell Research: A Path Not Worth Taking. *The American Journal of Bioethics* 2008; 12: 18–32.

[65] R. Steinbrook. Egg Donation and Human Embryonic Stem-Cell Research. *New England Journal of Medicine* 2006; 354: 324–326; and D. Magnus & M.K. Cho. Issues in Oocyte Donation for Stem Cell Research. *Science* 2005; 308: 1747–1748.

[66] S.L. Minger. Interspecies SCNT-Derived Human Embryos — A New Way Forward for Regenerative Medicine. *Regenerative Medicine* 2007; 2: 103–106.

ethical and social implications of creating such embryos for research.[67] The license decision was placed on hold pending the results of the consultation, which followed a legislative proposal to ban the use of hybrid embryos and chimeras in research.[68] This in turn led to a report by the House of Commons Science and Technology Committee, calling for regulation rather than prohibition of the activity.[69] Recently published draft legislation to amend the Human Fertilisation and Embryology (HFE) Act (1990) also states that any inter-species embryos created will be subject to regulations with regard to the HFE Act,[70] and both the *HFEA Scientific and Clinical Advances Group* and its *Ethics and Law Committee* argued that cytoplasmic hybrid embryos should be classified as human embryos. The HFEA recently announced its intention to license cytoplasmic hybrid research, but only in cases where the research is deemed 'both necessary and desirable'.[71] The first sentence of the HFEA decision statement illustrates the complexity of this issue:

> 'The decision on how the HFEA should approach the licensing of human-animal hybrids and chimera research has presented a particular challenge as this research is so novel in legal, scientific and ethical terms'.

The HFEA consultation documents include the arguments that such work undermines human dignity; that it may lead to research using true hybrid embryos (those in which nuclear genomic DNA from humans and

---

[67] HFEA. 2007a. *Hybrids and Chimeras: A Consultation on the Ethical and Social Implications of Creating Human/Animal Embryos in Research*. London.

[68] Department of Health. 2006. *Review of the Human Fertilisation and Embryology Act: Proposals for Revised Legislation (Including Establishment of the Regulatory Authority for Tissue and Embryos). Cm 6989.* London: The Stationery Office.

[69] Science and Technology Committee. 2007. *Government Proposals for the Regulation of Hybrid and Chimera Embryos: Fifth Report of Session 2006–07, House of Commons Science and Technology Committee*. London: The Stationery Office.

[70] Department of Health. 2007. *Human Tissue and Embryos (Draft) Bill (2007). Cm 7087.* London: The Stationery Office.

[71] HFEA. 2007b. *Statement on Its Decision regarding Hybrid Embryos*. London. 5 Sep.

non-human species are combined), or human chimeric embryos;[72] and that the creation of human/animal embryos is instinctively repugnant and/or unnatural. The relevance of such arguments to policy-making in this area has been much debated.[73] Robert and Baylis state that:

> 'A plausible "thin" explanation for the intuitive "yuck" response is that the creation of interspecies creatures from human materials evokes the idea of bestiality — an act widely regarded as a moral abomination because of its degrading character'.[74]

However, others argue that a strong case can be made for a research exemption to the creation of inter-species forms, 'when doing so serves important human needs...[as] the question of breaching species barriers is...less a matter of principle than a question of pragmatics and context'.[75]

A further key issue centres on the regulation of the human-animal boundary in the UK, namely which entities should be regulated as human embryos by the HFEA, and which should be regulated as animals by the Home Office. This arises from the boundaries between the 1990 Act, as amended by clause 17(2) of the draft Bill, and the Animals (Scientific Procedures) Act 1986. The Government initially chose 50% as a cut-off point as to whether an entity was 'human enough' to be regulated by the HFEA. However, the Joint Committee, appointed to consider and report on the Human Tissues and Embryos (Draft) Bill, states that the 50% rule

---

[72] HFEA. 2007a. *Hybrids and Chimeras: A Consultation on the Ethical and Social Implications of Creating Human/Animal Embryos in Research.* London.

[73] T. Caulfield & R. Brownsword. (2006) Human Dignity: A Guide to Policy Making in the Biotechnology Era? *Nature Reviews Genetics* 2006; 7: 72–76; T. Caulfield & A. Chapman. Human Dignity as a Criterion for Science Policy. *PloS Medicine* 2005; 2(8): 736–738; and R. Brownsword. Bioethics Today, Bioethics Tomorrow: Stem Cell Research and the 'Dignitarian Alliance'. *Notre Dame Journal of Law Ethics and Public Policy* 2003; 17: 15–51.

[74] J.S. Robert & F. Baylis. Crossing Species Boundaries. *American Journal of Bioethics* 2003; 3(3): 7.

[75] J.A. Robertson. A Response to 'Crossing Species Boundaries' by Jason Scott Robert and Francoise Baylis. *American Journal of Bioethics* 2003; 3(3): W64–W65.

was 'an essentially arbitrary attempt to draw a line between what qualifies as human and what as animal'.[76] Further, it noted its concern that 'there is a category of entities which would not be regulated under either the draft Bill or the 1986 Act'.[77] This ongoing debate highlights the profound difficulty of crafting acceptable legislative provisions governing scientific and clinical conduct that have enduring relevance, both scientifically and socially, particularly in such a morally contested area.[78]

In the next section of the chapter we turn to a discussion of some of the ethical issues raised by experimental treatments in current neuroscience in the fields of Motor Neurone Disease and Parkinson's Disease. These examples are further illustrations of the importance of multidisciplinary work, and will benefit from the combined expertise of our co-applicants from the disciplines of social science, ethics/law and bioscience/biomedicine.

Experimental Treatments: Motor Neuron Disease and Parkinson's Disease

Experimental neuroscience also raises a set of ethical, clinical, scientific and legal issues that mould, and are moulded by, the actual and emerging landscapes of experimental medicine for translational research. What are patients', scientists' and clinicians' views on the ethical issues raised by participation (or not) in experimental treatment/research? How is the boundary/overlap between experimental treatment and research in translational medicine drawn and justified? Which animal models of disease are considered necessary prior to human treatment/research in neurological diseases? How have legal, regulatory and ethical debates around

---

[76] Department of Health. 2007. *Human Tissue and Embryos (Draft) Bill (2007). Cm 7087.* London: The Stationery Office: 47. Josef Kure, in this volume, discusses the ontological confusion created in the current usage of 'chimera' and 'hybrid'.

[77] Ibid: 49.

[78] T. Caulfield. Clones, Controversy and Criminal Law: A Comment on the Proposal for Legislation Governing Assisted Human Reproduction. *Alberta Law Review* 2001; 39: 335–346; and F. Baylis. Animal Eggs for Stem Cell Research: A Path Not Worth Taking. *The American Journal of Bioethics* 2008; 12: 18–32.

animal models and experimental treatment/research shaped the field? Once again, these are all questions that our multidisciplinary research programme will address over the next five years.

In neurology, there is particular concern that what could be seen as experimental treatments might be introduced prior to adequate scientific testing. One key factor is that the diseases are often poorly understood, leading to pressure to develop appropriate animal models of the disease and treatments. In the UK, there is reluctance to carry out research on non-human primates, but it is argued that hESC treatments, particularly those which will be incorporated into the nervous system, necessitate this controversial use of animal experimentation. With such serious diseases which arguably threaten patients' sense of self; and where there is limited treatment, there is understandably a willingness from some patients to undergo experimental treatments. Key areas in neurological translational ethics to be explored in this theme include views on the ways in which new neurological therapies are being developed, tested, and translated into clinical practice. On what ethical grounds are animal experiments, particularly on non-human primates, being justified? What is the place of patient choice and practitioner preference in experimental medicine and what constitutes an ethical consent process? Who are the most appropriate patients to participate in experimental treatments and who decides? Does experimental neuroscience differ in any morally significant ways from other biomedical research? In summary, this neuroscience theme encapsulates broader ethical issues around animal experimentation, experimental medicine and changing what it means to be human and/or a person.

Translational research is often portrayed as a linear four-stage model: from molecules/genetics, to animal models, to experimental medicine, to clinical trials.[79] In our ongoing research programme we will examine the ethical complexities of this 'translational pipeline' by exploring the problems within and between these stages of the shift from basic science to clinical medicine. These issues are particularly pressing in the treatment

---

[79] S.P. Wainwright *et al.* 2009. Stem Cells, Translational Research and the Sociology of Science. In *Handbook of Genetics and Society: Mapping the New Genomic Era.* P. Atkinson, P. Glasner & M. Lock, eds. London: Routledge.

of degenerative neurological diseases, as many contend that it is the brain that most clearly defines us as human beings and persons. For example, it has been argued that a higher primate might have a claim to being a person in a way that a person robbed of all faculties by a degenerative neurological disease might not; and that an individual with a neurological disease might consider participating in experimental research as the only means of protecting their personhood. Hence, it is argued that neurological treatments can be understood as fundamentally different from other medical interventions,[80] given their potential to challenge our understandings of selfhood, personhood and the human species.[81] The creation of 'part-human beings', particularly in relation to non-human primates being used to test the developmental potential of human stem cells, has led to a number of ethical concerns including the potential transfer of human moral status to non-human animals and the effect of that on human — and animal — dignity;[82] and the moral status of such non-human animals as experimental animals.[83] As stated earlier, there is also concern about the creation and regulation of ever more ambitious transgenic and chimeric animals incorporating increasing amounts of human genetic material.[84]

One area that we are particularly interested in is experimental medicine in motor neuron disease (MND), a rapidly progressive, invariably fatal neurodegenerative disease that attacks the motor neurons responsible

[80] D. Weatherall. 2006. *The Use of Non-Human Primates in Research* [Weatherall Report]. London: The Academy of Medical Sciences, Medical Research Council, the Royal Society, and the Wellcome Trust.

[81] F. Baylis & J.S. Robert. 2006. *Primer on Ethics and Crossing Species Boundaries.* American Institute of Biological Sciences. Available at: http://www.actionbioscience.org/biotech/baylis_robert.html [Accessed 11 May 2009].

[82] M. Greene *et al.* Ethics: Moral Issues of Human–Non-Human Primate Neural Grafting. *Science* 2005; 309: 385–386.

[83] F. Baylis & A. Fenton. Chimera Research and Stem Cell Therapies for Neurodegenerative Disorders. *Cambridge Quarterly of Health Care Ethics* 2007; 16: 195–208; and L. Birke, A. Arluke & M. Michael. 2007. *The Sacrifice: How Scientific Experiments Transform Animals and People*. Purdue University Press.

[84] C.T. Scott. Chimeras in the Crosshairs. *Nature Biotechnology* 2006; 24: 487–490.

for controlling voluntary muscles.[85] 'Assisted Dying' requests from patients with MND are the highest relative to the numbers of people with the condition, due in part to high levels of hopelessness, which makes them a particularly vulnerable group in the research context.[86] There is understandably a keen search for experimental treatments by clinicians and scientists, and a demand for new treatments from patients. Some patients may even travel overseas for expensive 'stem cell therapies' which are widely publicised on the Internet, albeit with little scientific support for their effectiveness and safety.[87] When patients ask for advice, clinicians can be placed in an ethically difficult situation as there are no effective alternative treatment options, and patients may be keen to volunteer for such studies or 'treatments' in the hope of improving their condition, or for altruistic reasons. This is particularly the case where clinicians, who have usually developed close relationships with these patients, are also scientists working on developing new treatments (which is the case with one of our co-applicants).

A second case study that we intend to develop examines Parkinson's disease (PD), typically a slowly progressive and rarely fatal neurodegenerative disease mainly of dopaminergic neurons in the brain. Neuronal cell replacement can produce a significant clinical improvement for patients with PD,[88] but there are significant differences in patient outcome both between and within centres.[89] Several trials of foetal stem cell transplants, together with a growing body of experimental evidence (largely from animal studies), led the National Institutes of Health in the

---

[85] M.R. Turner *et al.* Prolonged Survival in Amyotrophic Lateral Sclerosis: A Descriptive Study from the King's ALS Database 1990–2002. *Journal of Neurology, Neurosurgery and Psychiatry* 2003; 74: 995.

[86] L. Ganzini *et al.* Attitudes of Patients with Amyotrophic Lateral Sclerosis and their Care Givers toward Assisted Suicide. *New England Journal of Medicine* 1998; 339: 967–973.

[87] M. Wasner, H. Klier & G.D. Borasio. The Use of Alternative Medicine by Patients with Amyotrophic Lateral Scelorsis. *Journal of the Neurological Sciences* 2001; 191: 151–154.

[88] O. Lindvall. Stem Cells for Cell Therapy in Parkinson's Disease. *Pharmacology Research* 2003; 47: 279–287.

[89] A. Björklund *et al.* Neural Transplantation for the Treatment of Parkinson's Disease. *Lancet Neurology* 2003; 2: 437–444.

USA to fund the first two RCT's of human foetal stem cell transplants for PD. However, these ethically contentious sham surgery-controlled trials showed only modest improvement.[90] Moreover, severe side-effects affecting 7% to 15% of patients led some neuroscientists to call for further animal studies.[91] This shift from experimental patient treatment back to animal studies illustrates just some of the ethical difficulties of experimental neurological translational research, including: what evidence is judged sufficient to move from animal to human trials; which patients should be selected, for example, those with the most severe symptoms who may be the least likely to show the benefit of the treatment but in some ways have 'the least to lose' — or those with the least severe symptoms, who run the risk of being made worse by the treatment; and the ethics of trials involving sham neurosurgery. Drawing on these two areas of neuroscience, we are beginning to explore the ethical landscape of animal models, experimental medicine and clinical trials, through a range of multidisciplinary research projects that examine scientists' and clinicians; patients and patient interest groups, and policy and regulatory perspectives on experimental neuroscience. In the final part of the chapter we reflect on our own programme of research and highlight some of the ways in which bioethics can, and should, become more multidisciplinary.

TOWARDS MULTIDISCIPLINARY TRANSLATIONAL ETHICS?

One of our particular interests lies in promoting multidisciplinary research on ethics, for instance through publishing multidisciplinary papers. In our own work this includes publications on stem cell translation

[90] C.R. Freed *et al.* Transplantation of Embryonic Dopamine Neurons for Severe Parkinson's Disease. *New England Journal of Medicine* 2001; 344: 710–719; and C.W. Olanow *et al.* A Double-Blind Controlled Trial of Bilateral Fetal Nigral Transplantation in Parkinson's Disease. *Annals of Neurology* 2003; 54: 403–414.

[91] O. Lindvall. Stem Cells for Cell Therapy in Parkinson's Disease. *Pharmacology Research* 2003; 47: 279–287.

co-written by sociologists and philosophers[92]; papers on PGD that combine sociology and ethics[93]; medicine and sociology[94]; and law, ethics and sociology.[95] We, and we hope our collaborators too, have found writing these papers aimed at different audiences with colleagues from different disciplines a challenging, stimulating and rewarding experience.

A second major area we wish to see increased attention and work on is the ways in which empirical ethics can be seen to have normative force. We suggest that the (stereotypical) poles of 'descriptive and normative' bioethics create an intermediary space where the productive conjoining of the empirical and the philosophical can be promoted.[96] For example, our previous research uses interviews conducted by social scientists followed by participation in multidisciplinary Ethics Discussion Groups facilitated by a health care ethicist, in order to provide a unique and constructive

---

[92] e.g., see S.P. Wainwright *et al.* From Bench to Bedside? Biomedical Scientists' Expectations of Stem Cell Science as a Future Therapy for Diabetes. *Social Science and Medicine* 2006a; 63: 2052–2064; and A. Cribb *et al.* Towards the Applied: The Construction of Ethical Positions in Stem Cell Translational Research. *Medicine, Health Care and Philosophy* 2008; 11: 351–361.

[93] K. Ehrich *et al.* Testing the Embryo, Testing the Fetus. *Clinical Ethics* 2007a; 4: 181–186; K. Ehrich *et al.* Choosing Embryos: Ethical Complexity in Staff Accounts of PGD. *Sociology of Health and Illness* 2007b; 29: 1091–1106; K. Ehrich, C. Williams & B. Farsides. The Embryo as Moral Work Object: PGD/IVF Staff Views and Experiences. *Sociology of Health and Illness* 2008; 30: 772–787; K. Ehrich & C. Williams. A 'Healthy Baby': The Double Imperative of Preimplantation Genetic Diagnosis. *Health.* In press; and C. Williams *et al.* Facilitating Choice, Framing Choice: Staff Views on Widening the Scope of PGD in the UK. *Social Science and Medicine* 2007; 65: 1094–1105.

[94] T. El-Toukhy, C. Williams & P. Braude. The Ethics of PGD. *The Obstetrician and Gynacologist* 2008; 10: 49–54.

[95] K. Ehrich *et al.* Social Welfare, Genetic Welfare? Boundary Work in the IVF/PGD Clinic. *Social Science and Medicine* 2006; 63: 1213–1224; and R. Scott *et al.* PGD: Health Professionals' Views on the Requirement for a 'Significant Risk of a Serious Genetic Condition'. *Medical Law Review* 2007; 15(3): 320–356.

[96] A. Cribb. 2005. *Health and the Good Society.* Oxford: Oxford University Press; A. Cribb *et al.* Towards the Applied: The Construction of Ethical Positions in Stem Cell Translational Research. *Medicine, Health Care and Philosophy* 2008; 11: 351–361; and J. Ives *et al.* Becoming a Father/Refusing Fatherhood: An Empirical Bioethics Approach to Paternal Responsibilities and Rights. *Clinical Ethics* 2008; 3: 75–84.

opportunity within which to discuss clinical and scientific ethical dilemmas posed by innovative medical technologies and identified by staff themselves.[97] Over the course of the 20 groups run to date, we have gradually increased the philosophical component of the groups, introducing a more critical, normative philosophical approach, thus extending the use of this methodology.[98] We are now extending and re-evaluating these methods and we anticipate that we will be able to further refine our recommendations about how best to bring ethics and social science into morally contested clinical and scientific settings and postgraduate education more generally as our new research programme develops.

All our empirical ethics publications to date are essentially contributions to the exploration of the ethical complexities inherent in particular social worlds (such as stem cell science and translational research). For some philosopher bioethicists such research lacks a normative dimension — it describes the complexities of ethical issues rather than offering guidance on what ought to be done. One typical riposte from sociologists to this potential objection is to argue that philosophical analysis is of little (or even no value) in helping 'real

---

[97] C. Williams, P. Alderson & B. Farsides. Dilemmas Encountered by Health Practitioners Offering Nuchal Translucency Screening: A Qualitative Case Study. *Prenatal Diagnosis* 2002; 22: 216–220; C. Williams, P. Alderson & B. Farsides. Too Many Choices? Hospital and Community Staff Reflect on the Future of Prenatal Screening. *Social Science and Medicine* 2002; 55: 743–753; C. Williams, P. Alderson and B. Farsides. Is Non-Directiveness Possible Within the Context of Antenatal Screening and Testing? *Social Science and Medicine* 2002; 54: 17–25; C. Williams, P. Alderson & B. Farsides. 'Drawing the Line' in Prenatal Screening and Testing: Health Practitioners' Discussions. *Health, Risk and Society* 2002; 4: 61–75; B. Farsides, C. Williams & P. Alderson. Aiming Towards 'Moral' Equilibrium': Health Care Professionals' Views on Working Within the Morally Contested Field of Antenatal Screening. *Journal of Medical Ethics* 2004; 30: 505–509; C. Williams. Framing the Fetus in Medical Work: Representations and Practices. *Social Science and Medicine* 2005; 60: 2085–2095; and C. Williams. Dilemmas in Fetal Medicine: Premature Application of Technology or Responding to Women's Choice. *Sociology of Health and Illness* 2006; 28: 1–20.

[98] P. Alderson, C. Williams & B. Farsides. Examining Ethics in Practice: Health Service Professionals' Evaluations of In-Hospital Ethics Seminars. *Journal of Nursing Ethics* 2002; 9: 518–531.

people in real settings' make ethical judgements as the complexities of the social world undermines the premises and assumptions of many philosophical arguments. The danger here, of course, is that our somewhat extreme versions of sociologists and bioethicists will talk at each other rather than with one another in what have been called 'ethics wars'.[99] However, our own experience is that once bioethicists and sociologists begin to engage in dialogue then ways can be found to leave the cul-de-sacs of the 'merely empirical' and the 'purely philosophical'. Sociologists and philosophers, including de Vries *et al.*[100] and Draper & Ives,[101] have argued that we should explore how philosophy and the social sciences could be brought together in happy, rather than dysfunctional, 'marriages'. In this spirit we have begun to argue that there are two ways that will enable our empirical ethics research to become more normative — although we also contend that 'descriptive empirical ethics' remains valuable in its own right.[102] First, with colleagues from philosophical ethics, we can begin to develop ethical frameworks, by drawing on a mix of our empirical data and philosophical arguments.[103] These ethical frameworks will provide a template for practitioners of, say, experimental biomedicine, to evaluate ethical issues and arguments against. Second, we (and others) can go a step further and begin to test such an empirically/philosophically grounded ethical framework against established 'hard cases' that are typically employed to evaluate purely

---

[99] K. Hoeyer. 'Ethics Wars': Reflections on the Antagonism Between Bioethicists and Social Sciences Observers of Biomedicine. *Human Studies* 2006; 29: 203–227.

[100] R. de Vries *et al.* Social Science and Bioethics: The Way Forward. *Sociology of Health and Illness* 2006; 28: 665–677.

[101] H. Draper & J. Ives. An Empirical Approach to Bioethics: Social Science 'Of' 'For' and 'In' Bioethics Research. *Cognition, Brain, Behaviour* 2007; XI: 319–330.

[102] S.P. Wainwright & C. Williams. 2008b. Sociological Reflections on Ethics, Embryonic Stem Cells and Translational Research. *Seminar, Centre for Biomedical Ethics Yong Loo Lin School of Medicine, National University of Singapore, Singapore.* 1 Dec; and S.P. Wainwright & C. Williams. 2008c. Sociological Reflections on the Ethics of Human Embryonic Stem Cells and Translational Research. *Seminar, Values, Ethics and Law in Medicine (VELiM), University of Sydney, Sydney Australia.* 15 Dec.

[103] M. Parker. Ethnography/Ethics. *Social Science and Medicine* 2007; 65: 2248–2259.

philosophical ethical reasoning.[104] We hope others who want to see increased dialogue and research between, for example, the empirical and the philosophical, will take up these suggestions for a continuum of normative empirical ethics of *exploration*, *framework*, *testing*, and that this will help lead to a new and productive era of interdisciplinary bioethics.

ACKNOWLEDGEMENTS

This chapter is based on five research projects: ESRC Stem Cell Initiative RES-340-25-0003 and RES-350-27-0001; Wellcome Trust Biomedical Ethics Programme grant 074935 and 081414; Wellcome Trust Biomedical Ethics Strategic Award 086034. We thank all the co-applicants, collaborators and respondents that we have worked with who have stimulated and developed our thinking in these areas.

[104] H. Draper & J. Ives. An Empirical Approach to Bioethics: Social Science 'Of' 'For' and 'In' Bioethics Research. *Cognition, Brain, Behaviour* 2007; XI: 319–330; and J. Ives. 'Encounters with Experience': Empirical Bioethics and the Future. *Health Care Analysis* 2008; 16, 1–6.

6

RHETORIC, POWER AND LEGITIMACY IN PUBLIC DISCOURSE: A CRITICAL ANALYSIS OF THE PUBLIC DEBATE SURROUNDING THE REVIEW OF EMBRYO RESEARCH AND CLONING LEGISLATION IN AUSTRALIA IN 2005

Tamra Lysaght and Ian Kerridge

INTRODUCTION

In 1998, a team of scientists at the University of Wisconsin announced that they had successfully isolated the first embryonic stem cell (ESC) lines from human blastocysts.[1] This announcement followed another important paper a year earlier, reporting the first mammal to be cloned using a technique known as somatic cell nuclear transfer, or 'SCNT' (also called Cell Nuclear Replacement).[2] The two events prompted lay and professional speculation about the potential application of controversial technologies in biomedical science and clinical research, and attracted intense public scrutiny as it became clear that the use of ESCs and SCNT required the creation and destruction of human embryos.

---

[1] J.A. Thomson *et al.* Embryonic Stem Cell Lines Derived from Human Blastocysts. *Science* 1998; 282(5391): 1145–1147.

[2] I. Wilmut *et al.* Viable Offspring Derived from Fetal and Adult Mammalian Cells. *Nature* 1997; 385(6619): 810–813.

Stem cell research has continued to generate considerable public debate. For the most part, these debates have typically centred on the moral status of human embryos and the utility of stem cells. Opponents of stem cell research have generally argued that it is morally unconscionable to destroy human embryos for research, while its advocates have argued that the potential for substantial medical and therapeutic benefits outweighs concerns for the embryo. Out of this discourse, most industrialised countries have developed legislation to regulate the use of human embryos and SCNT in research.

There has been, however, enormous variation in the degree to which ESC research and SCNT has been permitted in different countries.[3] In some countries, specific legislation has been enacted to completely prohibit all research on human embryos. In others, there is either no legislation that explicitly allows research on human ESC lines, or research is only permitted on lines that already existed prior to a specified date. Australia has taken a relatively liberal approach to the governance of stem cell research and its related technologies.

Australian Stem Cell Policy Context

After protracted public and parliamentary debate in 2001–2002, the Australian Federal Parliament enacted the *Research Involving Human Embryos Act 2002* and the *Prohibition of Human Cloning Act 2002*.[4] Prior to the introduction of this legislation, the regulatory environment in Australia was confusing and inconsistent. Research on human embryos was overseen at a federal level under guidelines from the *National Health and Medical Research Council* (NHMRC); with regulations at the state level varying considerably between states — being non-existent in some states to comprehensive and restrictive in others.[5] Recognising the speed

[3] L. Walters. Human Embryonic Stem Cell Research: An Intercultural Perspective. *Kennedy Institute of Ethics Journal* 2004; 14(1): 3–39. Also see Chalmers, this volume.

[4] D. Nicol, D. Chalmers & B. Gogarty. Regulating Biomedical Advances: Embryonic Stem Cell Research. *Macquarie Law Journal* 2002; 2: 31–59.

[5] M. Slabbert. Cloning and Stem Cell Research: A Critical Overview of the Present Legislative Regime in Australia and the Way Forward. *Journal of Law and Medicine* 2003; 10(1): 511 530.

at which stem cell science was evolving, the potential clinical applications of ESC and SCNT research, and the degree of disagreement in the community over its acceptability, a three-year review was built into each Act.[6] The Acts required that an independent legislative review committee (called the LRC) consider the scope and operation of the legislation and make recommendations for amendments to the Council of Australian Governments and the Commonwealth.[7]

The six-member LRC, chaired by the late Honourable John Lockhart, submitted its report to the Federal Minister for Ageing, the Honourable Julie Bishop, in December 2005.[8] The Lockhart Report made 56 recommendations, which included: the continued use of supernumerary IVF embryos; the creation of SCNT embryos for research purposes; and maintenance of the prohibition of SCNT for reproductive purposes.[9] All but one of the committee's recommendations (relating to the creation of human-animal chimeras) were subsequently incorporated into a bill that was put before a conscience vote in Parliament.[10] In December 2006, the Parliament enacted the *Prohibition of Human Cloning for Reproduction and the Regulation of Human Embryo Research Amendment Act 2006* with changes going into effect in June 2007.[11] Most Australian states, with

---

[6] Ibid.

[7] Legislation Review Committee. 2005a. *Issues Paper: Outline of Existing Legislation and Issues for Public Consultation. Legislation Review of Australia's Prohibition of Human Cloning Act 2002 and Research Involving Human Embryos Act 2002*. Available from: http://www.lockhartreview.com.au/ [Accessed 5 Aug 2005].

[8] Legislation Review Committee. 2005b. *Prohibition of Human Cloning Act 2002 and the Research Involving Human Embryos Act 2002*. Available from http://www.lockhartreview.com.au/ [Accessed 20 Dec 2005].

[9] D. Cooper. The Lockhart Review: Where Now for Australia? *Journal of Law and Medicine* 2006; 14: 27–44.

[10] R. Ankeny & S. Dodds. Hearing Community Voices: Public Engagement in Australian Human Embryo Research Policy, 2005–2007. *New Genetics and Society* 2008; 27(3): 217–232; and O. Harvey. Regulating Stem Cell Research and Human Cloning in an Australian Context: The Lockhart Review. *New Genetics and Society* 2008; 27(1): 33–42.

[11] NHMRC. 2007. Stem Cells, Cloning and Related Issues. 10 Dec. Available from http://www.nhmrc.gov.au/research/embryos/stemcells/patterson.htm [Accessed 28 Aug 2008].

the exception of West Australia and Tasmania, have since enacted sister legislation to reflect the Commonwealth legislation. The current legislation is due to be reviewed again in 2010.

As was the case with the introduction of the original legislation, the 2006 policy episode attracted an enormous amount of media attention. And as was the case with stem cell debates in other contexts,[12] the Australian media tended to frame the public debate around the 'embryo question', and the potential impact of stem cells in translational medicine.[13] While this may be understandable given the penetrating moral subject matter, the concern is that by framing the public debate in this way, the issues surrounding ESC research are dichotomised and oversimplified to the extent that the complexity of the social, moral and political issues is lost.[14]

In this chapter, we draw on the results of empirical research conducted on public discourse surrounding the Australian 2005–2006 stem cell policy episode. This research used qualitative content and thematic analysis techniques to examine 109 opinion editorials published in Australian newspapers during the time, and 23 in-depth interviews with participants from the debate. From this research, we argue that debates around ESC research are characterised by: 1) contested notions of science, where scientific facts are construed and mobilised in public discourse rhetorically according to the value preferences of participants; 2) disputes over who is included, where participants compete to establish legitimacy; and 3) conflicts over who has authority to influence how the moral issues are framed

---

[12] M.C. Nisbet, D. Brossard and A Kroepsch. Framing Science: The Stem Cell Controversy in an Age of Press/Politics. *Harvard International Journal of Press/Politics* 2003; 8(2): 36–70; and S. Parry. The Politics of Cloning: Mapping the Rhetorical Convergence of Embryos and Stem Cells in Parliamentary Debates. *New Genetics and Society* 2003; 22(2): 145–168.

[13] R. Robins. 2005. Biomedical Innovation or Bioethical Precaution: The Stem Cell Debate in Australia. In *Crossing Borders: Cultural, Religious and Political Differences Concerning Stem Cell Research*. W. Bender, C. Hauskeller & A. Manzei, eds. Munster: Agenda Verlag: 391–410.

[14] C. Ganchoff. Regenerating Movements: Embryonic Stem Cells and the Politics of Potentiality. *Sociology of Health and Illness* 2004; 26(6): 757–774; and C. Williams, J. Kitzinger & L. Henderson. Envisaging the Embryo in Stem Cell Research: Rhetorical Strategies and Media Reporting of the Ethical Debates. *Sociology of Health and Illness* 2003; 25(7): 793–814.

and understood. Further, we suggest that it is only by understanding these factors that we can better see how science is deployed rhetorically in public discourse and the ways in which it may be applied in negotiating compromise between irreconcilable moral positions.

CONTESTED NOTIONS OF SCIENCE

> The biological fact about this cluster of cells is that it is human, with an entire and unique genetic code. The embryo may indeed be only a potential person, but it is a unique human being. *Opponent A*

> It comes back to the definition of when life begins…I personally have some problems about giving the same credence to something which is less than the size of full stop, comma, dot, or whatever, to put it colloquially, compared to someone like you or myself. Basically, I find it very difficult to see how you can equate the two together. One is a person that has a personality that you can communicate with and relate to. The other one, even if you believed that this was how life had begun, it certainly has the potential for life no question, but it's a cluster of cells. How can you possibly equate the two together? *Advocate A*

The public understanding of science is an integral part of a wider moral discourse. This discourse influences decisions that are made about the types of things/objects/people/actions that are determined as normatively good/bad, useful/useless, un/necessary, un/justified and so on. When claims are made about science in these contexts, they are framed in ways that strengthen or undermine moral arguments for or against particular policy options. Their framing, therefore, influences policy outcomes by investing key terms and concepts with ontological meaning. And because these 'science claims' are used to inform ontological judgments, it is clear that science itself is used by participants in debates about public policy as a means of achieving desired normative outcomes. For the most part, these participants tend to use science either to justify the pursuit of scientific research on the basis of its claimed benefits or prevent it on the grounds that its potential costs are intolerable by emphasising scientific facts and concepts that are normatively consistent with one of these arguments. The use of science claims, therefore, tends to correspond with the types of moral arguments participants make in support of a particular policy position.

Arguments relating to the creation and destruction of early human life often rest upon normative assumptions about the significance of certain biological and genetic characteristics as ontological determinants of moral status.[15] At times these assumptions are made explicit, but more often they are implicit in how participants use science to describe human embryos.

Generally speaking, moral status is diminished whenever advocates of ESC research use science in their material descriptions of human embryos. To them, embryos are often simply a 'cluster of cells' with no literal capacity to develop into a human being. In contrast, embryos are imbued with much greater status by opponents of ESC research, who tend to personify them as 'persons'. Claims such as those made by *Advocate A* in the statement shown above, attach moral significance to the size (a 'dot') and *remote* developmental potential of certain organisms, and thereby suggest that embryo research is justifiable because embryos are morally irrelevant.[16] They contrast with those made by opponents to ESC research, who often argue that ESC research is morally indefensible because embryos have moral status derived from their *intrinsic* developmental capacity.[17]

These types of claims reflect broader tensions between the biological reductionism of genetics and holistic approaches to human ontology.[18] They are also a potent reminder that science inevitably embodies and reflects culturally-defined norms about the meaning and status of entities, such as the embryo, and that while there is often broad agreement about these norms at times, they will often be deeply contested.

---

[15] M.A. Warren. 1997. *Moral Status: Obligations to Persons and Other Living Things*. Oxford: Oxford University Press.

[16] N. Agar. Embryonic Potential and Stem Cells. *Bioethics* 2007; 21(4): 198–207.

[17] C. Hauskeller. How Traditions of Ethical Reasoning and Institutional Processes Shape Stem Cell Research in Britain. *Journal of Medicine and Philosophy* 2004; 29(5): 509–532.

[18] D. Nelkin & S.M. Lindee. 1995. *The DNA Mystique: The Gene as a Cultural Icon*. New York: W H Freeman and Company; C. Waldby. Stem Cells, Tissue Cultures and the Production of Biovalue. *Health* 2002; 6: 305–323; and P. Wilberg. 2003. *Heidegger, Medicine and 'Scientific Method'*. Sussex, UK: New Gnosis Publications.

Therefore, in moulding the ontological meaning of objects such as the human embryo, science becomes a discursive tool that participants deploy in positioning themselves within a moral debate. In highly contested areas of science policy, their purpose is to reinforce assertions about the necessity, justification and permissibility of scientific research. Participants gain the moral high ground in policy disputes by drawing on a range of theological, philosophical and political resources. Of these resources, science is used preferentially because the status of scientific knowledge is privileged. Science, therefore, provides participants with a powerful rhetorical device that they may use to gain legitimacy and shape the meaning of terms used in public debate.

RHETORIC, POWER AND LEGITIMACY

> Nuclear transfer from a skin or muscle cell into an inactivated egg does not give an embryo; it gives cells that are genetically identical to the cells of the sick person from whom the cell was taken. These cells have none of the genetic uniqueness we associate with a child compared with his or her parents. *Advocate B*

> Science will tell us at what stage a developing embryo or foetus or newborn child demonstrates capacities like perception, sensation, language or rational thought. Those are questions that science can provide some information on. But it can't tell us what is the marker that really matters — that it's rationality that matters or sensation is what matters or just being a human organism is what matters. Those are essentially philosophical questions…those are questions which scientists don't bring any special wisdom to but count as like any other human being faced with those big questions *Opponent B*

Science has enormous rhetorical power in public discourse, and can be deployed in a number of different ways in order to gather support for a favoured moral position. Science claims may be deployed in order to reinforce the validity of one's arguments, to appeal to the emotional and logical disposition of public audiences, to build trust, and to establish the status of some participants in public discourse and discredit others. And through the mobilisation of alliances with technical experts, participants use science claims rhetorically to establish legitimacy in the public domain.

Participants in stem cell policy debates also make their case using appeals that are based in both emotion and logic. The Australian debate about stem cell research was no different with participants using a range of rhetorical tools including metaphors, analogies and similes to 'humanise' embryos as moral subjects, or 'dehumanise' them as biological tissue.[19] Opponents of ESC research, for example, often referred to the 'unique genetic code' of human embryos to remind the public of the human identity of embryos and stem cells and the loss of human potential that is an inevitable consequence of ESC research.

Advocates of this research tend to avoid using this type of emotive language, because it diverts attention away from the logical appeal of their argument, and particularly to the clinical and epistemological utility of stem cells.[20] Research advocates instead use rhetoric that either reduces the embryo to the sum of its biological parts, or in the case of SCNT, make a claim that SCNT embryos are not embryos at all or are ontologically different from gamete fusion embryos. For example, *Advocate B* above claims that SCNT embryos are not really embryos, because a cell fused with an 'inactivated egg' has 'none of the genetic uniqueness we associate with a child'. The logic of this argument, which is a form of genetic essentialism, is that if something isn't even an embryo, let alone human, then it need not be excluded from use in scientific research.

Genetic essentialism is a culturally-loaded discourse which derives most of its power from the authority of science and genetics, but has meanings that also reflect social, political and moral agendas.[21] The gene concept, which asserts that human identity, health and illness are

---

[19] C. Williams, J. Kitzinger & L. Henderson. Envisaging the Embryo in Stem Cell Research: Rhetorical Strategies and Media Reporting of the Ethical Debates. *Sociology of Health and Illness* 2003; 25(7): 793–814.

[20] S. Parry. The Politics of Cloning: Mapping the Rhetorical Convergence of Embryos and Stem Cells in Parliamentary Debates. *New Genetics and Society* 2003; 22(2): 145–168.

[21] D. Nelkin & S.M. Lindee. 1995. *The DNA Mystique: The Gene as a Cultural Icon.* New York: W H Freeman and Company.

genetically determined, is deployed in many science policy contexts, particularly in contested areas of the biological and biomedical sciences, as a means of simplifying complex scientific ideas.[22] However, ideas about human identity are neither agreed nor fixed, but vary over time and according to the values, interests and beliefs of the speaker. The place that science, particularly genetics, plays in relation to stem cell research is likely, therefore, to vary enormously.

Science plays an important rhetorical role in public debates because it provides participants with the discursive tools needed to explore the possible meanings of contested ideas.[23] Science also privileges the persuasive and effective use of argumentation.[24] Hence, the use of science in public debate is an effective means of generating different types of logical arguments and emotional appeals that support and refute various positions.[25] To do this persuasively, however, participants must first gain the trust of those whom they are trying to convince.[26] The effective use of science claims is, therefore, contingent upon one's trust in the character and credibility of those who speak in public discourse.

Those who use science claims in public policy disputes are generally only 'credible' if they are able to effectively demonstrate their knowledge of science and its policy implications. Scientists, who are educated and trained in the technical language of science, are well placed for this

---

[22] D. Nelkin. Molecular Metaphors: The Gene in Popular Discourse. *Nature Reviews Genetics* 2001; 2: 555–559.

[23] B.V. Lewenstein. 1995. Science and the Media. In *Handbook of Science and Technology Studies*. S. Jasanoff, G.E. Markle, J.C. Peterson & T. Pinch, eds. Thousand Oaks, CA: Sage Publications: 343–360.

[24] A. Gross. 1990. *The Rhetoric of Science*. Cambridge, MA: Harvard University Press; and M.D. Zulick. Generative Rhetoric and Public Argument: A Classical Approach. *Argumentation and Advocacy* 1997; 33(3).

[25] S. Toulmin. 1990. The Uses of Argument. In *The Rhetorical Tradition: Readings from Classical Times to the Present*. P. Bizzell & B. Herzberg, eds. Boston: Bedford; and C. Waddell. 1997. The Role of Pathos in the Decision-Making Process: A Study in the Rhetoric of Science Policy. In *Landmark Essays on Rhetoric of Science: Case Studies*. R.A. Harris, ed. Mahwah, NJ: Hermagoras Press: 127–150.

[26] C. Carey. 1996. Rhetorical Means of Persuasion. In *Essays on Aristotle's Rhetoric*. A. Rorty, ed. Berkeley: University of California Press: 399–415.

purpose. However, participants must also present themselves as honest and trustworthy speakers. If not, then doubt may be cast upon their integrity. Science is thus not only deployed as a means of appealing to the credibility of participants, but also of casting doubt onto the trustworthiness of others.

Scientists are trusted largely because there is a high degree of trust in the norms, ethos and method of science,[27] and so are privileged with expert authority in policy contexts on the basis of assumptions about their impartiality and disinterestedness.[28] For this reason, where scientists are thought to have a conflicting interest in a policy issue — be it economic, ideological or political — their scientific credibility and judgments are called into question as biased because they run counter to the rhetorical norms of value-neutrality.[29]

How effective scientists, and others who use science claims, are at maintaining trust and authority in policy debates depends on how effectively they deploy the rhetoric of science, particularly the idea that 'objective knowledge' is, and should be, distinct from the subjective beliefs, values and ideals of social actors.[30] The most successful rhetors in

---

[27] L.J. Prelli. 1997. The Rhetorical Construction of Scientific Ethos. In *Landmark Essays on Rhetoric of Science: Case Studies*. R.A. Harris, ed. Mahwah, NJ: Hermagoras Press: 87–104.

[28] R.K. Merton. 1942/1973. The Normative Structure of Science. In *The Sociology of Science*. N. Stoner, ed. Chicago: Chicago University Press: Vols. 267–278.

[29] I. Mitroff. Norms and Counter-Norms in a Select Group of the Apollo Moon Scientists: A Case Study of the Ambivalence of Scientists. *American Sociological Review* 1974; 39(4): 579–595.

[30] D. Atkinson. 1999. *Scientific Discourse in Sociohistorical Context: The Philosophical Transactions of the Royal Society of London*. Mahwah, NJ: Lawrence Erlbaum Associates; C. Bazerman. 1997. Reporting the Experiment: The Changing Account of Scientific Doings in the Philosophical Transactions of the Royal Society, 1665–1800. In *Landmark Essays on Rhetoric of Science: Case Studies*. R.A. Harris, ed. Mahwah, NJ: Hermagoras Press: 169–186; G.N. Gilbert & M. Mulkay. 1984. *Opening Pandora's Box: A Sociological Analysis of Scientists' Discourse*. London: Cambridge University Press; B. Latour. 1987. *Science in Action: How to Follow Scientists and Engineers Through Society*. Milton Keynes: Open University Press; and B. Latour & S. Woolgar. 1979. *Laboratory Life: The Social Construction of Scientific Facts*. Beverly Hills, CA: Sage Publications.

public discourse are those who deploy this rhetoric so effectively that it seems like they really are just 'stating the facts' and are not attempting to bias the debate towards their political and ideological preferences.[31] However, this is precisely what does happen as science may be conjured up by virtually anyone wishing to frame the debate in a way that portrays a preferred set of norms, values and ideals.[32]

Legitimation Processes

The effective use of science claims and deployment of science rhetoric in public disputes is best understood as a contest over authority, power and legitimation. When public policy disputes reach a point where participants seek to justify how they know what they claim to know, they are engaging in a process of justification that may be seen as a feature of a hierarchy of legitimation.[33] This model predicts that, at first, participants seek to legitimate a line of scientific inquiry in accordance with accepted norms, values and beliefs by reference to certain facts within a particular context. In the context of the stem cell debates, this means that ESC research is legitimated by reference to facts about the biology of human embryos and potency of stem cells. These claims are contested in the legitimation process by opponents to this research by reference to other facts about the genetic composition of embryos and the biological equivalence of stem cells. The aim of all participants at this stage is to show that the claims of those on the 'other side' of a dispute reflect their beliefs or opinions, and not the 'facts'.

Without an authority to adjudicate on matters of fact, public policy disputes then move into a second stage whereby the rules that justify science are legitimated by reference to its teleological implications. This process entails an examination of the research and how it accords with

---

[31] A. Gross. 1990. *The Rhetoric of Science.* Cambridge. MA: Harvard University Press.

[32] C.P. Toumey. 1996. *Conjuring Science: Scientific Symbols and Cultural Meanings in American Life*. New Brunswick, NJ: Rutgers University Press.

[33] M. Zelditch & A. Floyd. 1998. Consensus, Dissensus, and Justification. In *Status, Power, and Legitimacy: Strategies & Theories*. J. Berger & M. Zelditch, eds. New Brunswick, NJ: Transaction Publishers.

accepted norms and values. In the stem cell disputes, the focus was on the potential for benefits and the costs of destroying embryos in research. These justifications are contested in claims that challenge the consensus of utilitarian analysis and its legitimacy in providing consent for stem cell research. Participants at this stage aim to establish credibility for their justification claims while creating uncertainty and suspicion in others.

Where consensus is not reached and the disputes remain unresolved, participants then go through a meta-process of justifying the justification rules. At this point, dissension has given rise to a process in which the norms, values and ideals that participants follow in resolving a dispute are themselves contested. In relation to stem cell research, norms that determine how embryos are assigned status and how stem cell science is invested with value are challenged; and they are impugned in claims that dispute the ontological and epistemological resources participants use to validate and justify scientific research. The purpose of science claims at this stage is to challenge the legitimacy of different types of knowledge and determine who is to be given authority in providing consent.

Those who have authority in these processes control the shape and direction of scientific research.[34] Scientists are in a hegemonic position in these contexts because science culturally obscures and patronises the intellectual and moral substance of other epistemologies and ontologies through its institutional processes.[35] These processes are directed by norms and ideals that attach less status to other ways of knowing. unmeasurable constructs such as personal experience and narrative, for example, do not 'count' as valid evidence and, at best, are considered as anecdotes. Science exercises its authority by separating itself from the value conflict and positioning its meanings, practices and methods as being transfixed with universal reality, even when they are not.[36] It lays

---

[34] M. Zelditch & H.A. Walker. 1984. Legitimacy and the Stability of Authority. In *Advances in Group Processes (Vol. 1).* E.J. Lawler, ed. Greenwich, CT: JAI Press.

[35] M. Leach, I. Scoones & B. Wynne. 2006. Science, Citizenship and Globalization. In *Science and Citizens: Globalization and the Challenge of Engagement.* M. Leach, I. Scoones & B. Wynne, eds. London: Zed Books: 3–14.

[36] H.M. Collins & S. Yearley. 1992. Epistemological Chicken. In *Science as Practice and Culture*. A. Pickering, ed. Chicago: University of Chicago Press: 201–326.

claim to truth-knowledge based on evidence that is negotiated and subject to the values and ideals of the normative structure from which it emerges.[37] Thus, it is the ideology and normative framework of science that are contested when these types of disputes arise in public discourse.

What especially distinguishes science from all other knowledge types in these contexts is that the cultural embeddedness of its claims is so ingrained that they really do seem to represent an objective reality.[38] These claims are persuasive in modern policymaking contexts because they are empowered with norms that legitimate the rhetorical power of scientific facts.[39] When deployed in public discourse, science claims are, therefore, a rhetorical means of establishing legitimacy. However, when harnessed primarily as a means of asserting authority over others and winning at all costs, science becomes abused in policy contexts.

CONCLUSION

Science claims were used rhetorically throughout the Australian policy episode by participants as a means of achieving a desired moral outcome and were deployed strategically according to preferred norms and values. Those opposed to the liberalisation of Australia's stem cell policies used science claims to state their opposition in terms of the immorality of creating and destroying human embryos for research purposes. In contrast, supporters of this policy proposal used science claims to position their arguments within the ethical framework of medicine and the moral good of pursuing outcomes associated with medical benefit. The science claims used by participants to support either position contained facts and values that implied ontological meanings that varied according to their stated policy preferences.

Science claims were used preferentially throughout this debate because the status of scientific knowledge is privileged in Australia's

---

[37] T.S. Kuhn. 1962. *The Structure of Scientific Revolutions*. Chicago: University of Chicago Press.

[38] A. Gross. 1990. *The Rhetoric of Science*. Cambridge. MA: Harvard University Press.

[39] R. Weaver. 1985. *The Ethics of Rhetoric*. Davis, CA: Hermagoras.

policymaking contexts. Science has a special place in these and other policy contexts because it is posited as the most reliable and value-neutral source of truth and knowledge. This perception invests science with moral authority that participants in stem cell policy debates draw upon to invest their position with truth and integrity. The preferential use of science claims in the Australian debate surrounding stem cell research meant that the status attached to scientific knowledge was greater than other ways of knowing and that the personal narratives and stories of those most likely to be affected by the outcomes of the policy episode were marginalised.

The widespread use of science claims in the Australian stem cell debate stems from the desire of participants to harness the epistemic authority of scientific knowledge and the legitimacy of technical expertise. Participants, therefore, formed alliances with scientists on both sides of the debate to deploy the rhetoric of science effectively and persuasively. As a consequence, each side accused the other of misconstruing scientific evidence and corrupting the truth with vested interests, political ideals and social values. Attacks were aimed at undermining the trust and credibility of experts acting for each side and thereby challenging the legitimacy of their authority. The aim was, therefore, not *merely* to persuade, but to *win*. The use of science claims was thus not simply rhetorical, but eristic.

The enormous rhetorical power of science claims in this dispute was an artefact of the legitimation process. Participants were legitimated according to a normative framework in Australia that favours secular ideals and technological advancements in science and medicine. These norms influenced how the policy question was framed around the status of science and who would be authorised to speak on its behalf. This framing was also responsible for the public contests over who had authority to determine the ontological meanings of the claims participants used to describe embryos, especially those created using SCNT, and the status that was attached to different sources of stem cells. Had the debate simply been framed as a moral one, questions over the technical viability of stem cells and embryos may well have been considered to have far less relevance than other political concerns.

The priority given to science in morally contestable areas of research raises important questions about how advances in stem cell science and its emergent technologies are likely to shape future public debates. While the moral questions pertaining to stem cell science may be resolved or at least become clearer as more becomes known about the biology, potentiality and application of stem cells, this seems unlikely. In part, this is because the moral positions upon which the stem cell dispute is fought are fundamentally incommensurable. The moral arguments made in support of ESC research and SCNT are generally consequentialist. In other words, they are based on claims that because stem cell science has potential clinical utility, there is a moral obligation to pursue it. In contrast, arguments against the permissibility of ESC/SCNT research generally reject the importance of clinical benefit and instead emphasise the moral status of the embryo and the intrinsic 'wrongness' of actions that end in the destruction of the embryo.

Developments in stem cell science are also unlikely to resolve moral contest because technical solutions generally create new problems. For example, a number of important scientific developments have recently taken place that could potentially resolve some of the ethical issues surrounding ESC research. Recent research into induced Pluripotent Stem Cells (iPS) suggests that it may be possible to create embryonic-like stem cell lines without the need for human oocytes or embryos.[40] Subsequent studies have since suggested that this process may be used to create patient specific cell lines[41] and may be done safely without the need for viral vectors.[42] However, moral and political support for iPS research must not obscure the fact that these cells are yet to be widely tested in human safety studies and it remains unclear whether the cells are as plastic, as accessible

[40] K. Takahashi *et al.* Induction of Pluripotent Stem Cells from Adult Human Fibroblasts by Defined Factors. *Cell* 2007; 131(5): 861–872; and J. Yu *et al.* Induced Pluripotent Stem Cell Lines Derived from Human Somatic Cells. *Science* 2007; 318(5858): 1917–1920.

[41] J.T. Dimos *et al.* Induced Pluripotent Stem Cells Generated from Patients with ALS can be Differentiated into Motor Neurons. *Science* 2008; 321(5893): 1218–1221.

[42] K. Kaji *et al.* Virus-Free Induction of Pluripotency and Subsequent Excision of Reprogramming Factors. *Nature* 2009; 458; 771–775. Available from: http://www.nature.com/nature/journal/vaop/ncurrent/abs/nature07864.html [Accessed 05 Sep 2009]; and K. Woltjen *et al.* PiggyBac Transposition Reprograms Fibroblasts to Induced Pluripotent Stem Cells. *Nature* 2009; 458: 766–770. Available from: http://www.nature.com/nature/journal/vaop/ncurrent/abs/nature07863.html [Accessed 05 Sep 2009].

or as viable as ESCs. Thus, from a technical and scientific standpoint, research into iPS cells does not circumvent the necessity for continuing research with ESCs, at least not at this current time.

Perhaps more importantly, while iPS research shows enormous promise and may reduce the need for destructive embryo research and a supply of human oocytes, like all technological solutions to moral problems, it may not resolve fundamental ethical concerns, such as those surrounding the creation of human life, and may indeed create new problems. For example, adult cells may be induced into human gametes thus enabling the production of sperm and eggs from a single individual and so cloning (or asexual reproduction) without the need for SCNT. Other strategies that have been posited as a means of circumventing the moral issues associated with ESC research, such as deriving ESCs from human embryos in non-harmful ways or altering the genetic viability of embryos, are not only plagued by technical limitations and safety concerns but also fail to counter concerns regarding the creation of human life for research purposes.[43] Thus, while the public discourse surrounding stem cell research is likely to change as scientific developments emerge, the manner in which science is deployed in response to moral, social and political concerns will not.

In the years ahead, ESC research may lead to the development of regenerative medicine, provide new insights into the pathophysiology of many diseases and be widely applied in drug testing. At the same time, research will continue into the clinical application of adult somatic stem cells and the biology and potential utility of other non-embryonic sources of stem cells — notably iPS cells. While the relative merit of each of these areas of research is not yet known, it may be that ASCs will retain their value in clinical medicine, particularly in transplantation, and the real benefits of ESC research will be the therapeutic components and molecules produced by ESCs and the insights it is certain to provide into understanding human development.

Yet while many hope that the moral, political and economic investment in ESC research will provide clinical and epistemic benefits, it is likely that these outcomes will be interpreted and construed in public

[43] President's Council on Bioethics. 2005. *Alternative Sources of Pluripotent Stem Cells.* Washington, D.C.: President's Council on Bioethics.

discourse according to whichever moral position participants are committed to. For proponents of stem cell research, the generation of tangible clinical benefits would morally vindicate their position and provide justification to continue research into other applications. However, those who are committed to a deontological position which imparts a moral status to the embryo, are likely to view the outcome as being a derivative of research that could have been achieved without the destruction of embryos. Irrespective of the resulting benefits from ESC research, it is unlikely to alter their commitment to moral principles that consider the creation of human life for utilitarian purposes as morally unconscionable.

This issue may become the major point of moral contest in stem cell research as new scientific developments emerge and the need for human embryos is reduced. That is, the public debate is likely to shift away from destructive research and onto issues surrounding the capacity to create human life. This, in turn, reminds us that science is not value-neutral and does not occur in a political vacuum. It also reminds us that moral discourse itself is responsive to advances in biology and in science. Moral debate surrounding early human life, reproduction and abortion has been inscribed by our understandings of fertilisation and embryogenesis. Stem cell research is yet another example of how moral debate shifts in response to scientific developments, and also how the direction of science is reflexively shaped by the social, political and moral context in which it occurs.

7

NEW DEVELOPMENTS IN STEM CELL SCIENCE: iPS CELLS AND THE CHALLENGE TO CONSENT

Jonathan Mackenney and Benjamin Capps

INTRODUCTION

In late 2007, two separate research teams announced that they had successfully created stem-cell like entities from human skin cells.[1] The technique reprogrammed somatic cells to behave like human embryonic stem cells (hESC), ostensibly imbuing them with the same characteristics: the ability to differentiate into specialised cell types, and the capability of indefinite mitotic self-renewal. If this cellular reprogramming could reliably induce 'pluripotency' (a state from which a cell may be encouraged to differentiate into any of the body's tissue types), it would be a valuable addition to the canon of regenerative medicine.[2]

The creation of induced Pluripotent Stem Cells (iPS) from somatic tissue was hailed by some as a viable, ethically preferable alternative to their contentious human embryonic counterparts. Some determinedly proclaimed that society could finally dispatch controversies, such as the moral status of the embryo, therapeutic cloning, and chimera research, to

[1] K. Takahashi *et al.* Induction of Pluripotent Stem Cells from Adult Human Fibroblasts by Defined Factors. *Cell* 2007; 131: 861–872; J. Yu *et al.* Induced Pluripotent Stem Cell Lines Derived from Human Somatic Cells. *Science* 2007; 318: 1917–1920.

[2] S. Yamanaka. Strategies and New Developments in the Generation of Patient-Specific Pluripotent Stem Cells. *Cell Stem Cell* 2007; 1: 39–49.

the annals of history.[3] The proof-of-theory research was more cautiously welcomed by others; they argued that it was far too soon to talk of an end to embryo research in stem cell science — embryo research would still have its scientific and translational uses. In this chapter, we do not enter the debate as to whether iPS cell science can supplant embryo research — at the time of writing, it remains to be seen if iPS cell research will deliver on its tremendous promise. Our focus is on the contentious claim that such cells are 'ethically clean', requiring a simple biopsy for which consent can easily be given. We suggest that, in the bidirectional debate in respect to 'embryo-free' research, there has been a failure to scrutinise a new set of ethical questions relating to the significant challenges to informed consent that iPS science could pose.

Stem cell science's most hyped promise is to create personalised, self-compatible tissue for autologous transplant. A patient with hypertensive renal failure could, for example, provide her own skin cells, which, through iPS techniques, could then become healthy, genetically compatible kidney tissue. However, before that goal is realised, there will be a period during which scientists require human tissue for study, and which will involve establishing immortal cell lines. These cell lines can be derived from both informed and unwitting 'donors'; the latter, who, as patients, could be opportunistically sourced for research material. In a world where iPS techniques dominate stem-cell science, it is possible that the 'business' of regenerative medicine will challenge considerations of 'informed consent', and patients are the likely targets of this sea change. Here, consent functions as a defence against a breach of right or duty by withholding permission, and may create new rights and duties through authorisation. 'Informed' — despite the problematic raising of the procedural bar of legitimate authorisation — indicates the knowledgeable and contextual signalling of permission necessary for there to be a consented action.

[3] Additionally, unlike the derivation of embryonic stem cells, iPS cells do not require a high level of technical skill and an array of specialised equipment; see: D. Cyranoski. Five Things to Know Before Jumping on the iPS Bandwagon. *Nature* 2008; 452: 406–408.

Despite all clinical procedures requiring the informed consent of the patient involved, there is a contested area of research in which tissues are routinely collected, either through an additional biopsy, or from discarded tissue. This disregard for consent is possible because the action of taking a biopsy or appropriation of surgical tissue — actions that normally would constitute one of battery or negligence, if not consented to[4] — appear proximate to the procedural exchange which established authorisation for the medical procedure. Thus, while researchers cannot fail to get consent for biopsies taken as part of an overt research project, they may conflate research with a medical procedure; and in doing so, conceal their intentions. This deception is not without precedent, and the customary justification has been the importance of unimpeded research (thus, in effect to argue that the requirement for the patient's authorisation, or any rights to object they may have, are restricted for the 'good of science').

Our contention is the exclusivity of intimate access to the body by virtue of an ongoing physician-patient relationship ought not to endorse, nor be intentionally conflated with, research goals. The vindication of this research practice relies on an assumed acquiescence to take part in research, under a utilitarian justification for the appropriation of human biological material. *But*, if a patient is not told about the research aims, or is led to wrongly believe that excised tissue is for medically indicated procedures only, then she cannot very well be said to have consented to its use in research (regardless of the research's propinquity to the medical procedure). Furthermore, we consider that the patient continues to have an interest in excised cells by virtue of a set of privacy rights, and that this interest continues despite the transfer (consented to or not) of property. This interest perpetuates into the immortal cell lines, and therefore utilitarian considerations do not absolve the researcher from needing explicit consent. Without approbation (in any form), additional biopsies or collection of abandoned tissue require an unacceptable level of deceit or misinformation.

---

[4] S. Pattinson. 2007. *Medical Law and Ethics*. London: Sweet & Maxwell: Chap. 4.

THE PERPETUATION OF A GREAT MISTAKE: IMMORTALS IN RESEARCH

An iPS line can, in theory, be propagated indefinitely. The long-lasting implications of deriving immortal cell lines from a human source are illustrated in the following two cases.

The commercial exploitation of HeLa cells had little to do with the medical interests of Dr. Howard Jones's patient, Henrietta Lacks.[5] Lacks voluntarily underwent a number of biopsies assuming they were medically indicated, but she was unaware that the ultimate purpose was to develop an important cell line derived from the aggressive cervical cancer which afflicted her. Though she would never know because of her untimely death, the HeLa cell line would become an invaluable research tool, and the cells would find their way (sometimes inadvertently, such was the invasiveness and durability of the cancer cells) into laboratories worldwide.[6] It is believed that Lacks died altogether unaware of the research which led to the isolation of the HeLa cell line — her identity was rather clumsily obscured as 'Helen Lane' or 'Larson'; and it seems that her family only discovered her unwitting legacy many years later. The Lacks case raises consent as a central issue in respect to the appropriation of cells from patients: in a *New York Times* article, her youngest daughter is quoted as saying, 'I went into shock... Why didn't they just ask if they could use her cells?'[7] Lacks was probably not harmed by the additional biopsies which were carried out to obtain the cells; and there was no record that she objected to them being taken — but, it requires little conjecture to imply that this was likely because she was not informed of the doctor's intentions.

In the wake of HeLa Cells came the important legal case of John Moore, also involving the fixation and propagation of a cell line from a

---

[5] G. Gey, W. Coffman and M. Kubicek. Tissue Culture Studies of the Proliferative Capacity of Cervical Carcinoma and Normal Epithelium. *Cancer Research* 1952; 12: 264–265.

[6] M. Gold. 1986. *Conspiracy of Cells: One Woman's Immortal Legacy and the Medical Scandal It Caused*. Albany, NY: State University of New York Press.

[7] R. Skloot. 2001. Cells That Save Lives Are a Mother's Legacy. *New York Times* 17 November.

living human source. Moore was diagnosed with hairy cell leukaemia. His physician, Dr. David W. Golde recommended that his spleen be removed. But, on several occasions following this procedure, and under the supervision and direction of Golde, blood, blood serum, skin, bone marrow aspirate, and sperm were taken from Moore without any connection to his medical care. Unbeknown to the patient, Golde recognised a scientific, and moreover, financial importance in securing a potentially immortal cell line. Golde successfully established a cell line in 1979, and secured a profitable patent (with the Regents of the University of California) on the 'Mo' cell line in 1981. On becoming aware of the patent, Moore brought a case against Golde, in part on the grounds that he continued to own his cells following their removal from his body, at least for the purpose of directing their use, and that he never consented to their use in potentially lucrative medical research.[8] Moreover, Moore was under the impression that all of the doctors' actions were medically indicated, and therefore he did not consider that he consented to any additional procedures which contributed directly to the eventual commercial exploitation of his cells by Golde. It was only after he was asked to waive any rights that he or his heirs may have with respect to the cell line developed from his bone marrow that he became suspicious.

The *Moore* case showed that the custom of taking cells without permission was beginning to be questioned in contemporary society. The Supreme Court of California ruled that the intentions of the physician, Golde, had been in breach of his fiduciary duty (on this point the parties reached settlement) — the failure to disclose, and then to conceal the research interests was an intentional contravention of the trust relationship with his patient, and a breach of the physician's disclosure obligations. But, although Moore (the patient) had rights based in the physician's fiduciary duty, market forces, responsible for the 'contorted reasoning of *Moore*' (the case),[9] resulted in the exclusion of the patient's property rights, and with them, any further privacy interests in who accessed and

---

[8] *Moore v. Regents of the University of California*, 51 Cal.3d 120, 271 Cal. Rptr. 146, 793 P.2d 479, cert. denied 499 U.S. 936 (1991).

[9] S. Jasanoff. 2005. *Designs on Nature: Science and Democracy in Europe and the United States*. Princeton: Princeton University Press: 215.

used excised cells: Moore only had a right to know that the doctors might make a profit out of his splenic cells.[10] *But,* this issue of consent was buried in the discussion of property in cells that followed. The Court did not consider the conditions of consent in the final judgement; and concluded that it was not necessary to recognise Moore's property rights (or that he ought to authorise any future use) because there was nothing unique about his cells (everyone has cells which produce lymphokines), but rather curiously, that the cell *line* was unique and novel enough to be awarded a patent.[11]

Moore established a US legal precedent (which was to become influential in other jurisdictions), that a person cannot claim a property interest in cells that are *unobjectionably* excised from the body. To do so would introduce uncertainties that could be detrimental to the research industry.[12] But while this claim appears to be more justified when consent is signalled, it seems inexcusable to suggest that the lack of an objection, because the intentions for taking additional biopsies are cloaked, is equally, and ethically acceptable. Thus, the requirement to find additional reasons for allowing appropriation was to affirm that cells, whether taken in addition to a surgical procedure, or leftover from surgery, were a raw material which ought to be shared for some ideological 'good of humanity'. Furthermore, *Moore*, in part, set up the subsequent scientific culture in which there was to be no obligation for 'giving back' to the donor in the form of sharing benefits or compensation. Human endeavour had effectively changed Moore's cells beyond recognition, and made them the property, via a patent, of the researchers who transformed them. The latter were completely free to exploit any financial benefits (regardless if consent was given for the material), and were under no obligation to include Moore in a share of these.

The story of Henrietta Lacks, and the case of John Moore, suggest several topics for ethical discussion. We focus on one that has direct

---

[10] *Moore v. Regents of the University of California* (1990) 271 Cal Rptr 146, at 168.

[11] *Moore v. Regents of the University of California* (1990) 51 Cal.3d 120.

[12] Ibid: 161–163.

relevance to iPS research: that the exclusivity of intimate access to the body by virtue of an ongoing physician-patient relationship ought not to endorse, nor be intentionally conflated with, research goals. What, in effect, the judgement in *Moore* held, was that there were utilitarian reasons to allow the use of non-consented human biological material. Furthermore, the asymmetry in property interests ought to be maintained because patents encouraged research, while personal property interests would hinder the circulation of biological materials. But without approbation (in any form), additional biopsies or collection of abandoned tissue require a certain level of deceit or misinformation. Moreover, patients' rights are ignored without proper consideration of the proportion of risks the patient unwittingly takes on: the creation of an immortal cell line in which their interests may be perpetuated indefinitely. The judgment in *Moore*, therefore, left the stone of consent unturned. Our concern is the low importance that consent is accorded in markets of biological materials, and 'the fundamental right to decide whether and how one's body and its parts will be used in research'.[13]

Property in Cells: Implications for iPS Science

The stem cell revolution 'potentially represents a quantum leap in medical treatment as significant as the introduction of antibiotics'.[14] However, 'the explosion of private tissue and biobanks in the United States, Europe, and beyond has created vast storehouses of biological matter (and bio-information) with great potential for generating commercial value'.[15] Stem cell lines, it would appear, are fated to join a so-called 'hot property' list of

[13] R. Sade. Research on Stored Biological Samples is Still Research. *Archives of Internal Medicine* 2002; 162: 1439–1440.

[14] J. Savulescu. The Embryonic Stem Cell Lottery and the Cannibalization of Human Beings. *Bioethics* 2002; 16: 508–529.

[15] C. Hayden. Taking as Giving: Bioscience, Exchange, and the Politics of Benefit Sharing. *Social Studies of Science* 2007; 37: 730.

body parts[16]; and with this come more reasons to collect, store and use human tissues. Realising the promise may increase pressure for raw material, and thereby lead to an escalation in the biopsy of cells or encouragement for the routine 'scavenging' of waste tissue. We could hypothesise that a demand for rapid progress risks shrinking the social, ethical and legal impediments to procuring cells and tissues.[17] The risk is the expansion of the practice to appropriate cells unbeknownst to the source. Moreover, a sudden awareness of the practice of non-consensual cell appropriation risks a widespread backlash, and this may, for example, potentially affect many kinds of worthwhile cell and tissue collections.

Is there a valid reason to procure cells for undeclared purposes? The case of Lacks introduced the issue of appropriating cells without consent through maintaining a culture of silence. The *Moore* judgment starkly illustrated the issues at stake: asymmetrical property interests and the 'good of science'. We were offered an explanation exonerating such actions: that utilitarian ethics could deny a patient autonomy as an unwitting research subject. How does this effect iPS cell science?

Cells may be taken either during a medical procedure as an additional biopsy, or appropriated from material left over, either as abandoned or waste tissue. Any cell can potentially be induced to a pluripotent state, and therefore, propagated indefinitely. (We will exclude all other ways of procuring cells, because they demand direct misinformation or the use of

---

[16] The term is from: D. Nelkin and L. Andrews. Homo Economicus: Commercialization of Body Tissue in the Age of Biotechnology. *Hastings Center Report* 1998; 28: 30–39. We do not indicate this kind of property to mean that individual cell lines will become especially marketable, because the 'value' in a stem cell line is not personalised to anyone in particular. Skin cells, for example, are so ubiquitous that there will not be any demand that can outstrip the fantastic supply (unlike cord blood, for instance.)

[17] The Food and Drug Administration's *Guidance on Informed Consent for In Vitro Diagnostic Device Studies Using Leftover Human Specimens That Are Not Individually Identifiable,* states: it will 'exercise enforcement discretion [that is, refrain from enforcing the regulations] as to the informed consent regulations for clinical investigators, sponsors, and IRBs'. Available at: http://www.fda.gov/downloads/RegulatoryInformation/Guidances/ucm127033.pdf [Accessed 22 September 2009]. This policy change was described as 'a dramatic shift' by Clayton E. in: So What Are We Going to Do About Research Using Clinical Information and Samples? *IRB* 2004; 26: 14–15.

potentially harmful force on the body, and therefore are unquestionably beyond the conditions of consent.) We assume that the excised cells will normally have no use or value to the original source; but grant, however, that cultural traditions may place special value in certain tissues. Through endeavour, these cells may become a potentially commercially viable line; although the ultimate goal of iPS science would be to create regenerative tissue from a consenting donor for autologous transplant.[18]

Precedent shows that the research endeavour has an expedient, utilitarian justification, qua *Moore*, for appropriating cells without the direct authorisation of the source, and therefore that biotechnological innovation could trump other kinds of claims. One explanation (but often not directly given by researchers) to explain the practice of appropriating cells and tissues surreptitiously, is that they want to avoid stirring any interest from the source. As with the creation of the HeLa cell line, anonymisation can dupe the patient into thinking nothing is untoward. The reasoning, which is strongly suggestive of utilitarianism, argues that either the raw material will somehow dry up, or the originators of the cells may push for a stake in the profits, or at least make noises about fair compensation. Either way, recognising the interests of the patients would unacceptably restrict the ways in which scientists can exploit cellular tissue for commercial interests, and thus be a disincentive to the research endeavour. The way to avoid this is to ensure that the patient is unaware of the commercial interest in a cell line from their body; asking them would only hinder the business of research.

The construction of the argument begins from two premises: firstly, that an excised cell (or tissue biopsy)[19] is no longer attached to either the

[18] There can be little complaint with this action. As an established medical practice, the patient will stand to directly benefit from iPS therapy. The 'market' would effectively be fixed in the provisions stating the expectations of the procedure and associated medical charges. But, even at this stage, researchers may wish to retain and propagate the cell line after transplantable tissue has been created. Whether the original donor retains an interest in this cell line would depend, in part, on the conditions of their initial consent. Subsequent commercialisation would therefore be in breach of the conditions of authorisation, rather than an employment of deception as per Moore or Lacks.

[19] 'Tissues' remains a generic, but problematic term; we will interchangeably use tissues and cells to refer to the relevant material used to create iPS cells.

patient's direct or wider interests by way of her body. The cells are therefore 'abandoned' even if accrued through non-consented appropriation, because, it is alleged, this does not obviously harm the patient in any way (or any minor harm is at least outweighed by the benefits to research).[20] And secondly, that the patient cannot make use of the cells themselves, because they lack the scientific ingenuity and the necessary technology to do so: the cells, therefore, appear as 'waste' until scientists invest time to create a patentable product which is both novel and innovative.

A direct insult to the body, that is using force or even non-consensual touching to remove cells, would not be so easily shrugged off in the manner found in *Moore*. Thus, it has been customary to argue that cell appropriation by researchers does not fall into this category of assault, and thereby avoids the legal challenge of battery. The ploy has been, therefore to consider direct appropriation of cells as a separate class of action; but, and as exemplified in *Moore* and Lacks, what has actually happened is the intentional shrouding of cell appropriation under the clinical indication of a medical procedure. Escaping the crime of assault (*qua* bodily harm) is possible, so it would seem, by abandoning valid consent from the patient; but this ostensibly continues to be battery or even negligence, because the researcher's or doctor's actions leave the patient in ignorance of the real intentions. The doctor's actions are not vindicated because there is no ill-will or malevolence meant to the patient.[21]

The implications, if cell appropriation were brought under a criminal tort, could be that markets in cell transfer, routine in innovative research, would be subsumed into the restrictions on organ trading; thus opening it up to the resistance to human commodification — that is the transfer of economic value to something not previously considered in economic terms.[22] Organs, it is argued, cannot have a market value because they

[20] P. Van Diest. For and Against: No Consent Should be Needed for Using Leftover Body Materials for Scientific Purposes. *British Medical Journal* 2002; 325: 648–649.

[21] Pattinson, *op. cit.* note 4, s. 4.2.1.

[22] See generally: A. V. Campbell. 2009. *The Body in Bioethics*. Abingdon, UK: Routledge-Cavendish.

ought not to be considered as interchangeable with other goods; nor, for that matter, should body parts be considered under a socio-legal system which encourages the improper instrumental treatment of persons whom ought to have an intrinsic worth. Opposition to instrumentalisation is normally meant as a criticism of practices which do not take into account the intrinsic interests (or worth) of persons. But does the commodification of human cells invite similar responses?

The outcry that followed the British Alder Hey Hospital controversy showed that, without explicit (parental) consent, bodies should not be transferred to the possession of those with prescience to exploit research benefits. The human *body* and its constituents, it appeared, were neither abandoned, nor waste. Alder Hey set in motion an overhaul of the law on consent in the removal of organs and the passing of the UK's *Human Tissue Act* 2004;[23] and accordingly the Department of Health published a comprehensive guide for healthcare workers entitled: *A Reference Guide to Consent for Examination or Treatment*. But, therein, was an acknowledgement that 'the legal status of tissue (including clinical samples such as blood samples) which has been removed from a patient during the course of a procedure is at present unclear'.[24] The retained organs scandal reiterated the importance of control or 'ownership' in the body (how death might transfer ownership to others we shall not consider here). But, at that time there was little enthusiasm for other human biological material to be included as part of the response to the shame felt. For example, one of the responses to the *Retained Organs Commission's* Consultation Document stated:

> 'If procedures designed to satisfy the emotional requirements of handling post-mortem tissue were to be applied to all human tissue the

---

[23] It should be noted that cell lines themselves are excluded from the UK Act's regulatory purview, implying that they are not to be considered as human material. Department of Health. 2002. *Human Bodies, Human Choices: The Law on Human Organs and Tissue in England and Wales — A Consultation Report*. London: Department of Health.

[24] Department of Health. 2001. *A Reference Guide to Consent for Examination or Treatment*. London: Department of Health: 7.

result would be disastrous for teaching and research. This would work against the common good and hence damage the very individuals the regulations are attempting to protect'.[25]

If this position is at all representative of the research fraternity, there is an impression that some tissues ought to be considered as human materials excluded from trade embargos. It is not clear what materials this may include (since organs and bodies are also important for research and education); but we may be confident that the argument being made is that excised cells at least ought to be exempt from current prohibitions. By categorising cells and tissues outside organ market exclusions, it means that consent processes can be trumped for the benefits of scientific discovery.

The arguments used to reframe the cell market ground themselves in property interests: a feature that separates them from other human body parts still fixed to, or within, the body. One tactic is to deploy a kind of Lockean notion of property that is generated by investment of labour.[26] It is argued that the labour involved in preparing cell lines creates a property right and corresponding right to fiscal transfer.[27] Thus, any cell *line* cultivated from a donor's tissue, via effort and industry, becomes the researcher's property, and thereby imparts control in what subsequently

---

[25] Academy of Medical Sciences. 2002. *Retained Organs Commission Consultation: Unclaimed and Unidentifiable Organs and Tissue*. Available at: http://www.acmedsci.ac.uk/p100puid39.html [Accessed 22 September 2008].

[26] Locke argued that in the 'state of nature' all the world's bounty is held in common, and is in that sense public. But. 'every Man has a Property in his own Person', and everyone one can also acquire property by mixing one's labour with it. In such cases, common goods become one's private property; J. Locke. 1988. *Two Treatises of Government*. P. Laslett, ed. Cambridge: Cambridge University Press: Student Edition: The Second Treatise, s. 27. On this account, the labour argument for a proprietary right asserts that persons own themselves through the endeavours of living and giving authorship to one's life, i.e. that their body and thoughts belong to no other (this is therefore offered as the antithesis of slavery). Thus, individuals own, or have property in, the constituent parts of themselves as the products of labour.

[27] D. Price. 2007. Organs and Tissues for Transplantation and Research. 2007. In *Principles of Health Care Ethics*. R. Ashcroft *et al.*, eds. Chichester, England: John Wiley & Sons Ltd: 2nd edition: 475–481.

happens to the lines, including indefinite storage and use of it without authorisation from the source. A second property-type argument may also be employed: that is to make sure that surgically excised cells are, to all intents and purposes, *abandoned.* Thus, in doing so, researchers are able to negate any rights in that tissue that the source may think they have, and thereby ensuring that no inhibiting claim can be made to dissuade further use by the present holder.

Both of these arguments entirely bypass the need for consent, and extinguish any property interest the source may have. But, by claiming the authority to appropriate the cells through property, the physicians and researchers by association are, as we see it, abusing their intimate access to the patient. This ought to immediately signal a form of unauthorised trespass on the human agent, since the procurement of cells without consent uses the patient-doctor relationship to gain access to the body; and ought not to obscure, contra the property interests of the researcher, any of the physician's duties to that patient. There can be no conflation of the patient's interests with the utilitarian interests underlying economic pursuits.

However, we might consider a third argument: that human cells might be 'contested commodities'; not being entirely barred from the free market, cells ought to nevertheless be carefully managed.[28] According to Radin, property enables us to have control over the external world — and thereby claims on property may signal complex and intertwined ideas of personhood.[29] Ownership of all kinds of things (personal, tangible and intangible objects) is bound up with respect for persons; in this way, property (of different kinds) is part of the way in which we constitute ourselves as personal entities interacting in the world. Thus, property may also be part of a 'right to bodily integrity' (if anything is intimately linked to ownership and control, it would arguably include our own bodies), and thereby signals the patients' interests in ownership and control over excised tissue. Thus, unauthorised appropriation does jeopardise the interests of the source, because it removes

[28] M. Radin. Market-Inalienability. *Harvard Law Review* 1987; 100: 1849–1937.

[29] Margret Radin's main work on this particular idea is found in: 1993. *Reinterpreting Property*. Chicago. University of Chicago Press.

control: 'Moore was author of his destiny but not of his spleen'[30]; but on our reading, *qua* Radin at least, both autonomy *and* authority to direct what happens to body parts are uncompromisingly linked. Using Radin's property argument implies that the taking of any cellular tissue from a competent agent would be precluded. Importantly, this control could continue into the future access and uses of these 'commodities', because their disputed status (and questionable appropriation) continues to link them to our 'persons'. On the other hand, once cells are excised from the body *with permission* a similar attack on the 'person' seems less problematic; the patient is aware of what they have gotten into and may voluntarily extinguish any further interest they have in the cells. The surgical biopsy is relatively simple and risk free in itself (and any risky procedure is likely to be subsumed under the benefits of the medical operation); and if done properly and with care, there is little or no expected long-term harm to the body. Moreover, the cells will be replaced by normal regenerative processes. So, once the cells are excised with consent, we might engage a right to use, right of exclusion, and right of transfer (but the implications of these conditions, for some, might exclude organs) to benefit the endeavours of research.[31]

The first two property arguments encourage a practice of 'silent gifts' to which no strings can be attached; there is no need to even involve the patient, because there is little apparent harm to the source in using waste or abandoned material (or at most, an additional, but minor surgical procedure that the patient has to go through), and indeed, a great deal to benefit as scientific progress. Although much has been written in praise of Lacks' unwitting generosity in the battle against cancer, and the importance of denying Moore any proprietary right in the advance of scientific knowledge, neither gave their permission for the additional biopsies, endorsed any future uses (or who used them), or were even aware that the

---

[30] J. Boyle. 1996. *Shamans, Software and Spleens: Law and the Constitution of the Information Society*. Cambridge: Harvard University Press: 107.

[31] We do not have space to go into all of the kinds of use, exclusion and transfer possible; much has already been written elsewhere about the codification of incentives and inducements, reimbursement and payment.

excised cells would to be exploited downstream for profit.[32] But leaving the situation as it stands raises the ethical stakes in respect to iPS cell science. Following Radin, we see that there can be little justification to preclude consent; but moreover, her account shows that society does not need to prohibit the kind of monetary markets that incentivises research — patients may, through approbation, donate to the research endeavour, and by giving up further (but not necessarily all) interests, contribute without necessarily hindering further progress. There is no evidence that *asking* for cell contributions would result in an unwillingness to donate; moreover, there is little factual evidence to support the assertion that informing the patient that they would like to take further samples to use in research, would, contradictorily to the judgement in *Moore*, impede scientific research in any significant way.[33] This welcome outcome is dependent on the micro-event of donation, and therefore, for the remainder of this chapter we focus on this issue within the process of consent.

REAPPRAISING CONSENT: WHERE'S THE HARM IN iPS CELL SCIENCE?

Research using cell and tissue biopsies, routinely retained as a result of medical indications or amassed from that which is 'discarded', are not

---

[32] S. Holland. Contested Commodities at Both Ends of Life: Buying and Selling Gametes, Embryos, and Body Tissues. *Kennedy Institute of Ethics Journal* 2001; 11: 263–284.

[33] The UK Biobank website states: '366,989 people are already helping. 11pm Monday 21 September 2009'; see: http://www.ukbiobank.ac.uk/ [Accessed 22 Sep 2009]. Participants are made aware that ethically vetted researchers will have access to their data and samples, and that the researchers may derive financial benefits. In a 2008 study, almost all patients wanted to be asked about retaining tissue, with only 5% declining to consent to use of their stored tissue for research purposes; E. Vermeulen *et al.* Opt-Out Plus, The Patients' Choice: Preferences of Cancer Patients Concerning Information and Consent Regimen for Future Research with Biological Samples Archived in the Context of Treatment. *Journal of Clinical Pathology* 2009; 62: 275–278. In an earlier study, 96.3% of patients indicated that they would not object to their tissue being used in research; R. Bryant *et al.* Ownership and Uses of Human Tissue: What Are the Opinions of Surgical In-Patients? *Journal of Clinical Pathology* 2008; 61: 322–326.

primarily *material* risks to the original tissue provider's health; but rather represent a different set of adverse downstream consequences of procurement or acquisition. It is perhaps only after such events as Alder Hey that people are inclined to ask, and become anxious about, what happens to excised tissues and organs, biopsied cells, and other surgical 'waste'.[34] New technologies, particularly in the field of human genetics and cloning, have raised public awareness of stem cell science; but test tubes containing cell lines of scientific curiosity have little public significance beyond the personal interests of willing research participants in individual protocols and biobank initiatives.[35] The culture is therefore to maintain this ignorance, and to shield research from unwanted attention. The easiest way to do this is to make sure that patients are not asked to donate in research, and to subsume their interests into the greater good of science. We argue, conversely, that the patient has *continuing* privacy interests in

---

[34] In the Wellcome Trust Report (2000): *Qualitative Research to Explore Public Perceptions of Human Biological Samples*, it was reported: 'Use of samples in research was not a well-known practice; in principle it was considered acceptable if accompanied by informed consent. Awareness that surgical waste is used in research was very low, but once explained this was generally regarded as acceptable. Individuals suffering from diseases and those individuals' relatives tended to be better informed and more accepting of the use of samples in research'; p. 7.

[35] This may shift to wider interest: the potential successes in regenerative medicine suggests that it is conceivable that we may soon be dealing with repositories of 'visible' organs grown from cells and stored in 'banks'. Although autologous transplants are the goal of such research, it is plausible that allogenic transplants will also be used, since emergency organ failure may require an immediate replacement, and the economic marketability of ready-made 'factory standard' resources may benefit lower income individuals. It is noted that providing a patient with their own cells is inherently expensive due to logistical and manufacturing issues; see: R. Tubo. 2007. Fundamentals of Cell-Based Therapies. In *Principles of Regenerative Medicine*. A. Atala *et al.*, eds. London: Academic Press: 16–27. Tailoring iPS cells for autologous transplants will likely be limited by slow inducement, expansion, differentiation, and safety processes — it is expected that a functional cell line suitable for transplantation would take some time to create in each case. This may not only limit treatment to conditions which do not require prompt management, but also creates a potentially huge cost; see Cyranoski, *op. cit.* note 3.

any excised cells, and therefore, the risk that iPS cells may be created and stored indefinitely should refocus researchers on the act of taking of cells, rather than any 'higher' scientific interest.

One argument for appropriating cells without consent is found in the intention to anonymise the cells and subsequent cell lines.[36] There are at least two problems with this approach. Firstly, that the anonymisation of the cells does not necessarily eliminate obligations that the physician (or by association, any other linked person) has to the patient. Thus, if a cell sample is taken from the patient, or 'picked up from the theatre floor', then consent is required for the process of anonymisation itself.[37] Given that permission is necessary for anonymisation, the difficulty still transpires in articulating the transfer of authority that must occur between the source, who, through lack of volition or objection, gives up the cells, and the researcher who comes to be in possession of them. Secondly, anonymisation may be used as a way to avoid the regulatory burden of ethical review.[38] The current opinion, as per *Moore*, is

---

[36] The explanation given in the Common Rule (USA) notes that exception from the rules formulated as a result of the *Belmont Report* (1979) is justified if information will be recorded by the investigator in such a way that it cannot be linked to the subject.

[37] We can take guidance here from the United Kingdom, where the *Office of the Information Commissioner*, the regulatory authority established under the Data Protection Act 1998, has issued a guidance note on the concept of 'personal data', which states that, although anonymous data may fall outside the remit of English law, the act of anonymisation does not. Two exceptions are made in the 1998 Act to allow anonymisation without consent: (1) if an equivalent duty of confidentiality can be established, such as where the person is a health professional. But, in iPS cell research, the cells will often be passed to specified researchers in non-hospital labs. (2) It is not immediately obvious that the appropriation of cells in this way mitigates any and all 'substantial damage or substantial distress that is, or is likely to be, caused to any data subject'. We come to this second point further below. 2002. *Data Protection Act 1998 Legal Guidance*. London: Office of the Information Commissioner.

[38] See: National Bioethics Advisory Commission. 1999. *Research Involving Human Biological Material: Ethical Issues and Policy Guidance*. Rockville, MD: US Government Printing Office. The Commission argues that consent may not be necessary for IRB approval if research on coded samples is of minimal risk.

to recognise the public interest in research so as to absolve any researcher from an obligation to gain permission to use them. It has been noted that, in August 2004 the federal *Office of Human Research Protections (OHRP)*:

> '...sought to clarify its position regarding consent requirements when human biological specimens are used in research by "reaffirm[ing] OHRP policy...that, under certain limited conditions, research involving *only* coded private information or specimens is not human subjects research"'.[39]

The OHRP guidelines, as quoted by Kapp, are explicit that consent obligations can be extinguished if the samples are anonymised.[40] And it is apparent that the legal discussion of this has tended to return to the utility of allowing researchers an unhindered right to use cells in the interests of scientific discovery. What this seems to suggest is that *everyone* benefits from the unwitting 'donation' by patients.

---

[39] M. Kapp. Ethical and Legal Issues in Research Involving Human Subjects: Do You Want a Piece of Me? *Journal of Clinical Pathology* 2006; 59: 335–339. Also see: Office of Human Research Protection (OHRP), United States Department of Health and Human Services. 2008. *Guidance on Research Involving Coded Private Information or Biological Specimens* 16 Oct, which states: 'OHRP does not consider research involving only coded private information or specimens to involve human subjects...if the following conditions are both met: (1) the private information or specimens were not collected specifically for the currently proposed research project through an interaction or intervention with living individuals and (2) the investigator(s) cannot readily ascertain the identity of the individual(s) to whom the coded private information or specimens pertain. Likewise, the UK's *Human Tissue Act* 2004 exempts material: '...where the person carrying out the research is not in possession, and is not likely to come into possession, of information from which the person whose body the material has come can be identified'; paragraph 13.26.

[40] Kapp quotes the OHRP's 2004 Guidance document. The OHRP guidelines referenced in note 39, *supra*, replaced these. However, the substantive direction remains the same.

It is already evident that individuals are often unaware that biopsies are used for profit, and moreover, that patients are not notified when tissue is retained by researchers.[41] As Andrews & Nelkin argue:

> '...expanding commercial interests in the biotechnological age have reinforced a tendency on the part of biomedical researchers to focus on the possession and control of valuable tissue, while exhibiting obliviousness to its human source'.[42]

Many societies have already seen the impact of embryonic stem cell research to ways in which the materials for research are amassed — most notably in the demand for human oocytes to meet research needs.[43] We do not intend to pursue this analogy: the demand for organs and oocytes is about the outstrip of supply; a condition that somatic cell research will not confront. Furthermore, organ and egg harvesting entail more material risk to the donor than an additional cell biopsy or collecting abandoned surgical waste. And additionally, post-mortem tissue has greater emotional significance than samples removed from living patients.[44] But the absence of any donation process at all belittles the *non-material* consequences of propagating an immortal cell line.

---

[41] M. Katches, W. Heisel and R. Campbell. 2000. Donors Don't Realize They are Fuelling a Lucrative Business. Orange County Register, 16 Apr; Retained Organs Commission. 2004. *Remembering the Past, Looking to the Future. The Final Report of the Retained Organs Commission Including the Summary Accountability Report for 2003/2004.* London: Department of Health.

[42] L. Andrews and D. Nelkin. Whose Body Is It Anyway? Disputes Over Body Tissue in a Biotechnological Age. *Lancet* 1998; 351: 53–57.

[43] The demand for oocytes has led to a rapid change in the conditions in many jurisdictions for procuring eggs as marketable artefacts: women should be encouraged to donate eggs for 'the greater good', but should not be expected to be burdened with responsibility unconditionally.

[44] The Wellcome Trust and Medical Research Council. 2001. *Public Perceptions of the Collection of Human Biological Samples.* London: The Trustee of the Wellcome Trust and the Medical Research Council.

The idea that 'benefit-sharing' contributes to society despite an asymmetrical relationship has been recognised as unacceptable in areas such as bioprospecting and gene piracy. The UN recognised that communities targeted by biotech companies for their biodiversity and 'genetic resources' were due compensation and recompense in the form of funds for economic development and technology transfer.[45] The genetic exploitation of communities has led to the same concern for families with genetic peculiarities; and some high profile cases have shown the kind of questionable processes that are possible in this respect.[46] Thus, contrary to the utilitarian idea promulgated by the research fraternity to isolate cells and tissues from consent norms, the *Convention on Human Rights and Biomedicine* 1997 is clear about the status of blood and tissue.[47] Article 22 states:

> 'When in the course of an intervention any part of the human body is removed, it may be stored and used for a purpose other than that for which it was removed, only if this is done in conformity with appropriate information and consent procedures'.

Accordingly, the *Additional Protocol to the Convention on Human Rights and Biomedicine Concerning Transplantation of Organs and Tissues of*

---

[45] See: *UN Convention on Biological Diversity* 1992. Although it is argued that this Convention does not apply to human genetic resources, the subsequent *Bonn Guidelines* (2002) stated that benefit-sharing should include both monetary (fees, joint ownership of patents) and non-monetary measures (sharing of research results); Secretariat of the Convention on Biological Diversity (SCBD). 2002. *Bonn Guidelines on Access to Genetic Resources and Fair and Equitable Sharing of the Benefits Arising out of their Utilization.* Montreal, Canada: SCBD.

[46] K. Gerg. The Ethics of Benefit Sharing. *Clinical Genetics* 2001; 59: 240–243. A notable case is the patenting of a test for the Canavan Disease. After involving the parents of children with the condition in the development of a molecular probe, the scientists began marketing the genetic screening technology. The research was seeded by a donation from the Canavan Society; E. Marshall. Families Sue Hospital, Scientists for Control of Canavan Gene. *Science* 2000; 290: 1062.

[47] The *Explanatory Report to the Convention*, in paragraph 133, excludes 'hair and nails, which are discarded tissues, and the sale of which is not an affront to human dignity'. Noting that there is a difference between the human body and body parts, and these products, we do not wish to open up a debate on dignity here.

Human Origin 2002, explicitly notes the non-excludability of cells from its principled objection to human commodification (and that is intimately interwoven throughout the Convention and Additional Protocol). As explained in the *Explanatory Report to the Additional Protocol*:

> '...in many respects, transplantation of cells poses problems, particularly the consequences of testing and traceability, which are the same as those relating to the transplantation of tissues....In particular, the provisions concerning informed consent or authorisation by or on behalf of the donor, confidentiality, health and safety, and the prohibition of profit apply as for tissues'.[48]

Thus, excised cells should also be categorised as 'off-limits' to market forces because the dangers are potentially far-reaching and discouraging to participation, even in the absence of physical harm: 'In human tissue research, genomic technology has not only increased the demand for human tissue, but it has also increased the potential for tissue donors to be subjected to both psychosocial and economic harms'.[49]

For example, individuals, possibly already compromised by their health condition (the source of interesting, and potentially profitable cell lines to the researcher), are particularly vulnerable to the exploitation of concealed, non-clinical intentions. Some patients, in this respect, may consider that they have been denied an opportunity to willingly contribute to, what they see as, an important endeavour to find cures for those who will suffer the same condition in the future. Furthermore, there are wider interests at stake, such as the source's privacy (as we discuss below), or the involvement of one's cells in research that is morally objectionable (for example, employment of tissue for financial gain or disrespectful display of the tissue). Demanding a say in the fate of excised tissue also entails a sense (and loss) of control of the tangible objects

---

[48] Ibid. para. 20.

[49] T. Ashburn, S. Wilson and B. Eisenstein. Human Tissue Research in the Genomic Era of Medicine: Balancing Individual and Societal Interests. *Archives of Internal Medicine* 2000; 160: 3377–3384.

which are connected to one's interests (cf. Radin's property argument), and disregarding these potentially leads to the disempowerment, and thereby involuntariness, of an individual's decisions.[50] There is evidence that at least a significant minority of patients surveyed want to be informed in advance and afforded the opportunity to consent to, or refuse the use of their tissue for research purposes,[51] and often want their own authority to make choices to be respected.[52] But, as already stated above, wanting to be asked does not necessarily mean that they *would not* donate for research.

There continues to be little recognition of these risks in routine cell appropriation; but those taking note of the negative consequences describe the implications within the framework of the donor as a research participant, and suggesting that we may think about implementing a 'more direct, traceable (re)distribution of the fruits of research'.[53] Our focus on the potential for iPS cell research to increase disregard for the procedural aspects of consent in cell procurement, calls into question the freedom of scientific enquiry, the inherent 'good of research', and the protection of

---

[50] The implications of which are that an individual is forced or coerced to act in a certain way or to take on certain non-consensual burdens. Disempowerment, here, may be linked to an idea of 'dignity', and as such is used to rebuke the subjugation of the intrinsic worth of persons in terms of their rights; see: D. Beyleveld and R. Brownsword. 2001. *Human Dignity in Bioethics and Biolaw*. Oxford: Oxford University Press.

[51] M. Goodson and B. Vernon. A Study of Public Opinion on the Use of Tissue Samples from Living Subjects for Clinical Research. *Journal of Clinical Pathology* 2004; 57: 135–138. This paper failed to specify the kinds of uses of 'tissue or organs' that those asked would object to. It is likely that specifying the kinds of cells, tissue or organs (hair, as distinct from a heart) will elicit different responses.

[52] E. Clayton. Informed Consent and Biobanks. *Journal of Law, Medicine and Ethics* 2005; 33: 15–21. We wish to stress that although some people want to be asked to donate, there is a higher level of disinterest in what happens to the samples once they are donated: cf. 'only a small number [of patients supplying tissue specimens] report their information levels to be of particular importance when biobank based research is assessed in relation to other issues pertaining to research politics and ethics'; K. Hoeyer *et al.* The Ethics of Research Using Biobanks: Reason to Question the Importance Attributed to Informed Consent. *Archives of Internal Medicine* 2005; 165: 97–100.

[53] C. Heyden. Taking as Giving: Bioscience, Exchange, and the Politics of Benefit-Sharing. *Social Studies of Science* 2007; 37: 738.

individual inviolability. Society cannot even enter the debate about benefit-sharing if the source is ignorant that cells have been taken and used.

Procedural Consent

The current utilitarian justification for cell appropriation without authorisation jars with consent theory, which places a much greater weight on the decision making authority of the individual: 'Out with this principle goes its principal actor — the instrumentalised, autonomous individual — and in comes something/someone else: the collectivity as sovereign ethical subject'.[54] Consent is a means to control access and the use of information about oneself, and which is found in both the research[55] and clinical[56] settings. Our focus is on the micro-event of the transfer of consented biopsy, or appropriation of 'discarded' or 'waste' cells, into the possession of the researcher (and the loss of preclusionary control by the donor).

The Declaration of Helsinki *Ethical Principles for Medical Research Involving Human Subjects* notes that consent is unequivocally protected under Principle 24: 'The potential subject must be informed of the right to refuse to participate in the study or to withdraw consent to participate at any time without reprisal'. Looking to the grounding of this principle, we may turn to Beyleveld & Brownsword who consider the jurisprudential idea of consent as a procedural, rather than a substantive justification for altering relationships between agents: 'while consent can function as a defence against a breach of right or duty, it can also function to create new

---

[54] Ibid: 744.

[55] Cf. consent includes disclosure of 'possible conflicts of interest, institutional affiliations of the researcher, the anticipated benefits and potential risks of the study and the discomfort it may entail, and any other relevant aspects of the study'; World Medical Association, *Declaration of Helsinki* 2008. Section 24, p. 3. Available at: http://www.wma.net/e/policy/b3.htm [Accessed 22 September 2009].

[56] Legal augmentation of this position can be found in the UK's landmark case *Sidaway*. This case was important because it established that the adequacy of information provided to a patient should be judged in the same way as every other standard of care, using the so-called 'Bolam test' to avoid claims of negligence. *Sidaway v Board of Governors of the Bethlem Royal Hospital* [1985] AC 871.

rights and duties'.[57] In this way, consent serves to isolate legitimate claim rights, and thereby ascertain justifiable other-regarding duties; but importantly, it also can be used to nullify any breach of rights under a competent waiver, and thus allow actions to be performed that would otherwise be impermissible. This suggests that, at a minimum (nominally under the conditions of communicative action),[58] the potential research participant/donor can signal her authorisation within an agent-agent transaction, and thereby provide a valid consent, that is:

(1) free from coercion;
(2) made while in possession of adequate capacity to make such a decision; and
(3) provided with adequate information about the proposed research (this relates to the idea of informed consent; we refer to informed consent as that which is voluntarily given or refused in response to a prior, explicit disclosure, detailing the proposed action).

If any of these criteria are unfulfilled, meaningful consent cannot be signalled by the participant, nor, of course, obtained by the researcher. On this understanding, the powers of the authorising donor become paramount, and largely dependent on the information provided. One of the major sources of 'harm' from research on immortalised human tissue is the unforeseen, unpredictable and unprecedented nature of the research that will be carried out in the distant future. When facing uncertain future avenues of research, how does a researcher reach the desired standard of *informed* consent?

In our case of appropriating cells from competent agents, it may be enough to disclose that their cells will be used in *unspecified* research. *Informed* consent is unlikely to ever be possible, because precise information regarding subsequent use may not be available at the time, and cell lines will persist in repositories and laboratories over years, potentially

[57] D Beyleveld and R Brownsword. 2007. *Consent In The Law.* Oxford: Hart Publishing: 7.
[58] Cf. N. Mason and O. O'Neill. 2007. *Rethinking Informed Consent.* Cambridge: Cambridge University Press.

being used by many different researchers for countless different purposes. Furthermore, as research develops, new avenues may come to light, and which were not, and indeed, could not be consented to at the point of procurement. However, certain members, for example, of a religion, may object to their cells being used in reproductive research (creating functional gametes from iPS cells); or whilst some may be happy to donate cells for iPS research, they would object to subsequent commodification of a cell line created from their donated cells. In such cases, a narrow use of consent may be called for, but which concurrently restricts the freedom of researchers, hampers progress by demanding barriers to research, or requires re-contact with the source.

Any relaxation of the need for informed consent tends to appease the research community. But at the same time, this also conceals the physicians' or researchers' real intentions. At the extreme, a failure to disclose any research intentions wrests control from the source as to the use of cells disassociated from their bodies; a point not lost in the EU's *Tissues Directive*:[59]

> '[information]...must cover: the purpose and nature of the procurement, its consequences and risks; analytical tests, if they are performed; recording and protection of donor data, medical confidentiality; therapeutic purpose and potential benefits and information on the applicable safeguards intended to protect the donor'.[60]

Notably, however, some consent procedures, such as that of the UK Biobank, have developed far more open forms. This serves a particular function in biobank governance: maintaining its goal of meeting a stated 'public good', while not disadvantaging research to the extent that it becomes a disincentive to use the resource. UK Biobank reasons that the

---

[59] *Directive 2004/23/EC of the European Parliament and of the Council of 31 March 2004 on setting standards of quality and safety for the donation, procurement, testing, processing, preservation, storage and distribution of human tissues and cells* (Final Act OJ L 102 7.4.2004 48).

[60] Ibid. Annex. A. *Living Donors*. 3.

long term commitment must depend on a strong motivation to assist in the project, and a high level of trust in the organisation. According to Campbell, this enduring commitment is a function of '(1) genuine participation and partnership; (2) independent scrutiny; and (3) public openness and accountability'.[61] While this recognises a continued interest in the samples participants donate to the project, any rights must stop short of giving them *control* of the biobank; therefore, participants are not permitted to direct who will have access to their data and samples, and for what purpose. This condition is part of the consent taken at the outset of participation, which also includes that participants can expect no financial gain, even though researchers may stand to make substantial profits, and that the participant is free, within certain bounds, to withdraw from the imitative. To date, UK Biobank has been successful in attracting participants. So why is there animosity within certain sectors of the research industry to the principle of consent?

The depth and breadth of the UK Biobanks authorisation/waiver is important, and central to the initiative's purpose is to 'seek active engagement with participants, research users and society in general throughout the lifetime of the resource'.[62] Researchers needing samples, and acting on their own volition, will not have such a public role; there is no intention to strike up a relationship with donors, and therefore they may piggyback on the consent necessary for the medical procedure. In this way, the patient cannot imply a permission/waiver to the use of residual tissues, because they don't know about it. The researcher is free of any fiduciary duties. But, in Moore and Lacks, research was a separate event, requiring a discrete consent despite its close juxtaposition to the medical indications. Research and therapy occur in different places, are often done by different people, and entail different dealings and affairs. While sharing some characteristics of one another, they should not be confused as a single intention; and therefore consent to one ought not to be assumed as consent to the other. Thus, anything that happens subsequently or that is

---

[61] A. V. Campbell. The Ethical Challenges of Genetic Databases: Safeguarding Altruism and Trust. *King's Law Journal* 2007; 18: 241.

[62] UK Biobank Ethics and Governance Framework. Version 3.0 (October 2007). p. 3.

distinct from the medical procedure ought not to be conflated as *medically* indicated. Tests, analysis or investigations may be conducted without implicit consent in terms of diagnosis, because they are of direct benefit to the patient — part of the medical role to which the patient has consented; and this includes an implicit authorisation for any further actions *to this end*. However, if biopsies are taken for research purposes, then this may be either entirely without benefits to the donor, or may benefit them indirectly through improved knowledge or management of the condition. Even if cells fall onto the theatre floor, they have been removed as part of a medical procedure — not for research; why, then, should it be appropriate to assume that the patient has no objection if the cells are picked up and used?

The degrees of separation between medical and indirect benefits (even the benefits of research in general) should not be conflated. What is at stake is the level of care given by clinicians involved which is itself harmed by disingenuous intentions. The trend for patient-centred care has established the requirement of the medical professional to provide information about any 'significant risk which would affect the judgment of a reasonable patient'[63] before undertaking a procedure. Failing to get consent represents an innate betrayal, embodied in the abuse of the fiduciary doctor-patient relationship. This relationship, it would appear, is inconsequential to the distinctly utilitarian justification of these actions when linked to research (expounding the interests society has in such research).

Privacy Interests and iPS Cell Research

At this point, we can start to draw the threads of this debate together: if individuals are to be *donors* in iPS work, they should be expected to consent — that is authorise the collection and use of those cells by researchers, based on the information they are given. This argument appears to hold only as long as the source maintains control of the cells and tissues after they have been surgically excised from the body, with the

[63] *Pearce v United Bristol Healthcare NHS Trust* [1999] P.I.Q.R. 53, at 49.

removal itself being separately consented to as medically indicated. The argument that consent is not necessary employs terminology to characterise cells and tissues as 'abandoned' or 'waste'; but this is at odds with a continued-interest thesis. It is not enough to maintain a proprietary interest, because property is transferable; and as such, any right to withdraw, contra to UK Biobank, would be defunct.

Even if a procedure does not directly harm an individual though pain or inconvenience, we find that privacy is a meaningful interest to prohibit non-consensual intrusions.[64] Privacy has been a mainstay of the idea of *proprietary* rights, and has been used to create a protected sphere about oneself and tangible objects; privacy, as such, defines what may be 'owned' and controlled within a defined territory. Objects may be stolen or misappropriated when accessed and used without permission, or transferred to the ownership of others with consent. Thus, if a biopsy is taken without consent there is a trespass on the person. The insult is not only to the physical person (thus precluding non-consensual biopsies), but also to their wider privacy interests, in the sense that samples can be quickly processed and profiled — a record of that person can be created, exposing genetic conditions, disease states, and peculiarities that others have an interest in knowing. The implications of a proprietary interest in excised tissue preclude scientists from taking samples for their own benefit or the 'good of humanity'. A continued interest is noticeably absent in utilitarian theories of property, because this allows the complete reassignment of rights to the present holder, even if transfer is achieved furtively. This underhandedness is perhaps intentional, because it invests *all* control with the researchers (*qua Moore*), and it would be problematic to assign interests in the source of appropriated tissue if the utility of scientific progress is to be realised.

Radin's idea of the person extending into their property, however, draws out a more extensive privacy interest; one that continues to resonate even when property interests have been severed. This right remains even if authorised transfer extinguishes any further property interests in the

[64] Beyleveld and Brownsword, *op. cit.* note 50.

source, and thus generates the need for withdrawal clauses. This condition of research is not unusual; as Caulfield *et al.* notes, the Canadian policy on tissue research explicitly allows that 'even in the context of tissue collection, the right to withdraw consent endures and could include the destruction of the research material'.[65] The same condition exists in the governance of UK Biobank.

The UK Biobank reasons that it is a steward, and the retention of samples is governed by a willingness, within practical bounds, to allow withdrawal from the initiative: the participant retains an interest in genetic samples, despite property rights being transferred. The Bank articulates this commitment in rules which do not become an impasse to continued research, but it still guarantees the main principle behind this option, i.e. that there will be no further use of the samples by researchers.[66] But to effect this procedure, the *Ethics and Governance Framework* (that details the various roles and responsibilities which UK Biobank will observe with respect to the participants' consent) states:

> 'UK Biobank would destroy your samples (although it may not be possible to trace all distributed sample remnants) and would only hold your information for archival audit purposes'.[67]

Thus, even if, as per the UK's *Nuffield Council on Bioethics*, biological material is considered as 'abandoned' in the context of surgical biopsy, it is not a simple and complete transference to the researcher.[68] This clearly

---

[65] T. Caulfield, U. Ogbogu and R. Isasi. Informed Consent in Embryonic Stem Cell Research: Are We Following Basic Principles? *Canadian Medical Association Journal* 2007; 176: 1722–1725.

[66] See: UK Biobank Ethics and Governance Council: Recent Activity, at: http://www.egcukbiobank.org.uk/recentactivity/index.html [Accessed 22 September 2009].

[67] Ibid. In this case, however, the UK Biobank found that the 'No further use' option (that is participants asserting their right to discontinue use of their data and samples) becomes problematic, because it was not possible for it to destroy all of a participant's health-related information and samples held in the project's back-up and audit system.

asserts an intention to allow a *continued* but limited degree of control on the part of the donor, a sentiment we can similarly find in Radin's work. What this amounts to is a paradigm shift, as others have written, which may actually strengthen the novel idea of 'benefit-sharing' by channelling the research endeavour *to recognise the contribution of research participants.*[69]

In UK Biobank, there is a *prima facie* right of use and transfer emanating from the donor, but which also extends to those bodies in possession of the samples (if an ownership interest can be identified with the researcher, hospital or biobank). These potentially competing rights signal a second privacy interest which remains with the originator after an object has been legitimately transferred to another's control, and thus allows the participant to actuate his right to withdraw from the initiative. These separate, non-proprietary privacy interests are established from *generic privacy rights* — so-called because they are derived from one's status as an agent *per se.*[70] This privacy interest, separate from the proprietary interest, is conceptualised beyond property (thus negating the thesis that privacy *is only* a property right), and empowers people to make decisions about the purposes that they consider as important (using reason, agents are able to reflect and control their behaviour with a view to attaining these ends), and to use the available means to achieve them (under the conditions of voluntariness). Generic privacy reflects a bundle of rights which are necessary for purposive action in a communal world (if some things are no longer private, then it is unlikely that one can

---

[68] Section 9.14.1 of their Report states: 'It will be entailed in any consent to treatment that tissue removed in the course of that treatment will be regarded in law as having been abandoned by the person from whom it was removed'; Nuffield Council on Bioethics (NCB). 1995. *Human Tissue: Ethical and Legal Issues*. London: NCB. The implications of the NCB statement is that tissue is abandoned if it is excised as part of therapy, but this is not clear. There is no reference to whether consent is necessary for tissue removed during a procedure but is not part of the therapy itself.

[69] Cf. J. Merz *et al.* Protecting Subjects' Interests in Genetic Research. *American Journal of Human Genetics* 2002; 70: 965–971.

[70] For a detailed approach to doing just this, see: B. Capps. (forthcoming, 2009). Privacy, Rights and Biomedical Data Collections. In T. Kaan and C. Ho, eds. *Genetic Privacy in Singapore. Science, Ethics and Law*. Singapore: World Scientific.

attain one's purposes), and which allow an individual to attribute worth to her purposes.[71] Empowerment, which gives purposes a certain worth, shows that at least some privacy interests, despite the legitimate transfer of proprietary interests, remains with the source. The authorised *or* unauthorised transfer of cells lines continues the potential threat of disempowering people for insidious ends; that is not only to infringe upon their rights, but also obliterates their worth as human agents. Any cell sample remains linked to the person in this way, and this means that they maintain certain rights of control; they do not give up all interests, so that access by others, especially for a utilitarian purpose, is ethically contestable.

Generic privacy rights justify rules of withdrawal of permission to use a transferred object, because even if a cell line is readily given up, or is unconsciously transferred to another, there continues to be an interest in what happens to these cells. Consent may modify the access that others have to cells, but to dictate future use of them, all interests cannot be sold or transferred: it makes little sense to talk about *owning* this sustained, but 'invisible' proprietary interest, because ownership has been, for all intents, constructions, and purposes, given up. (Whether such conditions are met in the future is a moot point, and often will come down to a complaint made in respect to a contract, if such a document is in existence.) Such intangible privacy interests are beyond the harms caused by theft, intrusion, or the like, but they also demand a level of privacy protection from zealous or disproportionate actions.

Naturally, this has ramifications in iPS science: donated, modified cells could be propagated for many years in the interests of research. Two questions arise in relation to this: should the original donor be allowed to withdraw a previously consented material transfer at all; and if so, should there be limits to this right?

Despite the lack of ambiguity in the declaration of Helsinki's assertion of the participant's right to withdraw *at any time*, many national guidelines, for example, with respect to hES cell research, effectively curtail the right to withdraw consent to a small window of opportunity before

---

[71] The idea of generic rights is derived from: A. Gewirth. 1978. *Reason and Morality*. Chicago: Chicago University Press.

research has begun in earnest.[72] We have reason to suppose that a similar policy should operate in the iPS settings.

We have argued that for someone to be harmed through research on human tissue, she must have a privacy interest in that tissue. If a tissue sample is taken without consent, even when there is a utilitarian justification, there is a sustained privacy interest that works in 'recognition of the right of individuals to exercise control over their own person, property and privacy, and to say "yes" or to say "no"'.[73] One is property based; the other is derived from rights that maintain an agent's control over things that affect her, and despite such objects not being strictly owned. However, if the conditions of procedural consent have been met, then this second generic privacy interest is thinned. Given the dynamic nature of stem cell science, the benchmark of informed consent is unlikely to ever be met; therefore we foresee the bar being set fairly low in respect to the informational interests of the patient, and that general consent would normally suffice (if a patient is at all concerned about the unspecified research goals, then they would be prudent to deny research use altogether). Our argument is that a generic privacy interest still remains in unadulterated cell lines, thus disqualifying unauthorised access beyond the condition of consent.

However, in order to withdraw consent, the original donor must maintain an interest in 'person', so as to actuate authorisation (that is, signal their wishes to the appropriate agent) for the further use of samples currently being used in research. So, if the researcher gains a stronger interest in these terms, it seems reasonable that she should supplant the initial donor as the person in a position of decision-making authority with regard to the research tissue. This condition would be important to limit the donor's claim on cells unobjectionably excised; patients would not be allowed to make property claims (and therefore a share of profits) downstream if such an agreement is not struck from the outset. A two-way agreement should be arrived at: if researchers are to ask for cells, then

[72] Cf. J. Mackenney. Should Gamete Donors be Allowed to Withdraw Consent from Embryo Research? *Asian Bioethics Review* 2009; 1(2): 89–107.

[73] R. Brownsword. Regulating Nanomedicine: The Smallest of Our Concerns? *NanoEthics* 2008; 2: 73 86.

patients should give permission, but without the authority to impose later, unstated conditions (thus, nominally, giving up property interests). But this also requires that the generic privacy interests are diminished at some future point, and where scientific endeavour supplants the donor's interests. Although a stem cell created from somatic cells (as in iPS science) would contain a person's entire genome, its cellular apparatus, function and behaviour could be completely different from those of the originally donated tissue: it could it be so different as to be beyond the decision-making jurisdiction of the original donor on our previously stated generic privacy rights. If this line of reasoning can be maintained, the donor's withdrawal of consent for the use of her tissue is meaningless: the tissue has already been used and now ceases to exist. If a donor maintains no enduring authoritative interests in the modified tissue, the consent process cannot continue to loom over the research: withdrawal would not be an option available to the donor beyond a certain point.

CONCLUSION

iPS science avoids the need for embryos in stem cell research and potential therapy. However, even without having to consider the moral position of the embryo, we have envisaged a number of challenges that stem cell science poses to the consent process in the context of immortalised cell lines. Lessons have been learned from scandals where tissue, appropriated through undeclared intentions, has been retained and used without express consent. We have argued that efforts to bypass consent for the 'good of humanity' do not remove any obligations that researchers have to ethical norms, and it is therefore necessary to get additional consent for any procedure that is not part of the medical procedure. However, the requirement to provide adequate information to donors poses a further challenge in iPS science: here, as with biobanks, the downstream uses of the donated tissue are not all foreseeable at the point of donation. The solution for UK Biobank is to get a general consent, but to ensure that the donor retains some control over the cells and which materialises as a right to withdraw. We argue that such a position is sound because of a remnant privacy interest, but that this right of withdrawal from a project is extinguished at the point at which a cell line is developed.

While it may obviate the need to consider the role of the embryo in further stem cell research, iPS cells are attended by all the ethical problems that potentially already plague long-lasting or stored tissue; as clinicians, ethicists and researchers, we would be sensible to consider the implications of appropriating and modifying human tissue for this purpose.

ACKNOWLEDGEMENTS

The authors would like to thank Alastair Campbell, Alvin Chew Kiah-Sian and Theodora Kwok Hui Xuan for their insightful comments on earlier drafts of this chapter. Needless to say, the responsibility for any mistakes remains with the authors.

Jonathan Mackenney was a visiting fellow at the Centre for Biomedical Ethics, National University of Singapore, during the initial inception of this chapter (November–December 2008).

8

'REASONABLE SUFFERING': THE APPLICATION OF STEM CELL TECHNOLOGIES TO NON-HUMAN ANIMALS

James Yeates

INTRODUCTION

Stem cell science has prompted a considerable volume of bioethical debate and commentary. This debate has prioritised the analyses of the use of human stem cells in the laboratory context and the medical applications of stem cell therapies to humans in the clinical context. It therefore seems worthwhile addressing the omission of non-human animals from the discussion of the ethics pertaining to stem cell therapies (SCTs).

This omission is despite the fact that non-human animals are not ignored in the bioethical literature or the public consciousness. The advent of stem cell technologies has been against a backdrop of concern about the use of increasing numbers of non-human animals in the laboratory context. Animal welfare, which scientifically addresses the suffering of non-human animals, is becoming increasingly conscious and analytic of its ethical premises, and the welfare-based 3Rs, discussed later in this paper, have become increasingly prevalent as a compromise that avoids the polarised debate between human needs and animal rights. Meanwhile, veterinary ethics is beginning to develop its own approaches and principles, and concern has been expressed by veterinarians and animal ethicists alike about issues such as the appropriate relationship of quality and quantity of life in questions over the treatment of animals beyond what would be in their interests. Addressing the omission of stem cell therapies in non-human animals in the bioethical literature therefore seems to be an ethical imperative.

In terms of the application of stem cell therapies to animals, there are two contextual decisions that are of especial relevance:

(1) What experimental stem-cell therapies is it acceptable to inflict on non-human animals in the laboratory context?
(2) What clinical stem-cell therapies is it acceptable to 'inflict' on non-human animals in the veterinary context?[1]

In this chapter, these interests are addressed with reference to the interests of the animals themselves; and are taken to concern primarily life and suffering; and the value of (animal) life and suffering are assumed to be at least partly reciprocal to one another. This paper posits a specifically instrumental value to life, leaving open the question of whether there might additionally be an intrinsic value. Life is instrumentally valuable for an animal because it permits it to have 'positive' ends: enjoyable, eudaimonic states (and it is these that have intrinsic value). Thus life is valuable to an animal if it affords sufficient positive value to outweigh any negative value: this is a life worth living (LWL). The desirability of a state of positive welfare is categorically valuable and this affords an instrumental value to life.

Suffering is what it is desirable to avoid *per se*. It is a 'negative' end, with a quality that one would be better off avoiding, even at the expense of experiencing no other actual state in its stead. An animal is better off having no state whatsoever than the state of suffering. A desire to avoid suffering a negative end is a 'conditional desire' in the sense used by Bernard Williams[2] — it can be achieved by either the replacement of the suffering with a positive welfare state that is worth living, or by the termination of the animal's life. A life that has suffering that is not outweighed by any positive welfare is a life not worth living (LNWL). A

[1] Of course, some clinical interventions will occur in the laboratory, e.g. treatment of sick animals where specified in the study. There may also be laboratory interventions in the veterinary clinic, for example where a veterinary surgeon takes a sample under the Animals (Scientific Procedures) Act 1986 rather than the Veterinary Surgeons Act 1966. A clinical trial might also be conceptually (though not legally) considered a combination of these two contexts.

[2] B. Williams. 1973. *Problems of the Self.* Cambridge: Cambridge University Press.

life that is of equal value to not living at all (if such a thing is possible), is termed an indifferent life. Such a life is neither worth living nor not living and we may say that it is a life worth zero (and abbreviate to LW0).[3] Since they are defined with reference to the specifics of the being's own ends, these concepts of suffering and LNWL can be pluralistic concepts, open to a number of 'conceptions of the good', both in terms of the being's own goods and in terms of axiological positions.[4]

This paper firstly describes the laboratory and veterinary contexts. It describes the context in more detail, then analyses the current, and in part very recent, UK legislation as a framework for each (the part of this pertaining to the laboratory context is not dissimilar to the EU legislation that is in draft form at the time of print), looking at the interests in terms of harms and compromises reached in each. These analyses reveal a number of relationships that can be considered unfair either to the animal itself or in balancing between interests. As a solution to this problem, the paper then sketches an extension of a Rawlsian approach to these contexts. It firstly address the use of stem cells in the veterinary context of animal patients. The conclusions from this context are then extended to the laboratory context and the balance between patients in the medical context and animal subjects in the laboratory context.

THE CONTEXTS

The Laboratory Context

The use of non-human animals in experimentation and in the development of therapeutic technologies and products has a long history. The most famous example is probably the understanding of diabetes mellitus and

---

[3] If an intrinsic value to life is posited in addition to the instrumental value described here, the definitions of LWL, LNWL and LW0 are likely to be more complicated, and (on the assumption that this intrinsic value posited will be positive) permit more suffering in lives classified as LWL or LW0, than if these definitions were calculated by welfare assessments alone.

[4] It does consider suffering as an essentially teleological concept, but only in the weak sense in which the legal system and, as I shall argue, Rawls's system, make every salient concept teleological.

the development of treatments based firstly on canine pancreas products. Even now insulin is produced that is of bovine or porcine origin. In the context of this paper, animals are increasingly used as models of disease for the development of stem cell therapies. For example, non-human animals are used as models for osteoarthritis,[5] osteochondral defects,[6] tendon injury,[7] bone fractures,[8] myocardial infarction,[9] cerebral infarction,[10] neurological disease,[11] retinal disease,[12] muscular dysfunction,[13] Crohn's fistulas[14] and

[5] J.M. Murphy *et al.* Stem Cell Therapy in a Caprine Model of Osteoarthritis. *Arthritis and Rheumatism* 2003; 48: 3464–3474.

[6] S. Nathan *et al.* Cell-Based Therapy in the Repair of Osteochondral Defects: A Novel Use for Adipose Tissue. *Tissue Engineering* 2003; 9: 733–744.

[7] H.A. Awad *et al.* Autologous Mesenchymal Stem Cell-Mediated Repair of Tendon. *Tissue Engineering* 1999; 5: 267–277.

[8] S.P. Bruder *et al.* The Effects of Implants Loaded with Autologous Mesenchymal Stem Cells on the Healing of Canine Segmental Bone Defects. *The Journal of Bone and Joint Surgery: American Volume* 1998; 80: 985–996; S.P. Bruder *et al.* Mesenchymal Stem Cells in Osteobiology and Applied Bone Regeneration. *Clinical Orthopaedics and Related Research* 1998; 355 Suppl: S247–256; C.M. Cowan *et al.* Adipose-Derived Adult Stromal Cells Heal Critical-Size Mouse Calvarial Defects. *Nature Biotechnology* 2004; 22: 560–567.

[9] B. Assmus *et al.* Transplantation of Progenitor Cells and Regeneration Enhancement in Acute Myocardial Infarction (TOPCARE-AMI). *Circulation* 2002; 106: 3009–3017; J. Herreros *et al.* Autologous Intramyocardial Injection of Cultured Skeletal Muscle-Derived Stem Cells in Patients with Non-Acute Myocardial Infarction. *European Heart Journal* 2003; 24: 2012–2020.

[10] J. Chen. Therapeutic Benefit of Intravenous Administration of Bone Marrow Stromal Cells After Cerebral Ischemia in Rats. *Stroke; A Journal of Cerebral Circulation* 2001; 32: 1005–1011; O.Y. Bang *et al.* Autologous Mesenchymal Stem Cell Transplantation in Stroke Patients. *Annals of Neurology* 2005; 57: 874–882.

[11] S.A. Goldman & S. Natesan. A Niche-Defying Feat: Induced Oligoneogenesis in the Adult Dentate Gyrus. *Cell Stem Cell* 2008; 3: 125–126; M.S. Windrem *et al.* Neonatal Chimerization with Human Glial Progenitor Cells Can Both Remyelinate and Rescue the Otherwise Lethally Hypomyelinated Shiverer Mouse. *Cell Stem Cell* 2008; 2: 553–565.

[12] A. Otani *et al.* Rescue of Retinal Degeneration by Intravitreally Injected Adult Bone Marrow–Derived Lineage-Negative Hematopoietic Stem Cells. *The Journal of Clinical Investigation* 2004; 114: 765–774.

[13] M. Sampaolesi *et al.* Mesoangioblast Stem Cells Ameliorate Muscle Function in Dystrophic Dogs. *Nature* 2006; 444: 574–579.

[14] D. Garcia-Olmo *et al.* A Phase I Clinical Trial of the Treatment of Crohn's Fistula by Adipose Mesenchymal Stem Cell Transplantation. *Diseases of the Colon and Rectum* 2005; 48: 1416–1423.

various autoimmune disorders.[15] In addition, stem cell therapies are developed and tested for safety in non-human animals, despite the differences between human and non-human stem cells.[16] In the future, even larger numbers of animals are likely to be used in research, especially given the anticipated concomitant developments in genetic modification technologies, cloning and use of chimeras, which may be all the more prevalent given the likelihood of a lack of ethically-sourced human oocytes for this research.

In the laboratory context, animals are used to discover information, which can be generalised and applied in a clinical context for the benefit of human patients. For many, especially those working in utilitarian frameworks, such benefits can justify the use of some non-human animals. Laboratory interventions can be categorised according to the direct applicability of the knowledge expected to be gained. Some projects can be loosely considered as aiming to discover 'fundamental' scientific knowledge, for example basic biology or psychology. Other projects concern applications of more basic knowledge, for example, toxicological studies, efficacy testing and product development, and the garnering of tissues or progeny for various purposes such as transplantation and the production of therapeutics.

Much of the popular and academic literature has tended to concentrate on the fundamental scientific experiments, but there are meaningful differences between the two sub-contexts, especially when balancing interests. One salient difference concerns the identifiability of the beneficiaries. Fundamental science has an instrumental value that is vague and uncertain — nobody can know with much certainty how valuable a fundamental science project will be. It is uncertain whether an experiment will produce any meaningful results and, if so, whether they will confirm

---

[15] S. Pluchino & G. Martino. The Therapeutic Use of Stem Cells for Myelin Repair in Autoimmune Demyelinating Disorders. *Journal of the Neurological Sciences* 2005; 233: 117–119; A. Uccelli *et al.* Stem Cells in Inflammatory Demyelinating Disorders: A Dual Role for Immunosuppression and Neuroprotection. *Expert Opinion on Biological Therapy* 2006; 6: 17–22.

[16] I. Ginis *et al.* Differences Between Human and Mouse Embryonic Stem Cells. *Developmental Biology* 2004; 269: 360–380.

or deny the null hypothesis, end up published, be read and stimulate further research. It can be even less clear how any results might be directed into therapies; how and to whom those products might be applied; the benefits and risks of such applications and the perception of the products amongst consumers, health care workers and the general public. The opacity in who will benefit makes balancing the harms and benefits speculative and vague.

As products move towards applications their target is increasingly identifiable. Predictions promise more accuracy in terms of the form and substance of the final products and in identifying how, why and who the products may benefit and harm. Despite this, the failure to address how interests are balanced is continued in the rarer analyses of the toxicological and efficacy research. Thus even products that may benefit few humans only mildly and have negligible risks are nonetheless developed and tested using non-human animals.

This subsection does not analyse the use of animals and embryos in fundamental stem cell science. This is partly because of the focus of this book. It is partly because the context of applied research has benefited from less ethical analysis than the fundamental science context. It is also because the focus on fundamental research has allowed both sides to avoid explicit comparisons between the interests of humans and animals. A focus on the applied context allows more explicit analysis on the methods by which human and non-human interests are balanced.

The Veterinary Context

The other context analysed in this paper is that of veterinary work. This is taken to mean the use of medical interventions on animals for direct effects on those animals. Veterinary interventions are (thought to be) legitimised by their benefits to the animals themselves. Veterinary medicine may lessen animals' suffering or extend their lives. However, this is not always the case. Some veterinary interventions, such as post-mortems and reproductive technologies, may benefit other animals. Other veterinary interventions are arguably not for the benefit of animals at all, but are aimed at improving human interests, such as increasing a horse's racing performance or keeping alive a suffering companion animal for the benefit of the owner.

As with the laboratory context, there are subdivisions within the veterinary context, which can have very different ethical landscapes. Animals in the companion animal, 'sports' animal (such as a racing horse), farmed animal and laboratory animals (when medically treated outside of the experimental aims) contexts, are each thought of differently by their owners, by veterinarians and the law. As this paper shows, the legislation affords some protection to all these, but this protection varies between contexts. This variation leads to significant unfairness within and between the different contexts and suffering of some animals far in excess of that of others.

Given the increase of research in stem cells on animal models, especially with the use of canine models, and the results from studies on stem cell therapies in joint and tendon injuries, it was inevitable that the use of stem cell therapies began in the veterinary context. Dogs have had stem cell therapies for osteoarthritis[17] and it can be expected that this will be followed by uses of stem cell therapy for heart disease, liver disease, kidney disease, muscular disease, neurological diseases and immune-mediated diseases. Currently, veterinary STCs provided by only one US company, which 'would like to ensure that this treatment modality is utilized with diligence and integrity'.[18] Because of the increased veterinary budgets and the family-linked nature of relationships to humans, companion animals are likely to have expensive and cutting-edge interventions performed upon them. This, combined with the use of dogs as models for several conditions, is likely to promote the development of SCTs for canine applications.

In the context of sports horses, work is underway developing SCTs for laminitis, neurological diseases and chronic obstructive pulmonary disorder. But by far the greatest use is in race horses. Autogenous stem cells

---

[17] J. Bickett. 2008. Stem Cells Being Used to Treat Animals. *My Fox Austin*. Available at: http://www.myfoxaustin.com/myfox/pages/News/Detail?contentId=7839521&version=1&locale=EN-US&layoutCode=VSTY&pageId=3.5.1 [Accessed 8 December 2008].

[18] J.A.R. Johnson. 2008. *Dear Doctor.* Available at: http://www.vet-stem.com/images/6505-0002-001%20SA%20Client%20Letter%20to%20Vet_Web.pdf [Accessed 26 February 2009].

therapies have been used in treatment of tendon, joint and ligament injury and more than 2000 horses have been treated since 2003.[19] Future uses might include the development of induced pluripotent stem cells both as models for disease and potentially as clonal replacements.

Current stem cell interventions use autogenous, rather than allogenous stem cells. This makes them, in many respects, not dissimilar to current practices not based on stem cells. For example the extraction, conditioning and incubation of autologous serum to derive interleukin-1 receptor-antagonist protein which is reinserted into the horse's joints or the collection of plasma for anti-clotting factors then used to treat liquidising corneal ulcers might be similar from a horse treatment perspective to future stem cell therapies. Perhaps consequently, the report of the first randomised, blinded, placebo-controlled clinical trial reporting on the effectiveness of stem cell therapy in dogs reported that 'autologous adult stem cells...have no ethical issues related to their use'![20]

THE LEGAL STATUS QUO

The UK legislation on animals represents a (roughly utilitarian) compromise between human and animal interests. Historically, it allowed the use of one's own animal property in any way one saw fit and without government interference (with some exceptions, such as letting one's animal harm another person and activities which blur species boundaries such as bestiality). With 19th century reforms such as Martin's and Pease's Acts and the Protection of Animals Act in 1911 came increasing prohibitions on certain acts of cruelty, especially where there was insufficient benefit in such treatment; and became the model for the current legislature in the laboratory and veterinary contexts. In general terms, the laws pertaining to the laboratory context prescribe harms that are legal if there are

---

[19] Vet-Stem Regenerative Veterinary Medicine. Available at: www.vet-stem.com [Accessed 10 Dec 2008].

[20] L.L. Black *et al.* Effect of Adipose-Derived Mesenchymal Stem and Regenerative Cells on Lameness in Dogs with Chronic Osteoarthritis of the Coxofemoral Joints: A Randomized, Double-Blinded, Multicenter, Controlled Trial. *Veterinary Therapeutics: Research in Applied Veterinary Medicine* 2007; 8: 272–281.

justificatory benefits; the laws in the veterinary context proscribe harms that are not legal if there are not justificatory benefits.

The Laboratory Context Legislation

The use of stem therapies in the laboratory contexts is regulated by the European Directive 86/609/EEC[21] (based on The Council of Europe's 1986 European Convention for the Protection of Vertebrate Animals used for Experimental and other Scientific Purposes) and the Animals (Scientific Procedures) Act 1986[22] and its secondary legislation produced by the Home Office.[23] These protect scientists from prosecutions and protect animals from unnecessary suffering. The EU Directive is currently under review,[24] as is the way in which it is implemented in UK law.[25]

The A(SP)A defines a regulated procedure as any 'scientific procedure...which may have the effect of causing that animal pain, suffering, distress or lasting harm'.[26] It also permits animals to be caused suffering and thereby subjected to a state potentially considered as not worth living. Animals can be used in stem cell research with a 'substantial severity band', which can involve a 'major departure from health or well-being' in licensed experiments. For example, in an applied experiment[27] three-quarters of the mice on which a stem cell intervention was used died from neurological disease; not counting the control group who received no

[21] Though animals used in 'fundamental' research are not included within the scope of this directive.
[22] As amended by the Animals (Scientific Procedures) Act 1986 Amendment Regulations 1998; hereafter, referred to as the A(SP)A.
[23] A(SP)A, s21(4).
[24] A draft revised directive was sent by the European Commission to the European Parliament in 2007.
[25] See Home Office. 2008. *Animals in Scientific Procedures: Better Regulation.* Available at: http://scienceandresearch.homeoffice.gov.uk/animal-research/better-regulation [Accessed 26 Feb 2009].
[26] A(SP)A, s2(1).
[27] M.S. Windrem *et al.* Neonatal Chimerization with Human Glial Progenitor Cells Can Both Remyelinate and Rescue the Otherwise Lethally Hypomyelinated Shiverer Mouse. *Cell Stem Cell* 2008; 2: 553–565.

treatment, and who therefore had no opportunity to improve from the disease. It also explicitly allows killing. The killing of an animal is not considered a 'lasting harm'. This is clear from the wording of the Act, and was confirmed in a recent judicial review case which failed (though other arguments were successful) to satisfy the court that death should be considered 'a lasting harm'.[28] In fact, the Act in many cases mandates that at the end of an experiment an animal is killed.[29] The A(SP)A would also permit the prevention of the development of a non-human embryo, its perpetuation and its use while in an embryonic form.[30]

But it does not allow any suffering. Scientists experimenting on stem cells therapies should minimise 'pain, distress [and] discomfort',[31] by causing the least harm to the lowest number of animals.[32] This is in some ways a consensus between those who oppose animal experimentation from an animal rights or animal welfare position and those who wish for animals to be legitimately exploited for human benefit, since everyone should agree that unnecessary suffering is unnecessary. It is well captured in Russell and Burch's[33] 3Rs — Replacement, Reduction and Refinement.[34] Replacement involves eschewing animal experiments for studies using tissue cultures, models or clinical trials. Reduction involves using fewer animals, by performing fewer experiments, smaller groups with tighter statistical analysis and not duplicating experiments. Refinement involves the amelioration of suffering, by using anaesthetics and analgesics or improving husbandry. There are also legal provisions for stem cell therapy developers to preferentially use animals with 'the lowest neurophysiological sensitivity'.[35]

---

[28] *R (BUAV) v Secretary of State for the Home Department.* QBD 27 Jul 2007.

[29] European Directive 86/609/EEC, Article 9(1), (3)(b); 15(1).

[30] A(SP)A, s1(2): 'Any such vertebrate in its foetal, larval or embryonic form is a protected animal only from the stage of its development when — in the case of a mammal, bird or reptile, half the gestation period for the relevant species has elapsed'.

[31] A(SP)A, s10(1)(b).

[32] A(SP)A, 5(5)(b) & s10(1)(a).

[33] W.M.S. Russell & R.L. Burch. 1959. *The Principle of Humane Experimental Technique.* London: Menthuen.

[34] Applied in both European Directive 86/609/EEC and A(SP)A.

[35] European Directive 86/609/EEC, Article 7(3); Animals (Scientific Procedures) Act 1986, 5(a).

The compromise represents a balance between the competing interests of animals and humans and which is explicit in the Act itself: '[i]n determining whether and on what terms to grant a project licence the Secretary of State shall weigh the likely adverse effects on the animals concerned against the benefit likely to accrue as a result of the programme to be specified in the licence'.[36] For example, some harms; such as the use of great apes[37] or the Lethal-Dose 50 test in the safety-testing of a stem cell product[38] are considered generally unjustifiable, and some benefits such as testing cosmetic products[39] and ingredients[40] are regarded as insufficient to justify stem cell research on animals.

However, this compromise might be considered unfair, because, firstly, the balance of costs and benefits is biased enormously towards human benefits. Suffering that is not necessary to the study should be minimised, as per the 3Rs, but this still allows projects to proceed that are of dubious necessity overall; and perhaps not sufficient value to warrant the suffering they involve, even if that suffering is necessary for the project. Secondly, even where the suffering represents a balance of interests, it could be argued that this very act of balancing represents unfairness. Decisions to excessively exploit one being for the benefits of another may sometimes be inherently unfair. To illustrate this, cost-benefit analysis, which underpins much of the compromise in the laboratory context, was

---

[36] A(SP)A, s5(4).

[37] Select Committee on Animals in Scientific Procedures. 1997. *Select Committee on Animals in Scientific Procedures Report*. 1.5. Available at: http://www.publications.parliament.uk/pa/ld200102/ldselect/ldanimal/150/15004.htm [Accessed 19 Dec 2008].

[38] Animals Procedures Committee (APC). 1999. *Press Release: LD 50 Test — Changes to Licensing Procedure*. Available at: http://www.apc.gov.uk/press_releases/991021 [Accessed 11 Dec 2008]. (In actual fact the LD50 test can still be licensed where there are no alternatives.)

[39] Animal Procedures Committee. 1997. *Press Release: Cosmetic Product Testing on Animals Ends Today*. Available at: http://www.apc.gov.uk/press_releases/971106.htm [Accessed 11 Dec 2008].

[40] A *de facto* ban since 16 November 1998. Select Committee on Animals in Scientific Procedures. 1997. *Select Committee on Animals in Scientific Procedures Report*, 1.5. Available at: http://www.publications.parliament.uk/pa/ld200102/ldselect/ldanimal/150/15004.htm [Accessed 19 Dec 2008].

originally developed by economists to determine how much humans harmed by a project should be compensated in order to redress any unfairness. But non-human experimental subjects are not compensated at all — they are only harmed.

The Veterinary Context Legislation

The veterinary context is controlled in the UK by the Veterinary Surgeons Act 1966 (VSA) and the Animal Welfare Act 2006 (AWA). The latter protects animals in various ways, notably against being caused unnecessary suffering in section 4,[41] against non-exempted mutilations in sections 5 and 6, and against failure to ensure their needs are met in section 9.[42]

Any interventions that are part of the 'art and science of veterinary surgery and medicine' come under the Veterinary Surgeons Act 1966 and subsequent amendments. These regulate who can perform such interventions, by limiting it (with some derogation[43]) to registered members of the Royal College of Veterinary Surgeons (RCVS). The conditions of membership include academic qualifications and an undertaking to adhere to a professional code, which mandate that the welfare of animals under a veterinarian's care is their primary aim.[44] The VSA, like the 3Rs, represents not so much a compromise as a consensus, since it is intended to advantage all parties. The animals benefit from skilled clinicians acting under a professional ethics, so long as this ethics is of sufficient rigour. The clinicians benefit from a level of privilege. The clients benefit from the assurance afforded by a regulated profession.

Section 4 of the AWA builds on the offences of causing suffering implemented in the 19th century. This is effectively an offence of cruelty,

---

[41] This used to be part of an offence of cruelty under the 1911 Act, but the AWA no longer uses the word (and given that the Protection of Animals Act 1911, s1-3; Protection against Cruel Tethering Act 1988 and Animals (Cruel Poisons) Act 1960 are now repealed under AWA Schedule 4, the word has effectively disappeared from UK legislation).

[42] AWA, s9.

[43] VSA, s19(3) and Schedule II, Part I; VSA, Schedule III, Part I; The Veterinary Surgeons Act 1966 (Schedule 3 Amendment) Order 2002 under The Veterinary Surgeons Act 1966, s19(5).

[44] RCVS, 2008, *Guide to Professional Conduct*, § 1.B.1a.

since a series of precedent defined cruelty not just as 'wanton' cruelty, but as causing unnecessary suffering. The *actus reus* of a section 4 offence involves causing or allowing suffering to be caused. Suffering includes 'pain, distress or tribulation',[45] i.e. both physical and mental suffering.[46] Sections 5 and 6 of the AWA prohibit mutilations, which are defined as interference with the sensitive tissues or bone structure of the animal, otherwise than for the purpose of its medical treatment. Some mutilations are then exempted from this section under secondary legislation[47] made after consultation with representatives of interested parties.[48] Many permissible interventions must be performed by a veterinary surgeon, outside of the laboratory context, but there are derogations for many agricultural mutilations on juveniles. Like the A(SP)A, the AWA and VSA not only allow killing but mandate it when it is the only way to protect against suffering.[49] Again paralleling the A(SP)A, the AWA affords no legal protection to embryos.[50]

Indeed, the AWA parallels A(SP)A yet again by allowing suffering. As previous courts had stated, 'infliction of...extreme pain, is manifestly not by itself sufficient' for an offence.[51] What is relevant is whether the suffering was 'necessary'. 'If the suffering inflicted is necessary, it may be inflicted'.[52] The VSA says nothing to limit the causation of suffering so long as it is part of an act of veterinary practice.

This causes risks in the application of stem cell technologies. The aforementioned affection and finances of dog owners can lead them to

---

[45] *Patchett v Macdougall.* 1984. SLT 152, 154.

[46] M. Radford. 2001. *Animal Welfare Law in Britain.* Oxford: Oxford University Press: 243.

[47] AWA, s5(4).

[48] AWA, s5(5).

[49] This and the above citations concerning the A(SP)A can be taken as a legal affirmation of the characterisation of suffering in the introduction. Since all these laws regulate that, in the animal's interests, an animal that is suffering must be killed, this suggests that suffering is considered worse than non-existence for the animal. (As in other cases, suffering may be deemed 'necessary' for the benefit of others and so legitimise that animals be kept alive while suffering.)

[50] AWA, s1(2).

[51] *Ford v Wiley.* 1889. 23 QBD 203, 209, *per* Lord Coleridge CJ.

[52] *Ibid.*, 215.

use extreme and novel treatments to keep their animal alive in conditions of suffering. There is a real danger that veterinary stem cell technologies will be used, without sufficient ethical reflection, to extend lives that are not worth living. For example, the treatment of canine cardiac problems is likely to be a major veterinary use of stem cell technologies. Cardiac disease sufferers will typically be older or more inbred animals. Such animals are likely to have concomitant problems, such as arthritis, obesity, bronchitis and genetic conditions. If sufficient safeguards are not in place to prevent it, there is a danger that well-meaning veterinarians, acting as agents of well-meaning owners, will perpetuate lives of such low quality that the animal would be better off not living. Perpetuating these lives may gain some benefits to the owners, but only at the great cost to the animals themselves. Similarly, the use of stem cell technologies might also lead to suffering of sports animals. For example, it is often said that a risk factor for catastrophic injury during races is previous injury. If more horses are repaired and raced again, this may lead to injuries, suffering and consequent killing.

The UK might also permit the use of products of one animal in the treatment of another. Previously, the code of practice for vets under the VSA does not allow the storage of blood for transfusions or kidney transplantation for fear that these would lead to unfair exploitation of some animals at the expense of others. But these have now been made permissible[53] and a similar pattern might be expected for stem cells. The removal of embryonic or gamete tissue from an animal for use in the treatment of human being is exempted from the VSA,[54] and mutilations to isolate embryos are often exempted or considered acts of veterinary surgery.

Not all suffering is allowed in the veterinary context: inflicting *unnecessary* suffering is considered as cruelty: 'we have neither the moral nor the legal right to inflict it, a conclusion not of sentiment but of good sense'.[55] In the courts and the AWA s4, the question of necessity is partly

[53] RCVS, *op. cit.* note 44, §3.
[54] VSA, s19(4).
[55] Coleridge, *op. cit.* note 51, p. 215.

a matter of whether the suffering was for a reasonable benefit. Courts may seek to determine whether a harm was for a legitimate purpose (ss3c); whether the suffering could have been reduced (ss3a) and whether it was proportionate to the benefits (ss3d).

This is conceptually very similar to the A(SP)A — and this balance may be similarly unfair. Firstly, it may be biased. Francione, reviewing US cases, argues that the current compromise involves normative considerations which allow almost any animal interest to avoid suffering to be 'trumped' by the most trivial human interests.[56] In the UK, raising white veal calves[57] (before it was specifically legislatively outlawed[58]) and not treating fly-strike and footrot in sheep[59] were deemed non-prosecutable because courts felt unable to comment on husbandry systems.[60] Other examples include many interventions to improve sporting performance, productivity or fertility and reproductive technologies, such as embryo transfer in farm animals and horses. The main motivation for treating such horses is probably not their own interests. It is to get them racing again, or for breeding purposes, and this is in the interests of the owner and trainer. As the law can allow that even extreme pain may not be an offence if it is sufficiently justified, this may be considered unfair in that animals may be caused severe suffering for the benefit of their owners. Secondly, it might again be argued that the very act of balancing, even if justifiable on utilitarian grounds, might sometimes be unfair to those exploited.

---

[56] G.L. Francione. Animals, Property and Legal Welfarism: 'Unnecessary' Suffering and the 'Humane' Treatment of Animals. *Rutgers Law Review* 1994; 46: 721–770.

[57] *Roberts v Ruggiero.* QBD 3 Apr 1985.

[58] Welfare of Calves Regulations 1987, SI1987/2021. See also more recent Welfare of Farmed Animals Regulations 2007.

[59] *Drury v Northamptonshire Country Council.* 2005 (court transcript).

[60] While in theory, according to *Waters v Braithwaite* (1914) 78 JP 124, traditions cannot be used to justify any conduct, courts have proved almost completely reluctant to comment on the necessity of any overall system that involves suffering, concentrating instead on whether suffering is necessary within that context— thereby further paralleling the judgements described above under A(SP)A.

UNFAIRNESS

The unfairness in the laboratory and veterinary contexts can be characterised in different ways. Some unfair differences are between individuals. Some owners may spend far larger sums of money on some animals than they would on other animals or than other owners would. Different companion animals are loved to various degrees and owners vary in their wealth or pet's insurance status. Different racehorses may be treated depending on their performance or expected value at stud. But also, there can be more 'systematic' unfairness between animals of different species or in different contexts, based on the socio-politics aspects of human treatment of non-humans.

The differences in how species are treated are most obvious in a comparison of human and non-human animals, although other taxonomic classifications also affect animals' treatment. The Human Rights Act 1998 applies only to human beings. The AWA applies only to vertebrates (and human beings are specifically excluded), and A(SP)A applies only to vertebrates and, arbitrarily, *Octopus vulgaris*. Thus, a human child is treated differently from a chimpanzee, which is treated differently from a cat, which is treated differently from a chipmunk, which is treated differently from a catfish, which is treated differently from a cuttlefish. Some of this differential veterinary treatment can be justified by properties of the animal. If a juvenile rat has only a three-year life-expectancy, it may seem less appropriate to subject it to radical surgery than a juvenile dog with a ten-year life-expectancy. But other differences that are independent of the animal's properties may be unreasonable.

Individual animals within the same species are also treated differently according to their individual 'social position'. Pet dogs often have far larger sums of money on their treatment than laboratory dogs or racing greyhounds might. This may be because, unlike other 'products', whose instrumental status somewhat precludes sympathy,[61] the benefit of companionship requires that owners treat their animals with some respect and value. Companion animals are often considered as

[61] J.A. Serpell. Factors Affecting Human Attitudes to Animals and Their Welfare. *Animal Welfare* 2004; 13: S145–151.

family-members[62] and pet owners are less sure of the human-animal moral divide.[63] People with pets tend to have more love,[64] more stringent assessments of suffering[65] and high 'fortune in the distribution of assets'.[66] Consequently, many would spend 'any' amount on their companion.[67] This has lead, in Western countries at least, to increasingly technological and expensive veterinary therapies being performed on companion animals compared with their farmed counterparts. Even if inter-specific differences may be based on fair reasons, it is less clear that differences in the treatment of animals of the same species in different contexts can be fair. If the animals are similar in morally-relevant ways, then basic principles of fairness, such as equity and appropriateness, demand that they are treated similarly. The differential treatment of laboratory and pet rabbits cannot be defended by claiming higher properties of the one over the other.[68]

---

[62] J. Bryant, L. Baggott la Velle & J. Searle. 2005. *Introduction to Bioethics.* Chichester: Wiley.

[63] B.K. Boosgaard, S.J. Oosing & B.B. Bock. 2006. Importance of Emotional Experiences for Societal Perception of Farm Animal Welfare: A Quantitative Study in the Netherlands. In *Ethics and the Politics of Food.* M. Kaiser & M. Lien, eds. Wageningen: Wageningen Academic Publishers: 512–517.

[64] A. St. Yves *et al. Psychological Report* 1990; 67: 1067–1075.

[65] Boosgaard *et al., op. cit.* note 63.

[66] N. Endenberg, H. Hart & H.W. de Vries. Differences Between Owners and Non-Owners of Companion Animals. *Anthrozoos* 1992; 4(2): 120–126.

[67] A. Albert & K. Bulcroft. Pets and Urban Life. *Anthrozoos* 1987; 1(1): 9–25.

[68] In fact, the (unfair) use of therapeutics and application of knowledge derived from individuals of the same species is often presented as an argument that the use of animals in research is *fair*. This argument has dubious validity. It is not clear that the animal subjects in a laboratory context can be considered compensated in any way by the recipients being also non-human. It is as if the animal parties might be thought to be recompensed by this: as if a reasonable mouse representative might say, 'O, my suffering is benefiting other *mice*. Well, why didn't you say? Go ahead then'. (In fact, even if we imagine some species-based justice, it still seems unfair, since, mice are almost certainly the most studied animal in stem cell research, but it is unlikely that many will benefit from stem cell therapies.) It instead might be argued more weakly that the existence of benefits to non-human animals from animal research at least suggests that the cost-benefit analysis is less biased, but this argument is also invalid. The animals benefited are the animals we care about, and at the cost to those about whom we care less. Mice in laboratories are harmed for benefits to dogs we care for. Dogs in laboratories are harmed for dogs we love. In a way, then it is even less defensible, since at least the human–non-human comparison could claim some populist metaphysics.

It is not merely that certain animals of different species or in different contexts experience differing quality of life. Different animals experience different *minimum guaranteed* quality of life. The minimum ensured within the laboratory context differs from that in the companion animal context; the minimum for a dog differs from that of a dogfish. Certain species, in certain contexts, have no opportunity to reach anywhere near the minimum in other contexts. Some will unavoidably suffer. For example, GM animals that are increasingly bred as disease models may have no opportunity for a quality-of-life experienced by primates; indeed many do not even have an opportunity to have a LWL.

These different types of unfairness are not contingently unfair states of affairs (as for example, when different owners spend different amounts of money on animals they love more or ones which perform better). The differential contexts *cause* the differences in minimum guaranteed quality of life. Animals in the laboratory context are caused to have a lower minimum quality of life *in order to* elevate the quality of lives of companion animals and owner. Companion animals and sports animals benefit from the research that harms laboratory animals and from products 'farmed' in other animals. It is this unfair compromise that means many animals in the veterinary and laboratory contexts suffer a LNWL.

The balance of interests may be considered unfair from many perspectives, not least the liberalist perspective. The current legal status, based predominantly on utilitarian concepts of unnecessary suffering and balance between cost and benefits, can reduce but not avoid suffering and it cannot avoid unfairness. In fact, as Rawls and others have pointed out, from a point of social contract theory, utilitarianism in general has no inherent method to avoid unfairness. Rawls criticised utilitarian compromises based on balancing the interests of different inter-contextual beings, in which some are advantaged at the expense of others. He argues at length that this is manifestly unfair.

A PROPOSED SOLUTION: RAWLS AND FAIRNESS

In order to address this unfairness, it is necessary to look elsewhere, and for this Rawls can provide a worthwhile approach. As part of his critique, Rawls repeatedly and explicitly compares his own thesis, Justice as Fairness (JAF), with other approaches that aim to balance interests (usually utilitarianisms), finding the former to lead to fairer states of affairs. His approach is a heuristic tool that aims at establishing a method by which one could test the legitimacy of institutions.

Rawls argues that one can get nearer to a concept of natural duty of justice (and of an ideal state) by certain thought experiments. Rawls asks us to imagine legislators located in a certain imaginary scenario — called the original position (OP). This 'models what we regard — here and now — as acceptable restrictions on the reasons on the bases of which the parties, situated in fair conditions, may properly put forward certain principles of political justice and reject others'.[69] The conditions of this original position can be defined by using intuitive principles of justice, tested by a process of reflective equilibrium. One set of conditions Rawls proposes are epistemic. Parties are allowed 'the general beliefs and forms of reasoning found in common sense, and the methods and modes of science, when not controversial'.[70] Participants are not allowed specific beliefs about which members of the society they represent, in terms of their actual social position, fortune in the distribution of assets, abilities and intelligence, likes and wants and concept of the good. The intent of this ignorance is to 'nullify the effects of specific contingencies which put men at odds and tempt them to exploit social and natural circumstances to their own advantage'.[71] Other conditions are normative. Rawls specifies that the legislators are aiming at a democratic constitution[72] (i.e. following Rousseau); that they are rational (following

---

[69] J. Rawls. 2001. *Justice as Fairness: A Restatement.* New York: Harvard University Press: 17.

[70] *Ibid.*, 90.

[71] J. Rawls. 1971/1999. *A Theory of Justice.* Oxford: Oxford University Press: 136.

[72] *Ibid.*, viii [NB: A minor point relevant to the UK is that, unlike almost every other country, there is no constitution. Rawls argues that the OP process should work out the basic structure and then the constitution before considering issues of legislation. While this is a common method that has been employed at some point in most countries' histories, it is not one that the UK has used. I think it would be unlikely that Rawls or anyone would argue that the UK is especially a less ideal democratic state for this omission. It may be that this provides a real-life counter-example to his argument for this process. It may be equally reasonable for the contractors to work out the basic structure and then move straight on to fundamental legislations and omit any constitution. Consequently, and since this paper is based on UK law, it considers only the basic structure of society and legislation, and omits any mention of the place of non-humans in a democratic state's constitution.]

Kant);[73] and that they are inspired by self-interest (following Hobbes).[74] Rawls then asks us to hypothesise the form of the contract that rational contractors would choose from such a position, generating both concepts and principles, with lexical priority, which would determine the construct of an ideal state. The next step is to compare these results with our intuition, i.e. a process of reflective equilibrium, to check that the conclusions do not conflict with our intuitions. If the OP were not to yield intuitively-acceptable principles, then the reflective equilibrium interpolation could change the OP until it did.[75]

With this scenario in mind, Rawls speculated that such contractors would choose principles of justice (revised following critical comments by Hart) which prescribe that:

> 'a) each person has the same indefeasible claim to a fully adequate scheme of equal basic liberties, which scheme is compatible with the same scheme of liberties for all; and
> b) social and economic inequalities are to satisfy two conditions: first they are to be attached to office and positions open to all under fair conditions of fair equality of opportunity; and second, they are to be to the greatest benefit of the least-advantaged members of society (the difference principle)'.[76]

It is a basic assumption of this paper that Rawls' approach is reasonable but not perfect. (From his writings it seems likely that Rawls would agree

[73] Rawls says he follows Kant: *op. cit.* note 71, p. 252 though this can only be the case if his justice as fairness is considered as heuristic only since, while Kant may appear contractualist, he considers contractualism as 'trivial' [I. Kant. 1785/1902. Grundelgung zur Metaphysik der Sitten (Groundwork of the Metaphysic of Morals) in *gesammelte Schriften*. I. Kant. Berlin: Walter de Gruyter: Vol. IV: 387–463].

[74] T. Hobbes. 1651/2005. *Thomas Hobbes Leviathan: A Critical Edition*. Edited by G.A.J. Rogers & K Schuhmann. London: Continuum International Publishing Group: Part 1, Chap. 15. This point is argued in: M. Brown. 1996. *The Quest for Moral Foundations: An Introduction to Ethics*. Washington, DC: Georgetown University Press: Part Three.

[75] Rawls, *op. cit.* note 71, p. 20.

[76] Rawls, *op. cit.* note 69, p. 42. [NB: Rawls specifically does not insist that the fair equality of opportunity should have lexical priority over the difference principle of vice-versa.]

entirely.) Thus the original position, and justice as fairness more generally, is not a concept that is immovably fixed in 1970s or 1990s America — we can interpret it in light of other developments in normative theory. In so doing we can develop both the concepts of reasonable basic structure and consider how it might be applied into stages beyond this. This paper proposes several simultaneous extensions to Rawls's thesis that are required for this analysis. One is to include non-human animals. A second is the explicit status of suffering and of death in Rawls's thesis.[77]

Rawls's 'Putting Aside' of Non-Human Animals and Suffering

Rawls is ambivalent and inconsistent in his consideration of non-human animals, but in general he appears to consider that human 'conduct towards animals is not regulated by these principles [of justice], or so it generally believed'.[78] His system, as he describes it, affords non-human animals no rights. This is effectively based on the idea that dates back through Christian and scholastic philosophy that because animals are incapable of justice, they cannot be recipients of it. Indeed, Rawls explicitly endorses the Christian view of animals as being legitimately used.[79]

Three basic conditions can be identified that all need to obtain to explain this exclusion. The first is that non-human animals are not included as hypothetical legislators in the original position. The OP is sometimes characterised as a place where representatives agree on a reasonable system. Animals cannot be contractors in the OP because they do not have a concept of justice. The second is that the contractors are legislating selfishly. A condition of the OP is that the representatives of each party have no direct concern for the interests of other parties. Human legislators contracting selfishly would not contract according to non-human interests. The third condition is that legislators know that they are representing the

---

[77] The position of the embryo and duties pertaining to creation are also not considered in Rawls. Rawls assumes a set population. Rawls does speculate that public law should 'properly regulate the institutions through which society reproduces itself'.- Presumably whether citizens are created is important for the society.

[78] Rawls, *op. cit.* note 71, p. 441.

[79] J. Rawls. 1993. *Political Liberalism.* New York: Columbia University Press.

interests of humans and not of non-humans. For Rawls this is based on a principle of reciprocity that being 'capable, to a certain minimum degree, of a sense of justice' is a necessary condition of receiving justice,[80] so that only '[t]hose who can give justice are owed justice'.[81]

Furthermore, Rawls's reflective equilibrium condition states that where principles conflict with intuitions, the OP should be redefined; and since he appears to consider it a shared intuition that non-human animals' interests should not be included in concerns of justice, it seems inevitable that his system would not include them, since if his system were somehow to afford interests to non-human animals, he would argue for further reformulation. This means that an argument to include animals' interests would not only have to refute the above conditions, but also assume different 'intuitive' principles,[82] at least enough to challenge the *a priori* exclusion of non-human interests as an unfair 'fix' of the structure of the OP.[83]

As well as not being concerned with non-human animals, Rawls does not explicitly consider suffering. He is concerned with 'primary goods', which are defined politically rather than in any other way. In fact Rawls is explicit that 'fair shares of primary goods are not intended as a measure of citizens' expected overall psychological well-being, or of their utility'[84] Rawls's writings may suggest that suffering is important in JAF only insofar as is contingently important for political activity. For example, he asserts that parties are not 'moved to protect only the material and physical desires of those they represent, say...for food and drink' but rather 'are trying to guarantee the political and social conditions for citizens to pursue their good'.[85] Thus it may be that avoiding suffering is valuable only insofar as to allow citizens to exercise the moral powers and cooperate in society.[86] Given the (theoretical) possibility that citizens could function

---

[80] J. Rawls. The Sense of Justice. *Philosophical Review* 1963; 72: 284.

[81] Rawls, *op. cit.* note 71, pp. 510'511.

[82] Or challenge either the reflective equilibrium condition.

[83] A similar criticism has been made of other aspects of Rawls's approach, e.g. by R.M. Hare. 1975. Rawls's Theory of Justice. In *Reading Rawls.* N. Daniels, ed. New York: Basic Books; B. Barry. 1973. *The Liberal Theory of Justice.* Oxford: Oxford University Press.

[84] Rawls, *op. cit.* note 79, pp. 187–188.

[85] *Ibid.*, 76.

[86] Rawls, *op. cit.* note 69, p. 58

politically while suffering, this suggests that JAF is not intrinsically concerned with suffering.[87]

Rawls also provides little guidance on matter of maintaining life more generally. He appears to assume a completely healthy population, and his theory of justice is applied only to 'normal, active and fully cooperating members of society'.[88] Life is presumably a basic need for a person and thus presumably contractors would consider some efforts to ensure citizens stay alive. Rawls does also argue in a passing comment on abortion that public law should 'show an appropriate respect for human life' (despite reiterating his argument against including comprehensive moral doctrines).[89] More specifically, Rawls's writings do not help us understand how JAF should value non-human life (beyond briefly commenting that Political Liberalism, with its idea of public reason, does not rule out as a reason the good of wildlife achieved by protecting its habitat[90]).

Before addressing non-human animals and suffering separately, it is useful to point out that Rawls does not deny that we have any duty to non-human animals or any duty regarding suffering or life. Given that humans generally appear to intuitively think that cruelty is to be avoided, for Rawls's account to reach reflective equilibrium, it must include, or at least not exclude, some duty of non-cruelty. Rawls indeed recognises that animal sentience and capabilities may necessitate 'duties of compassion and humanity'.[91] It is not clear whether he means wanton cruelty or the causation of unnecessary suffering, as cruelty has been defined legally in the UK.[92] But since it would be hard for contractors in the OP to legislate for citizens' mental states, it seems more likely that they would be

---

[87] We may suspect Rawls of a slight-of-hand in this matter, ensuring that his theory affords basic 'utility' without actually respecting it, perhaps due to an effort by Rawls to further distinguish his position from that of restricted utilitarianism, but this might be unfair and is, anyway, besides the point, since we argue below that this implicit inclusion or legitimate extension alters the Rawlsian position, if not Rawls's own opinion.

[88] Rawls, *op. cit* note 71, p. 168.

[89] Rawls, *op. cit.* note 69, p. 117.

[90] *Ibid.*, 152.

[91] Rawls, *op. cit.* note 71, p. 512.

[92] *Bernard v Evans* 1925 2 KB 794, defined cruelty as causing unnecessary suffering.

legislating against cruelty as defined in many democratic legislations, i.e. causing unnecessary suffering. However, as Regan argues, if duties (of justice) apply only to persons, which non-human animals are not, then it is inconsistent for duties of cruelty to apply to non-human animals.[93] It may be that, as this chapter argues, citizens have duties of justice to non-human animals. If not, then, as Regan argues, either the duty of non-cruelty must be excluded or both duties included in justice as fairness (this paper favouring the latter).

Extending JAF to Non-Human Animals and Suffering

Despite his own view endorsing the Christian view of animals as being legitimately used, Rawls recognised that 'some will not accept these values as alone sufficient to settle the case'.[94] He specifically pointed out that the question of what is owed to animals is one of the 'problems of extension' of JAF.[95] Thus, even from Rawls's perspective, it appears to be an open question whether and how animals can be included in JAF, which further work needs to evaluate. This section challenges the three basic conditions for the exclusion of non-human animals.[96]

To challenge the first condition that non-human animals are not included as hypothetical legislators in the original position, one might note that the original position uses representatives. Rawls's system of interpolation is a heuristic device to ascertain 'objective' principles, rather than an actual model of what should be done. As Rawls stated, 'the parties [in the OP] are artificial persons, merely inhabitants of our device of representation: they are characters who have a part in the play of our thought-experiment'.[97] There is no condition specified that representatives must be representative in the scientific, rather than political sense (i.e. they need

[93] T. Regan. 1983. *The Case for Anima Rights*. Berkeley: University of California Press: 167.

[94] Rawls, *op. cit.* note 79, p. 245.

[95] *Ibid*: 21.

[96] It is sufficient for anyone not to obtain for animals to be permissibly included.

[97] Rawls, *op. cit.* note 69, p. 83.

not be members of the class each represents). These representative characters can represent members of society that are not perfectly just. Indeed Rawls is at great pains to note that his theory is not entirely idealistic in its representation of a well-ordered society.[98] For example, one aspect of such a society is to promote any necessary values of justice,[99] which is an activity completely unnecessary if it applied only to just beings. This means that whether or not non-human animal are capable of justice, there is scope for them to have animal representatives that are capable of justice.

To deal with the second condition, Rawls takes it for granted, rather than proves or necessitates, not only that agents behind veil of ignorance would choose principles of justice that served their own interests; but that they would be so selfish. In fact, it might be better to avoid this selfishness, for example by positing a principle of equality in deliberations in the OP. Rowlands has applied this line of reasoning at some length to argue that Rawls's principle of equality, insomuch as it is meant to allot benefits/opportunities regardless of 'undeserved', morally-arbitrary differences, would mean that cognitive abilities are undeserved, hence equality should be extended to beings regardless of their rationality.[100]

One might challenge the third condition by arguing that it is arbitrary that the contract should apply only to humans. Rawls conflates legislators and recipients, but one can differentiate between legislators and subjects. Indeed, by definition representatives do not have strict identity with the subjects themselves — no actual humans perform any contracting. Kant could fall back upon metaphysical claims of *a priori* knowledge; but Rawls can make no such move, because the impartiality sought for by Rawls's methodology is not one of Platonic objectivity, but rather one of consensus, albeit an impartial consensus. So legislators and subjects cannot necessarily share the same properties. This is fortunate, since otherwise JAF would exclude those humans who are incapable of

---

[98] Rawls, *op. cit.* note 69, §3, pp. 8–9; §58–59, pp. 192–198.

[99] Rawls, *op. cit.* note 69, pp. 56, 146.

[100] M. Rowlands. 1998. *Animal Rights: A Philosophical Defence.* Basingtoke: Palgrave MacMillan.

justice.[101] This means that species-membership is just another of the 'contingencies which put "men" at odds' and, as Tom Regan has argued, '[t]o allow those in the original position to know what *species* they will belong to is to allow them knowledge no different in kind from allowing them to know what race or sex they will be. If knowledge of these latter details must be excluded by the veil of ignorance, in order to assure a fair procedure in the selection of principles of justice, then knowledge of the former detail must be excluded as well'.[102] To do otherwise risks that 'specific' contingencies 'tempt contractors to exploit social and natural circumstances to their own advantage'.

The reflective equilibrium condition can also be satisfied. Global 21st century intuitions are very different from those of 1970s America. They certainly appear more 'animal friendly', if only on the evidence of the introduction of the A(SP)A and the AWA. The intervening period has seen the work of ethicists, welfare scientists and animal-interest groups within and outside governments and internationally. This should at least entail that animal interests should not be excluded *a priori*. Indeed, there have been arguments that their interests should be included.[103]

One objection is worth considering. The idea of including animals opens the door for the inclusion of other beings — if animals, then why not plants, rocks, books? But in fact it does not matter. Those beings are included whose inclusion matters: those beings who have interests that can be represented. To be more precise, beings are included if it is relevant to them to be included. If they have no interests then their inclusion or exclusion is literally irrelevant, and their inclusion is relevant only to

[101] Rawls 'take[s] it as obvious, and accepted by common sense, that we have a duty towards all human beings, however severely handicapped' [Rawls, *op. cit.* note 69, p. 176] but he 'puts aside' the question of marginal humans that 'can never be normal contributing members of social cooperation' [Rawls, *op. cit.* note 69, p. 170]. He leaves it, along with the same task regarding non-human animals, as a future task for future researchers to 'see whether justice as fairness can be extended to provide guidelines for these cases; and if not, whether it [justice as fairness] must be rejected rather than supplemented by some other conception...as an essential complementary part' [Rawls, *op. cit.* note 69, p. 176].

[102] Regan *op. cit.* note 92, p. 171.

[103] E.g. D. VandeVeer. 1979. Of Beasts, Persons and the Original Position. *Monist* 62: 368–377.

the 'workload' of the parties in the OP. This group of represented beings includes, as a sufficient criterion, those that can suffer. As noted before, the requisite idea of suffering might need to be pluralistic, but it seems relatively uncontroversial that beings should be included if there is something that it would be desirable for them to avoid *per se*. This fits with our other consideration of suffering in JAF.

Having demonstrated the possibility (if not the necessity) of including non-human animals, we may turn to considering the omission from JAF as described by Rawls, of suffering. Rawls partly anticipated such an extension: 'Provided due precautions are taken, we can, if need be, expand the list [of primary goods] to include other goods, for example...certain mental states such as freedom from physical pain'.[104] Physical pain is, of course, one type of suffering (including as defined legally), and freedom from pain is, in animal welfare, an exemplar negative end.

In fact, it may be that concern for suffering is implicit rather than explicit in Rawls's approach. Rawls asserts that '[w]hat counts as primary goods depends...on various facts about human needs and abilities, their normal phases and requirements of nurture...and much else'[105] and he includes health care and public health measures ('if need be') in the index of primary goods.[106] In the quotation above, he describes parties as moved to protect political and social conditions and 'not...only' material and physical desires.[107] The primary good of freedom of movement and occupation is considered 'against a background of diverse opportunities, which opportunities allow the pursuit of a variety of ends'[108] and the primary good of income is to be 'understood as an all-purpose means...generally needed to achieve a wide range of ends whatever they may be'.[109] He assumes that human existence and the fulfilment of basic human needs and purposes are good'.[110] Here, note that, unlike primary goods, 'ends'

[104] Rawls, *op. cit.* note 79, pp. 181–182.

[105] Rawls, *op. cit.* note 69, p. 58.

[106] *Ibid.*, 172; J. Rawls. Fairness as Goodness. *Philosophical Review* 1975; 84: 536–555.

[107] Rawls, *op. cit.* note 79, p. 76, *emphases added.*

[108] Rawls, *op. cit.* note 69, p. 58.

[109] *Ibid.*, 58–59.

[110] *Ibid.*, 139.

and 'purposes' are not defined politically.[111] There is also evidence of Rawls bearing in mind a salient concept of utility, such as his suggestion that the adjustment of the minimum in restricted utility may be actually guided by the difference principle[112] and that 'in this case the utility principle does not offer a genuine alternative to the difference principle'.[113]

It is my contention that Rawls should include avoidance of suffering in his system. Contractors representing parties would be foolish to legislate for basic structures of legislation that caused significant suffering, even if they were concerned about a political subject. A central aspect of reasonable pluralism is that should allow agents to avoid what they will want to avoid — to fulfil their conditional desires to avoid negative ends. And since suffering is what is undesirable *per se*, it is something that they will want to avoid. This is a part of their liberty to achieve their own good, which is due political protection.[114] One may posit that in the OP parties will not know what will cause suffering, but an epistemic condition that parties do not know that those they represent will want to avoid suffering is absurd (and impossible to imagine). Firstly, such a condition would run contrary to the condition that parties are allowed commonsense knowledge, since knowledge of suffering is common knowledge. Secondly, such ignorance would be a contradiction anyway, if suffering is defined as above as being what one wants to avoid *per se* — to not know that one would want to avoid suffering is impossible.[115] To deny society's members the liberty to avoid their negative ends is to deny them half their liberty.

If JAF should include negative ends of suffering, it is an obvious extension for it to be concerned with whether a life is a LNWL. If primary goods should include the avoidance of suffering, as an end intrinsically

---

[111] It could also be argued that this political-apolitical distinction is fallacious, but the fact that the OP has epistemic conditions at least means that there is a distinction, albeit a synthetic one, between political (about which is known in the OP) and apolitical (about which OP parties are ignorant).

[112] Rawls, *op. cit.* note 71, §49, pp. 278–281.

[113] Rawls, *op. cit.* note 69, pp. 127–128 fn 47.

[114] Rawls, *op. cit.* note 79, pp. 337–378.

[115] Or possible only if one is epistemically incapable of beliefs about 'want' or 'avoid' and conditions that were to make the contractors incapable of such beliefs would make them incapable of legislating

worth avoiding, then it should include the avoidance of a LNWL, as something intrinsically worth avoiding. This fits with Rawls's derivation of primary goods from the idea of beings' 'life prospects' (their prospects over a complete life).[116] Such life prospects must include avoiding states worth avoiding. If life affords negative ends, then this provides a reason under JAF (though not necessarily a determinative one) against that life being continued. This position can fit with a positive instrumentalist value of life. Life is an 'all-purpose means...generally needed to achieve a wide range of ends whatever they may be' and should be respected when so.[117] When negative ends of avoiding suffering or a LWNL make life an *impediment* to fulfilling those ends, then life has a negative value and should be avoided.

Having established that JAF can — and indeed should — include non-human animals and suffering, it is apodictic that JAF would *at least* include the provisions currently in UK legislation to avoid unnecessary suffering in animals. This would allow the duty of cruelty to non-human animals specified by Rawls to be consistent with the rest of his thesis, thereby addressing the accusations of inconsistency described above. But as we have seen, this duty of cruelty is insufficient to preclude the systematic unfairness in the applications of stem cell therapies to non-human animals. Granting the inclusion of pain and suffering also allows us to explore in more detail the further requirements of JAF in terms of fairness between animals.[118]

---

[116] Rawls, *op. cit.* note 69, p. 40, see also *op. cit.* note 71, §16.

[117] Thus, instrumentally valuing life in JAF need not entail an absolute respect for life, or even an equal distribution of life, but should include its consideration in the overall calculation of liberty.

[118] It is not possible here to determine everything that contractors in the revised original position would legislate. It might be possible to argue for the application of principles of JAF other than the difference principle. For example, (in order of lexical priority), it might be possible to use the basic liberties to challenge ideas of property; use the principle of equal opportunity to ensure ability to perform motivated behaviours and it might be possible to ensure a maximin higher than LW0. It might also be the case that including non-human animals in the OP considerations would alter which principles are generated. For example, the two-way comparison between Rawls's two principles and restricted utilitarianism might be decided the other way around, in which case a utilitarian society would be legislated. (If this was the case, then the arguments of this thesis would largely pertain).

Non-Human Animal Suffering and the Difference Principle

One such detail explored in this section concerns the application of Rawls's maximin or Difference Principle.[119] While Rawls's thesis generated several concepts and principles (and some with higher lexical priority than this one), the analysis of this principle is especially relevant to consideration of non-humans in the laboratory and veterinary contexts. The difference principle, simplified is that 'the higher expectations of those better situated are just if and only if they work as part of a scheme which improves the expectations of the least advantaged members of society'.[120] Following on then, 'the maximin rule tells us to rank alternatives by their worst possible outcomes: we are to adopt the alternative the worst outcome of which is superior to the worst outcomes of the others'.[121]

It should be noted that the difference principle does not include any obvious reason why its likelihood of being adopted would change if non-human interest were included. If it is true[122] that contractors would rationally opt for a maximin distribution of resources if they were only anthropocentric, there seems no reason to believe that including the interests of non-human animals would change this.

The difference principle could be applied to a number of 'primary goods', either as adapted from Rawls, or using the list of capabilities provided by other theorists with similar ideas, such as Nussbaum.[123] These include life, except in the case of euthanasia; health; absence of cruelty and neglect; harsh treatment; avoidance of non-beneficial pain and

---

[119] These are slightly different in terms of conditions of application: the former is a matter of reciprocity; the latter a method for decisions under uncertainty. Because of the similarities in substance and the confusion between the two, as well as the uncertainty at what stage of the deliberative process these concepts would apply and how much information the contractors would have, the distinction is not important in this paper.

[120] Rawls, *op. cit.* note 71, p. 65.

[121] *Ibid.*, 133.

[122] It is of course not a necessary truth, and a matter of debate, whether such contractors would opt for a maximin distribution.

[123] M.C. Nussbaum. 2004. Beyond Compassion and Humanity: Justice for Non-Human Animals. In *Animal Rights: Current Debates and New Directions*. C.R. Sunstein & M.C. Nussbaum, eds. New York: Oxford University Press: 299–320.

control of their environment. This paper focuses on the one already addressed: the primary good of absence of suffering.

If the maximin rule was applied, it is posited here that it would preclude any being having a LNWL. It would certainly be irrational for any contractor to opt, *ceteris paribus*, to have a maximin that was lower than an indifferent life (a LW0). For any being, non-existence is by definition better than a LNWL. Thus, if on one system the least advantaged citizens would have a LNWL, then these citizens would be better off not existing. Thus for these citizens, a system or distribution of resources that involved their non-existence (even if that required everyone's non-existence) would fare better in a two-way comparison with a system in which some beings had a LNWL. Therefore legislators in the OP would be expected to contract to it in preference. This would occur in all two-way comparisons which involved some citizens suffering a LNWL. This would effectively elevate the maximin to the upper end of LNWL, i.e. LW0. (It of course would need further specification to determine whether the maximin would be LW0 or higher than this).[124] This relatively simple and obvious conclusion that JAF would not allow non-human animals to have a LNWL can now be applied to the two contexts with which we were originally concerned: the veterinary context and the laboratory context.

APPLICATION TO SCTs IN THE VETERINARY CONTEXT

The task of detailing how JAF would be applied to the veterinary context is an extension far beyond Rawls's thoughts. As well as not applying JAF

---

[124] An issue that this paper has ignored is whether the stem cells themselves might be worthy of respect under JAF. It is likely to come down to the definitions of individuals, parties, opportunities and existence. Rawls comments briefly on abortion and children, but he gives little guidance, since his ideas stem mainly from the act that human embryos might potentially become political citizens; the same is not true for non-human animals. The analysis of non-human embryos is therefore better deferred until the issue of human stem cells has been investigated. As a brief sketch, it seems not implausible that they might be included as represented parties, but that since embryos that are not allowed to develop cannot have a LWL, it might follow that their inclusion would entail that the maximin is no higher than a LW0, which, given the considerations in this thesis that it should be no lower, it would follow that the maximin across all contexts would be LW0.

to non-human animals (or marginal humans) or suffering, Rawls also originally failed to apply it to human medicine. He appeared to assume a healthy population of humans — as Daniels' noted, 'there is no distributive theory of healthcare because no-one is sick!'[125] But there is some, albeit limited, guidance on how veterinary treatment might be included in JAF. Daniels has worked out Rawlsian principles in more detail in *Just Health Care.*[126] Rawls himself gave some comments in *Political Liberalism.* Campbell, applying Rawls' principles, suggests that the first of Rawls's principles prevents any 'over-simplified emphasis on life-saving at any cost'[127] and, by considering also the difference principle, this can be extended very specifically to non-human animals.

One piece of guidance from Rawls is that the specifics of health care matters (for humans) are 'to be decided at the legislative stage and not in the original position or constitutional convention'.[128] This is not because justice as fairness is inappropriate for such matters, but because the application of the principles depends in part on the prevalence and severity of the various illnesses, which information is available only at the legislative stage.[129] Thus this application is not limited by epistemic conditions of the OP. This allows, for example, that the evaluation of whether a given test of a specific stem cell technology should consider the rarity and severity of the diseases in patients as well as the numbers, severity and duration of the suffering of the animals used.

One general question, given the status of animals in society, is the extent to which principles of JAF can legitimately interfere with the human-animal relationships. All we can say here is that perhaps some human-animal relationships should not be *entirely* based on justice as fairness. A useful analogy here in the companion animal context might be with family-life given the treatment of pets as family-members. In this context, Rawls argued that 'we wouldn't want political principles of

[125] N. Daniels. 1985. *Just Health Care*. Cambridge: Cambridge University Press: 43.
[126] *Ibid.*
[127] A. V. Campbell *et al.* 2001. *Medical Ethics*. Oxford: Oxford University Press: 251.
[128] Rawls, *op. cit.*, note 69, p. 173.
[129] *Ibid.*, 173.

justice to apply directly to the internal life of the family. It is hardly sensible that as parents we be required to treat our children in accordance with political principles'.[130] Similarly, animal owners cannot and should not always be thinking as hypothetical contractors. But, it does not follow that JAF is irrelevant to human-animal relationships.

> 'A domain so-called, or a sphere of life, is not then, something already given apart from principles of justice...If the so-called private sphere is a space alleged to be exempt from justice, then there is no such thing...political liberalism...does not regard the political and the non-political domains as two separate, disconnected spaces, as it were, each governed solely by its own distinct principles. Even if the basic structure alone is the primary subject of justice, principles of justice still put essential restrictions on the family and all other associations'.[131]

So, 'the prohibitions of abuses and the neglect of children, and much else, will, as constraints, be a vital part of family law'.[132] It might further be considered that animals in less family-like relationships, such as sports and farmed animals, should be under tighter constraints. The activity of veterinary surgeons is also not a family-like relationship, and so might come under tighter control.

The principles of justice as fairness would prescribe that all animals should have a guaranteeable minimum opportunity. For pets, this should be regardless of their 'actual social position' and their owners' 'fortune in the distribution of assets'. Racehorses should similarly have a minimum level regardless of their 'actual fortune in the distribution of abilities', i.e. their performance. More generally, animals should have a guaranteeable level regardless of context and species, to ensure intra-contextual and intra-specific fairness.

---

[130] *Ibid.*, 165.
[131] *Ibid.*, 166.
[132] *Ibid.*, 165.

The difference principle would entail that no animal should be afforded a LNWL, even if that provides significant benefits to their owner. Stem cell therapies cannot be legitimately used to provide further companionship for an animal's owner, increase performance of sports animals or increase productivity of farmed animals, if that requires the animal having a LNWL.[133] Animals with diseases should be euthanatised if the treatment cannot avoid their having a LNWL. This is in accordance with the AWA, but explicit assessment is not always performed. A major fear with novel therapies is that they are implemented by clinicians enthusiastic about the novelty and progress, rather than about the interests of the animal itself. Since animals must, ceteris paribus, be killed if they are suffering, yet veterinary interventions may extend life, legitimate veterinary interventions should ensure that the animal's life is better than non-existence. Veterinary interventions, or at least those that extend life, should be ones that provide the animal with at least a LWL. Even if they may cause momentary or minor pain, the life they give the animal should be worth living.

These conclusions in the veterinary context seem intuitive and relatively uncontroversial. In fact, they are more radical than it immediately appears. The difference principle applied to an owner-animal dyad entails that if one animal is worse off than its owner already, then a vet cannot make it worse off to benefit the owner. Thus animals that are worse off than their owners cannot fairly be further disadvantaged to the benefit of the latter. Indeed, their lives should be improved *at whatever cost* to their better-off owners. The same principle would apply in the same way to animals and consumers — farm animals cannot be disadvantaged to advantage consumers, unless those consumers are originally worse-off, perhaps in cases of extreme poverty.

The application of the difference principle on a micro-scale may have an even more radical conclusion in the veterinary context if one believes that many animals, especially intensively farmed chickens, turkeys, ducks, pigs and fish, experience lives that are not worth living. If this is the case, then these animals should not exist at all.

[133] Unless perhaps in some situations where the owner's life is also LWNL, and worse than the animal's and cannot be euthanatised, and the animal is necessary to keep them from having an even lower quality of life.

APPLICATION TO APPLIED STEM CELL RESEARCH IN LABORATORY CONTEXT

The use of non-human animals in the development and testing of stem cells therapies and products intended for use on humans or in the veterinary context can be informed by the above. This might ensure that all living animals are provided with a LWL as a minimum, whatever the benefits, and/or that harms to the animals should be meaningfully compensated as well as possible. No laboratory animal should be caused a LNWL. Any animal that is suffering should be treated or euthanatised even if that means that the experiment is useless.

This would involve the refinement of studies to use anaesthetised animals instead of conscious animals, and the replacement of animals with clinical trials, computer models and tissue cultures, including stem cells lines. Stem cells have a LW0, and so are 'better off' than living animals suffering a LNWL. This lends extra import to recent work suggesting a scope for the 'farming' of stem cell products from non-human animals. Pigs stem cell lines might be cultured *in vivo* or *in vitro* for tissues or organs for transplantation.[134] This may allow the development of products such as ß-cells to produce insulin,[135] or even the development of stem cell products that do not use non-human products. The use of stem cells may decrease the use of non-human animal subjects in the laboratory context. For example, the use of human embryonic stem cells either *in vitro*, as described by Jiang *et al.*,[136] or *in vivo*, as described by Kroon *et al.*,[137] would decrease the requirement for animals as a source of insulin. Stem cells therefore provide an excellent opportunity to decrease the unfair

---

[134] V. Hall. Porcine Embryonic Stem Cells: A Possible Source for Cell Replacement Therapy. *Stem Cell Reviews* 2008; 4: 275–282.

[135] A.M. Holland & E.G. Stanley. Stem Cells and the Price of Immortality. *Stem Cell Research* 2009; 2: 26–28; E.E. Baetge. Production of Beta-Cells from Human Embryonic Stem Cells. *Diabetes, Obesity and Metabolism* 2008; 10(S4): 186–194.

[136] E. Jiang *et al. In Vitro* Derivation of Functional Insulin-Producing Cells from Human Embryonic Stem Cells. *Cell Research* 2007; 17: 333–344.

[137] E. Kroon *et al.* Pancreatic Endoderm Derived from Human Embryonic Stem Cells Generates Glucose-Responsive Insulin-Secreting Cells *In Vivo*. *Nature Biotechnology* 2008; 26: 443–452.

suffering of animals by replacement and, on this analysis at least, qualms about the status of the human embryo should not be legitimate cause to allow millions of animals to suffer. An embryo without basic neural structures cannot suffer, and therefore *ceteris paribus* cannot have a life worth living. Its life is always — from the embryo's experiential perspective at least — a LW0.[138]

Such a basic justice would risk foregoing significant benefits to humans (and other animals). If clinical trials were performed without a reduction in the amount of prior animal-testing that causes suffering currently, then fewer human patients might be given efficacious drugs or even riskier drugs, since the current testing, even if it has little value, at least has some. But, it should need no explanation that under JAF the benefits to other subjects would not legitimise keeping any subjects with a LNWL, any more than any other system which lowered the maximum for the benefit of any better-advantaged citizens. It would also follow that, unless there is a principle that overrides the Difference Principle, the use of *human* stem cells should be used instead of live animals.

The conclusions so far do not mean that animal subjects can never be caused short periods of suffering. If subjects are considered as individuals extended in stages through a lifetime, then short periods of LNWL might be balanced by periods of LWL. This would effectively be a refinement, but one focusing not on lessening pain but on increasing positive experiences as counterbalance. This is likely to be acceptable in the OP, since it would be rational to prefer such an existence to non-existence. If benefiting the better-advantaged subjects also benefited the least-advantaged, then benefits to the better-advantaged might be sought. Indeed, this would be necessary for the maximum to obtain. This would be completely in accordance with Rawls's approach and would better reflect the origins of the cost-benefit analysis used. Animals therefore could be used to benefit other animals or humans, but they would need to be compensated for this use. Effectively, they could be treated as means but not *merely* as means.

[138] This is not to say it is completely worthless *per se*.

Before we can bring these conclusions to a close, one objection needs to be considered both for this paper, and because it throws light on the issues of human euthanasia and nativity. The objection might run that if animals could be killed and humans couldn't (as per the legal status quo), then this would lead to different maximums for humans and non-human animals. Non-human animals would have a maximum of the value of non-existence because they could be euthanised below this point; but humans who could suffer such a life and not be euthanised, would have a lower maximum, i.e. a LNWL. This would suggest that the minimum is that of the least-advantaged human being. In order to raise this minimum to the maximum possible, it might be necessary to have some non-human animals with a LNWL in order to elevate that of the worst-off human with a LNWL that cannot be terminated. Of course, this objection would have to be argued in some way that did not mean that the humans are kept alive for their own good — since otherwise the account would be arguing that they have a LWL. Rather, it would have to be due to external reasons, such as the societal benefits of not killing. This objection if successful would allow the suffering of non-human animals for the benefit of those suffering humans.

This paper does not refute this objection, since it has specifically left open the question of whether life may have intrinsic value, and there are myriad reasons against human euthanasia.[139] More humbly, it points out only that the objection is not as potent as it sounds, once certain anthropocentric assumptions are removed. Even if the objection is granted, there are four considerations that still would radically change how animals are used in stem cell laboratories.

Firstly, the thesis of the paper, even if corrected to allow for this scenario, would still mean that non-humans could not be given worse lives than humans except if it so happened contingently that the best society was one in which it was a non-human animal's life that ended up

[139] One possible response worth mentioning is that if humans were allowed to be euthanatised if they suffered a LNWL, then this would re-elevate the maximin to at least LW0. Indeed, this might be mandatory, if the difference principle is to be applied thoroughly. This could provide a robust Rawlsian argument for active euthanasia of humans. It is not, however, the intention of this paper to answer this question.

least-advantaged. This would still represent an improvement for animals, since it would prevent their suffering the more serious harms that give them lives far worse than those of the worst-off human.

Secondly, this would not affect situations where humans are not killed but die. Causing animals a LWNL in order to keep humans alive would not be justified because the LNWL would be worse than non-existence. Therefore research for disease *cures* is not necessarily affected by these objections, but only research for palliative care. Given that most research is done on saving and extending lives (and comparatively little on palliative care), this would have a massive impact on what is allowed. In fact, given the legality of the Doctrine of Double Effect in UK law, and the general anaesthetics and analgesics available, this may mean no further testing, since suffering humans could be anaesthetised in preference to animal suffering.

Thirdly, this does not undermine the position that it is unfair to cause one animal a LNWL in order to benefit another non-human animal, however much benefit there is for the more-advantaged non-human animal. Causing laboratory animals to suffer a LNWL in order to improve the lives of companion animals or competition horses in the veterinary context is unjust.

Fourthly, this thesis would still argue for the use of stem cells and oocyte-chimeras, instead of live animal models. This includes human stem cells and it is unfair to mandate the suffering of animals that are already probably the worst off in preference to using embryonic stem cells, which ostensibly have at most a LW0, especially when this is at the behest of, and for the benefit of, healthy adult humans who are generally better off than animals.

9

ONTOLOGICAL STATUS OF HUMAN–NON-HUMAN EMBRYONIC CHIMERAS

Josef Kuře

INTRODUCTION: FROM THE MYTHOLOGICAL CHIMERA, TO THE CHIMERA IN BIOMEDICAL RESEARCH

Introductory Remarks

The possibility to transcend the limits of human life by transgressing species barriers has been a continuous fascination in human fantasy and a challenging human venture since antiquity. At present, this archetypical endeavour has been potentiated by biomedical research involving the creation of various combinations of human and non-human — mostly animal — entities. The goals for creation of such mixed entities called chimeras, hybrids, cybrids, mosaics, and the like, is the acquisition of new knowledge in the area of developmental biology and in basic research, with future applications in medicine. One area is the development of regenerative therapies using stem cells. The aim of this research is the development of cell and tissue replacement therapies for accidental damage and disease conditions, which are not treatable by the methods of contemporary medicine. Thus, there is significant justification for this kind of research; for if research on human-animal (embryonic stem cells) mixtures meets its expected goals, it would mean not only a gain of knowledge in developmental biology, which probably cannot be obtained by other means, but also a tremendous advance in clinical medicine. However, the public and the scientific community are not unified regarding the creation of human–non-human chimeras.[1] Indeed, the creation of entities that are mixtures of humans and animals does raise many moral concerns. These concerns are reflected in the governance of these novel entities, which challenge traditional categories and common conceptual tools, such as our notions of 'human' and 'animal'. With respect to the ontological status of 'human' and 'animal', this challenge is reflected in the social-legal demands arising from such categorisations.

In this chapter, I do not intend to provide a normative ethics of chimeras (i.e. what *ought* to be done with respect to such entities). Instead, I focus on the clarification of the ontological status of these novel entities created by present biotechnologies, from which the prescriptive judgements may follow. I argue that these entities do not fit completely into our traditional semantic scope: we have some common understanding of what is 'human' and what is an 'animal', but we do not have an established semantics and common conceptual understanding for these novel entities. In addition, the types, levels and rates of chimera crossovers are very distinct, and they naturally have to be taken into account; regulators, if they are to avoid ambiguity, have to distinguish if these mixtures are created at cellular, tissue or organ level; or if they are mixed species or subspecies crossbreeds. Furthermore they also have to consider the importance of the proportions of cells coming from human and animal, or whether the stage of their (biological) development makes any difference. All these diversities and complexities make ethical reasoning and regulatory assessment even more difficult should we not accept some dogmatic assumption of 'all-or-nothing' with respect to novel entities.[2]

So, in the first instance, the broader cultural context, scientific state of the art, and terminology used in this area, should be made clear. Since the clarification of the ontological status is necessary for any ethical considerations and appraisal (moral status), this chapter is an exploration of the ontological status of human–animal chimera(s). Not all possible combinations of human–non-human mixtures will be investigated. The emphasis

---

[1] Cf. N. DeWitt. Biologists Divided Over Proposal to Create Human-Mouse Embryos. *Nature* 2002; 420: 255.

[2] Cf. D. DeGrazia. Moral Status As a Matter of Degree? *The Southern Journal of Philosophy* 2008; 46: 188–190 and 195–196.

will be on the embryonic form of human-animal chimeras; especially as they appear in human embryonic stem cell (hESC) research. I begin from the presupposition that any ethical discussion is based on our ontological and (philosophical) anthropological hermeneutics. Rather than use the language of *moral* status, I use the concept of *ontological* status, because, as I will argue, before we make any moral statement regarding these new entities, we need clarity in knowing *what* we are talking about, and specifically, what a biotechnological chimera *is*. Only when we know what a chimera of this kind is, or more precisely, how it relates to all the various types and forms of chimeras there are, can we then discuss what our normative attitudes to these entities should be. Accordingly, we are then in a position to make an ethical assessment in respect to the creation and the use of these chimeras in biomedical research. Thus, this investigation of the ontological status of chimeras is a precondition for ethics of using chimeras in research.

The Mythological Chimera

The ideas of 'mixed creatures' — part human, and part animal — and the possibility of crossing-traditional human species boundaries have fascinated and influenced societies for thousands of years. In the mythology of ancient Egypt, Greece, and Rome, for example, there exist creatures such as the Centaur (man-horse mixture), Minotaur (man-bull mixture), Mermaid (woman-fish mixture), Harpy (woman-bird mixture), Pegasus (horse-eagle mixture), Griffin (eagle-lion mixture), Basilisk (cock-snake mixture) and Pan[3] (man-goat mixture). In Ancient Egypt and in Hindu religion, the majority of deities were mixtures of man and animal. Such mixed creatures are well known also in Asian and American cultures.[4]

[3] Pan (Παν) was the God of Shepherds (archaic 'pasture god'): a man with hindquarters, legs, and horns of a goat.

[4] There is a plenitude of human-animal and animal-animal chimeras in all world mythologies. The chimera, as a mixed creature, is one of the basic ideas on which the world mythologies are grounded. See: R. Willis, ed. 1993. *World Mythology*. New York: H. Holt; E.M. Thury & M.K. Devinney. 2005. *Introduction to Mythology: Contemporary Approaches to Classical and World Myths*. New York: Oxford University Press; M. Mayer. 2006. *Legendary Creatures of Myth and Magic*. New York: Madison Park Press.

These creatures were accepted as being *sui generis* and endowed with specific powers. Although not having been considered as being part of the human species, they were neither seen as being entirely animal. Their nature has been regarded as a composition of human and animal features ('natures'), human and divine features, or of animal and divine features. All chimeric mixtures in history and in world cultures bear witness to the ambition of human beings to extend their existing possibilities, and combine the outstanding qualities of different entities into a single creature of surpassing power. Indeed, their distinct and solitary status in mythology — for example, the primordial Greek mythological Chimera (Χιμαιρα) was a fire-breathing horrifying creature — resulted in them being sometimes rejected as (too) different and abhorrent; and often they were portrayed as lonely monsters.[5]

Beside mythology, chimeras also appear in music, games, logic, computing, and architecture.[6] A significant revival of the chimera concepts can be observed in literature, especially in the contemporary fiction and fantasy stories (e.g. the many distinct characters to be found in J. K. Rowlings' 'Harry Potter' series).

Chimera in Biomedical Research

In spite of their sometimes-terrible, mythological nature, chimeras did not lose their magnetism, but, as an archetypical form, they retained our

---

[5] Ancient chimeras would be called more properly hybrids, i.e. offspring of different species. However the ancient Greeks would probably be horrified by the term 'hybrids' (see note 55 in this chapter). The term 'Χιμαιρα' was reserved to the creature which was the mixture of different animal species (lion, goat, and snake), who was of divine origin, and had a deterrent nature — causing harm (breathing fire and devastating land) and who was finally slain by Bellerophon (with a help of another chimera).

[6] In the Middle Ages, all kinds of mixed creatures — fantastic, mythical or grotesque figures — were used in architecture for the ornamentation of churches in particular serving as gargoyles to scare away bad ghosts, having the practical function, as termination of spouts, to convey water from the roof away from the sides of buildings (e.g. chimeras at the Notre Dame in Paris). In modern architecture, chimeras or chimeric modes are used as cross-categorical couplings which transform the initial system into a system with completely new identity — on the base of affinities.

fascination over the centuries. And they remain a popular curiosity in the 21st century; although it is their utility, rather than human transcendence, which interests us.[7] In this section, a summary of the scientific state of the art with regards to human-animal embryonic chimeras will be presented. The aim of this summary is not to provide a state-of-the-art scientific overview, but to demonstrate the immense diversity of both already undertaken experiments, and possible future developments.

The intentions of scientists and physicians in generating human-animal mixtures are diverse. Some lines of research, such as studies of the embryology or ontogeny of mammals, serve to answer questions in basic biology. Others search more for clinical applications, such as regenerative medicine.[8] For studying human embryology and development, scientists transplant stem cells (SCs) from humans into embryonic or adult animals. These SCs can be derived from early embryos, and therefore they are pluripotent (so-called embryonic stem cells, or ES cells, that can differentiate into any of the cells of the mature being). They also can be derived from later embryonic-foetal stages with a pluripotent capacity. SCs are also present in some adult tissues, although they possibly exhibiting less developmental capacity — or multipotency (e.g. limited to specific cell lineages, such as neuronal stem cells).[9] This science is rich with examples of human-animal combinations. In clinical settings, human tumour cells are transferred routinely into immune-compromised mice in order to study their growth characteristics and to assess the therapeutic options.[10] In reproductive medicine, the techniques to investigate male fertility problems routinely involves the creation of animal-human mixtures, i.e. human sperm quality has been tested by its ability to penetrate hamster

---

[7] Cf. E. Bazopoulou-Kyrkanidou. Chimeric Creatures in Greek Mythology and Reflections in Science. *American Journal of Medical Genetics* 2001; 100: 66–80.

[8] Cf. F. Baylis & A. Fenton. Chimera Research and Stem Cell Therapies for Human Neurodegenerative Disorders. *Cambridge Quarterly of Health Care* 2007; 16: 195–208.

[9] Cf. A.G. Smith. Embryo-Derived Stem Cells: Of Mice and Men. *Annual Review of Cell and Developmental Biology* 2001; 17: 435–462.

[10] Cf. Summary, Conclusions and Recommendations. 2009. In *Chimbrids. Chimeras and Hybrids in Comparative European and International Research — Scientific, Ethical, Philosophical and Legal Aspects.* J. Taupitz & M. Weschka, eds. Berlin: Springer: 435.

eggs.[11] Cloning experiments have involved methods where animal host embryos are used for the transfer of human nuclei. In attempts to study the role of human genes in physiology and pathophysiology, single genes or whole chromosomes are transferred into early animal embryos, and the effect of the additional gene(s) is studied in the resulting transgenic or transchromosomic animals. The same technology is employed for the production of human proteins in farm animals for pharmaceutical purposes. Such genetically altered animals may also be created to serve as donors for the transplantation of organs into human patients, a procedure called xenotransplantation.[12] Such experiments and tests, although objectionable for some, serve a scientific purpose. However, there are other comparably contentious techniques of mixing human and animal embryos or gametes which are feasible but, as yet, are of no scientific interest.[13]

One of the many ways to generate (inter-species) chimera is the production of transgenic animals. Developed in 1981,[14] the technology involves introducing the genes of one mammal species into the zygotes of another. This technology has yielded thousands of chimeric animal models. Furthermore, employing the semantic presupposition that a chimera is an individual whose body contains different cell populations derived from different zygotes of the same or different species (discussed further below), intra-species chimeras occur in nature frequently. In fact, every mammal, including each human, is a (micro) chimera, since the maternal cells that circulate in the foetus can still be found in the adult organism.[15] Numerous intra-species human chimeras have been created by allogenic

[11] R. Yanagimachi, H. Yanagimachi & B.J. Rogers. The Use of Zona-Free Animal Ova as a Test System for the Assessment of the Fertilizing Capacity of Human Spermatozoa. *Biology of Reproduction* 1976; 15: 471–476.

[12] *Ibid.*

[13] Cf. Summary, Conclusions and Recommendations. 2009. In *Chimbrids. Chimeras and Hybrids in Comparative European and International Research — Scientific, Ethical, Philosophical and Legal Aspects.* J. Taupitz & M. Weschka, eds. Berlin: Springer: 437.

[14] K. Harbers, D. Jähner & R. Jaenisch. Microinjection of Cloned Retroviral Genomes into Mouse Zygotes: Integration and Expression in the Animal. *Nature* 1981; 293: 540–542.

[15] S. Maloney *et al.* Microchimerism of Maternal Origin Persists into Adult Life. *The Journal of Clinical Investigation* 1999; 104; 41–47.

blood transfusion between humans (such as through cord blood donation to treat blood diseases). Other examples of intra-species chimeras are common medical procedures, such as solid organ transplantation, bone marrow transplantation, and injection of stem cells into humans. While spontaneous chimerism in non-human mammals (e.g. chimeric cattle) is not exceptional, spontaneous human chimerism occurs extremely rarely. It implies the presence of two genetically different cell lines not only in cells of the blood and lymphatic system, but also in solid tissues.

> 'Spontaneous human chimerism can result from events like:
>
> — aggregation of two non-identical twin embryos in early stage of development;
> — suppression of second meiotic division and fertilisation of secondary oocyte and first polar body;
> — fertilisation of ovum and first/second polar body;
> — fertilisation of first two mitotic products of unfertilised ovum;
> — fusion of one mitotic product of fertilised ovum with second polar body; and
> — suppression of second meiotic division and fertilisation of secondary oocyte'.[16]

Conversely, inter-species chimeras, not occurring naturally, have only been artificially generated for scientific purposes. Usually specific technology is needed in order to generate inter-specific chimera in this way. Historically 'probably the first inter-species human chimera was a boy who got a blood infusion from a lamb in 1667 by Jean-Baptiste Denys and who survived this procedure'.[17] In 1931, Paul Niehans developed a method of creating human inter-species chimeras by injecting

---

[16] R. Schreiner, R. Klose & E. Wolf. 2009. Xenotransplantation — Aspects of Chimerism. In *Chimbrids. Chimeras and Hybrids in Comparative European and International Research — Scientific, Ethical, Philosophical and Legal Aspects.* J. Taupitz & M. Weschka, eds. Berlin: Springer: 489.

[17] M. Bader, R. Schreiner & E. Wolf. 2009. Scientific Background. In *Chimbrids. Chimeras and Hybrids in Comparative European and International Research — Scientific, Ethical, Philosophical and Legal Aspects.* J. Taupitz & M. Weschka, eds. Berlin: Springer: 22–23.

foetal or juvenile lamb cells into humans as anti-aging therapy ('Frischzellentherapie').[18]

At the embryonic level, the first intra-species chimeric animals, which were artificially generated by the fusion of two preimplantation embryos (called morula aggregation), were created in mice in the early 1960s.[19] Since then, the technique has been extended to different micro-surgical techniques (e.g. injection of embryonic stem cells into embryos at the blastocyst stage), and to other combinations, such as embryonic cells with teratocarcinoma cells, embryonic cells with other embryonic cells, embryonic cells with primordial germ cells, and embryonic cells with embryonic stem cells.[20] In the early 1970s, the first inter-species chimeras were produced by this technique. It is now possible to create inter-species chimeras between different mouse species, and bovine species, between mouse and rat, and sheep and goat.[21] The latest development in the use of this technology to generate chimeras can be found in embryonic stem cell science. Although first attempted using mouse blastocysts, it can also be used in other mammals, including humans. These cells 'are pluripotent and can be integrated into all tissues when injected into embryos of adult animals creating high expectations for their use in regenerative medicine'.[22]

---

[18] Cf. P. Niehans. 20 Years of Cellular Therapy. *Medizinische Klinik* 1952; 47: 1–16. Cited from M. Bader, R. Schreiner & E. Wolf. 2009. Scientific Background. In *Chimbrids. Chimeras and Hybrids in Comparative European and International Research — Scientific, Ethical, Philosophical and Legal Aspects.* J. Taupitz & M. Weschka, eds. Berlin: Springer: 23.

[19] Cf. A.K. Tarkowski. Mouse Chimeras Developed from Fused Eggs. *Nature* 1961; 190: 857–860.

[20] Cf. R. Schreiner, R. Klose & E. Wolf. 2009. Xenotransplantation — Aspects of Chimerism. In *Chimbrids. Chimeras and Hybrids in Comparative European and International Research — Scientific, Ethical, Philosophical and Legal Aspects.* J. Taupitz & M. Weschka, eds. Berlin: Springer: 489–490.

[21] Cf. M. Bader, R. Schreiner & E. Wolf. 2009. Scientific Background. In *Chimbrids. Chimeras and Hybrids in Comparative European and International Research — Scientific, Ethical, Philosophical and Legal Aspects.* J. Taupitz & M. Weschka, eds. Berlin: Springer: 23.

[22] *Ibid.*

With the generation of human embryonic stem cells in 1998,[23] the creation of animal-human chimeras has become an interest for research, and prospective therapy. This research could help us to extend our knowledge in developmental biology[24] and in basic research, and therefore could lead to the development of future therapies for many severe diseases. Many scientists consider research using human-animal chimeras to be indispensable for answering fundamental questions in stem cell research.[25] Experiments in embryonic chimeras are expected to become helpful tools to clarify, in particular, the following:

— the process of human embryonic stem cell differentiation;
— the regulation of differentiation *in vivo* (with regard to the research cloning);
— to test human embryonic stem cell pluripotency *in vivo*;
— to create animals carrying organs of human tissue as donor animals for transplantation (i.e. to develop "humanised organs"[26] as an alternative to xenotransplantation); and
— to create *in vivo* models for drug and toxicological testing.[27]

Research proposals, involving the creation of animal-human embryonic chimeras with the aim to study differentiation of human stem cells,

---

[23] J.A. Thompson *et al.* Embryonic Stem Cell Lines Derived from Human Blastocysts. *Science* 1998; 282: 1145–1147.
[24] Cf. A. McLaren. 1976. *Mammalian Chimeras.* New York: Cambridge University Press; P.P. Tam & J. Rossant. Mouse Embryonic Chimeras: Tools for Studying Mammalian Development. *Development* 2003; 130: 6155–6163.
[25] Cf. I. Hyun *et al.* Ethical Standards for Human-to-Animal Chimera Experiments in Stem Cells Research. *Stem Cell* 2007; 1: 159–163.
[26] Cf. S.P. Westphal. 2003. "Humanised" Organs Can Be Grown in Animals. *New Scientist.* Available at: http://www.newscientist.com/article/dn4492-humanised-organs-can-be-grown-in-animals.html [Accessed 12 February 2009].
[27] Cf. R. Schreiner, R. Klose & E. Wolf. 2009. Xenotransplantation — Aspects of Chimerism. In *Chimbrids. Chimeras and Hybrids in Comparative European and International Research — Scientific, Ethical, Philosophical and Legal Aspects.* J. Taupitz & M. Weschka, eds. Berlin: Springer: 492.

gives rise to many ethical considerations, such as crossing or transgressing species boundaries, 'unnaturalness', the moral status of embryo, and animal suffering.[28] Furthermore, the ethics transgresses into many aspects of scientific and social interactions, such as the patenting of procedures and technologies and justice in access to modern therapeutics.[29]

One can highlight the ethical dimension of this kind of research by recalling a research publication which described the engraftment of human neural stem cells into the brains of old world monkey embryos.[30] This experiment combined a number of critical issues in animal-human chimera ethics: the cell populations were transplanted at an early stage of development, resulting in widespread migration and distribution of foreign cells. Significantly, the pluripotent human stem cells were found in the brain (the cognitive abilities of resulting chimera might no longer

---

[28] Cf. M. Green *et al.* Ethics: Moral Issues of Human–Non-Human Primate Neural Grafting. *Science* 2005; 309: 385–386; Scottish Council on Human Bioethics. 2006. *Embryonic, Fetal and Post-Natal Animal-Human Mixtures: An Ethical Discussion.* Available at: http://www.schb.org.uk [Accessed 2 February 2009]; F. Baylis & J.S. Robert. Part-Human Chimeras: Worrying the Facts, Probing the Ethics. *American Journal of Bioethics* 2007; 7: 41–45; Human Fertilisation and Embryology Authority. 2007. *A Consultation on the Ethical and Social Implications of Creating Human/Animal Embryo in Research. Hybrids and Chimeras.* Available at: http://www.hfea.gov.uk [Accessed 2 February 2009]; BioCentre: The Centre for Bioethics and Public Policy. 2007. *The New Inter-Species Future? An Ethical Discussion of Embryonic, Fetal and Post-Natal Human–Non-Human Combinations.* Available at: http://www.bioethics.ac.uk [Accessed 8 January 2009]; The Danish Council of Ethics. 2008. *Human-Animal Crossbreeds. Man or Mouse? Ethical Aspects of Chimera Research.* Available at: http://www.etiskraad.dk/sw293.asp [Accessed 2 February 2009].

[29] Cf. R.M.T. Iwasaka. From Chakrabarty to Chimeras: The Growing Need for Evolutionary Biology in Patent Law. *The Yale Law Journal* 2000; 109: 1505–1534; D.B. Resnik. Patents on Human-Animal Chimeras and Threats to Human Dignity. *The American Journal of Bioethics* 2003; 3: 35–36; E. Check. Biotech Critic Tries to Sew Up Research On Chimaeras. *Nature* 2003; 421: 4; W.B. Hurlbut. Patenting Humans: Clones, Chimeras, and Biological Artifacts. *Science and Engineering Ethics* 2005; 11: 21–29; S. Rabin. The Human Use of Humanoid Beings: Chimeras and Patent Law. *Nature Biotechnology* 2006; 24: 517–519.

[30] V. Ourednik *et al.* Segregation of Human Neural Stem Cells in the Developing Primate Forebrain. *Science* 2001; 293: 1820–1824.

fit known categories) and the germ line (the resulting chimera might be able to produce human sperm or eggs) of the primate.[31]

> 'As the two species (human and old world monkey) are closely related, anatomical and physiological barriers to successful and consequence-bearing chimerism are low. For example, it is very unlikely that the structural complexity needed for any significant degree of humanlike mental capacity can be achieved under tight size limitations, e.g. in the skull of a mouse'.[32]

As a result of this research, some researchers began speculating about human-chimpanzee chimeras called humanzees (humanised animals or animalised humans). Would these chimeras be members of the specie *Homo sapiens* or of an animal species, neither of them, or both of them? Then, one might speculate, some fundamental questions would arise, such as the question of whether such a creature would enjoy 'human' rights, or if a humanzee would have to pass some kind of 'humanness' test to get its liberties. Some opponents may argue that we risk undermining our own integrity as biological species in the name of human progress; although it is probable that repeating the humanzee experiment is not a project that many researchers want to try, or one that would get support from an ethical review board given its questionable scientific merits and the moral concerns.

In animal breeding, successful generation of interspecific chimeras developing to adulthood has been conducted in the 1980s. These interspecific chimeras included combinations of *Mus musculus* X *Mus caroli*,[33]

---

[31] Recently the Guidelines of International Society for Stem Cell Research (ISSCR) have explicitly prohibited the interbreeding of animals likely to harbour human gametes and recommended experiments likely to result in extensive animal-human chimerism of the brain or the germline to be permitted only after strict SCRO review (Stem Cell Research Overview) — G. Daley *et al.* The ISSCR Guidelines for Human Embryonic Stem Cell Research. *Science* 2007; 315: 603–604.

[32] R. Schreiner, R. Klose & E. Wolf. 2009. Xenotransplantation — Aspects of Chimerism. In *Chimbrids. Chimeras and Hybrids in Comparative European and International Research — Scientific, Ethical, Philosophical and Legal Aspects.* J. Taupitz & M. Weschka, eds. Berlin: Springer: 493.

[33] J. Rossant. Interspecific Chimeras in Mammals: Successful Production of Live Chimeras Between Mus Musculus and Mus Caroli. *Science* 1980; 208: 419–421.

Bos taurus X *Bos indicus* and goat X sheep ('geep'); the latter resulted from the injection of caprine cells of the inner cell mass into ovine blastocysts and subsequent transfer to ovine recipients.[34]

To date, a number of human–non-human embryonic and foetal chimeras have been generated (although none were designed to be developed to the stages of independent life): mouse-human chimeras, rat-human chimeras, chick-human chimeras, pig-human chimeras, sheep-human chimeras, goat-human chimeras and monkey-human chimeras.[35] Shortly, I will discuss the significance of the whether these are considered as animal-human or human animal. Suffice to say that an animal-human chimeric embryo is one produced by unification as a result of aggregation of an animal embryo and human cells. The animal-human chimera has already been developed to stages of independent life by injecting human cells into the foetal rat, for example, and allowing it to develop. The human-animal mixture requires injecting animal cells into the human foetus or embryo and the subsequent development of the entity. Importantly, one may not have many objections for the transfer of a limited number of adult human stem cells into an animal embryo, but may have very certain opposition to the creation of a human-animal mixture capable of independent life.

Other experiments such as placing a non-human embryo into a human, or placing non-human sperm into a woman, are theoretically possible, though there is a strong ethical and scientific opinion that such experiments should be strictly prohibited (and indeed, is prohibited by law is some countries, such as the UK and Singapore).

---

[34] See M. Bader, R. Schreiner & E. Wolf. 2009. Scientific Background. In *Chimbrids. Chimeras and Hybrids in Comparative European and International Research — Scientific, Ethical, Philosophical and Legal Aspects.* J. Taupitz & M. Weschka, eds. Berlin: Springer: 28–29.

[35] For references see www.bioethics.ac.uk/index.php?do=event&rid=77 (BioCentre: The Centre for Bioethics and Public Policy of the UK. 2007. *The New Inter-Species Future? An Ethical Discussion of Embryonic, Foetal and Post-Natal Human–Non-Human Combinations* [Accessed 8 January 2009]).

Various modalities of human-animal embryonic chimeras are exemplified by the following cases:[36]

1) *Mouse-human embryonic chimera*
   Human embryonic stem cells have been engrafted in mouse blastocysts. As a result, mouse-human chimeric embryos have been generated and implanted in the uteri of foster mice. The developmental stage of the recipient animal was an early embryo. Most of the resultant (chimeric) embryos were developmentally abnormal.[37]

2) *Chicken-human embryonic chimera*
   Human embryonic stem cells were engrafted into early chicken embryos (around two days old). The result was that the human embryonic stem cells contributed to the neural cells of the developing chicken embryos.[38]

3) *Rat-human embryonic chimera*
   Human mesenchymal stem cells were injected into late rat embryos (11 days old). As a result, the whole-embryo culture gave rise to complex functional structures of the kidney.[39]

---

[36] These cases which illustrate the field of human-animal chimeras in stem cell research are taken from the final report of the project Chimeras and Hybrids (including references). See: R. Schreiner, R. Klose & E. Wolf. 2009. Xenotransplantation — Aspects of Chimerism. In *Chimbrids. Chimeras and Hybrids in Comparative European and International Research — Scientific, Ethical, Philosophical and Legal Aspects.* J. Taupitz & M. Weschka, eds. Berlin: Springer: 498–500 (Table Annex A.3).

[37] D. James *et al.* Contribution of Human Embryonic Stem Cells to Mouse Blastocysts. *Developmental Biology* 2006; 295: 90–102.

[38] R.S. Goldstein *et al.* Integration and Differentiation of Human Embryonic Stem Cells Transplanted to the Chick Embryo. *Developmental Dynamics* 2002; 225: 80–86.

[39] T. Yokoo *et al.* Human Mesenchymal Stem Cells in Rodent Whole-Embryo Culture are Reprogrammed to Contribute to Kidney Tissue. *Proceedings of the National Academy of Sciences of the United States of America [*further as *PNAS]* 2005; 102: 3296–3300.

4) *Monkey-human chimera*
Human neural stem cells have been transplantated into a foetal monkey brain. It was shown that the human neural stem cells had extensively incorporated and contributed to neural differentiation.[40]

5) *Sheep-human chimera*
Human haematopoietic stem cells were implanted into sheep foetuses. This experiment resulted in human haematopoiesis and in formation of functional human liver cells.[41]

6) *Pig-human chimera*
Human haematopoietic stem cells were implanted into the bone marrow of pig foetuses. As a result, three kinds of cells were found in the resulting piglets (pig cells, human cells and fully fused pig-human hybrid cells, in which the DNA of both species was mixed).[42]

7) *Mouse-human chimera*
Human embryonic stem cells were injected into the lateral ventricle of foetal mouse brains. This experiment resulted in rise of functional human neurons and glia cells within the adult mouse brain.[43]

8) *Goat-human chimera*
Human primitive haematopoietic cells were implanted into foetal goats; with the result that it led to chimerism in multiple organs.[44]

Another type of experiment which combines human and animal materials is that which involves human–non-human hybrid embryos. Embryos containing cells made up of both human and non-human chromosomes

---

[40] V. Ourednik *et al.* Segregation of Human Neural Stem Cells in the Developing Primate Forebrain. *Science* 2001; 293: 1820–1824.

[41] G. Almeida-Porada *et al.* Formation of Human Hepatocytes by Human Hematopoietic Stem Cells in Sheep. *Blood* 2004; 104: 2582–2590.

[42] B. Ogle *et al.* Spontaneous Fusion of Cells Between Species Yields Transdifferentiation and Retroviral Transfer *in Vivo*. *FASEB Journal* (official publication of the Federation of American Societies for Experimental Biology) 2004; 18: 548–550.

[43] A. Muotri *et al.* Development of Functional Human Embryonic Stem Cell-Derived Neurons in Mouse Brain. *PNAS* 2005; 102: 18644–18648.

[44] F. Zeng *et al.* Multi-Organ Engraftment and Differentiation of Human Cord Blood CD34+Lincells in Goats Assessed by Gene Expression Profiling. *PNAS* 2006; 103: 7801–7806.

have been created, for example, experiments which resulted in frog-human hybrid entities (human nuclei were inserted into non-human eggs), or mouse-human hybrid entities (as a result of human–non-human chromosome transplant).[45] Also human–non-human cytoplasmic hybrids have been produced.[46] In these experiments, human nuclei were inserted into non-human eggs stripped of their chromosomes, and gametal cow-human and rabbit-human hybrid embryos were created.[47]

CHIMERISM AND SEMANTICS: Problems With Terminology and Definitions

What once was a mythical entity, the Chimera (Χιμαιρα) has become a reality; produced not by 'divine stock',[48] but by human technological endeavour. However, in modern biotechnology, the notions of 'chimera', and references to other animal-human combinations, have led to an ill-defined usage. Chimera refers to a multitude of various types and kinds of entities and combinations, which are in different stages of development. So, prior to any ethical discussion on chimeras in general, and specifically in the area of human-animal chimera research, one has to clarify the terminology to be used. A general lack of knowledge of the potential development of science in this area, and a lack of understanding of the potential consequences of mixing human and animal biological material, has generated the need for a broad reflection, which presupposes semantic clarification.

Paradoxically, while the mythical chimera had a clear denotation and meaning — in Classical Greek, χιμαιρα stands for a mythical, imaginary being — the modern, biotechnological chimera has developed an equivocal and diverse definition.[49] The Greek adjective, χιμαρικος means

[45] *Ibid.*

[46] F. Li *et al.* Activation of Human Embryonic Gene Expression in Cytoplasmic Hybrid Embryos Constructed Between Bovine Oocytes and Human Fibroblasts. *Cloning Stem Cells* 2008; 10: 297–305.

[47] F. Zeng *et al.* Multi-Organ Engraftment and Differentiation of Human Cord Blood CD34+Lincells in Goats Assessed by Gene Expression Profiling. *PNAS* 2006; 103: 7801–7806.

[48] The Chimera in Homer's Iliad (VI.) 'was of divine stock, not of men'.

[49] Cf. H. Bok. What's Wrong With Confusion? *The American Journal of Bioethics* 2003; 3: 25–26.

'chimeric', 'unreal', 'fantastic', 'impossible', or 'utopian'. However, the English language has developed a use of 'chimera' which is associated with a notional being: like 'phantasm', 'phantom', 'delusion', 'illusion', or 'apparition'. In English, it can also refer to, as in the Greek adjective form, a more vague reference — a 'pipe dream', 'a castle in the air', 'unreal ambition', 'fanciful scheme', 'unreality', or a fantastically impracticable plan or desire. In this sense of use, it signifies any (futile) attempt to illustrate or action an impossible idea, concept or theory.

There are significant differences between the ancient and contemporary understanding of chimera: the ancient chimera existed in mythology only, while the contemporary chimera is a real entity; the ancient chimera was a mixture of individuals of various species, the contemporary chimera is a mixture formed predominantly on the cellular level. From a semantic point of view, the term chimera is highly inadequate for current biotechnological products called 'chimeras'.[50] The only way to prevent linguistic confusion is not to use the term chimera for entities that are interspecies mixtures in reality. To avoid confusion and to provide a matter-of-fact correctness, and provide a morally neutral description, some semantically more appropriate terms have been proposed. This includes: 'transgenic creatures',[51] 'novel being', 'novelty', 'mixtures' or 'composed

[50] If these meanings are sustained, chimeras, as biotechnological products, are not 'chimeras' at all: they are not 'utopian' or 'chimeric' — they are real entities with a clear biological status. Under a basic semantic assumption that terms (words) have to symbolise things that the words stand for, the use of the word chimera for entities (biotechnological products), such as a pig with human blood, or a mouse with human brain, does not fit into our common semantic scope. A pig with human blood is neither 'chimeric' nor 'horrendous'; a mouse with one per cent of human brain cells is neither a 'phantom' nor a 'monster'. To call these entities chimeras, semantically, does not make sense. Otherwise, in each individual case when we use the term 'chimera', we have to explain that, in fact, we do not mean 'chimera', though we are saying 'chimera', and that we are using this term for a kind of an interspecific combination. This seems not to be very helpful in a standard communication.

[51] L.M. Glenn. When Pigs Fly? Legal and Ethical Issues in Transgenics and the Creation of Chimeras. *Physiologist* 2003; 46: 253–255 (here 254).

entities'.[52] However, such alternatives are used rather as secondary or explanatory terms and, in the meantime, the word chimera became a *terminus technicus.* Unfortunately in some languages, in those Non-Indo-European ones in particular, the difficulty exists in finding an appropriate word (character) denominating the meaning of this *terminus technicus*.[53] In the following, I attempt to clear the water in the further use of chimera-terminology in modern bioscience.

First, the term 'chimera' should be distinguished from the term 'hybrid'. Both these terms are used in many different ways, in various disciplines and contexts, and denoting diverse entities — even among scientists these terms are not used univocally and lack exact definitions in experimental biology. Moreover, these terms may be used interchangeably by some biologists; and 'the distinction between chimeras and hybrids is sometimes not acknowledged, or the terms are used in the wrong context'.[54] The fact that 'hybrid' and 'chimera' are disparate terms has implications: firstly, for ontological status discussions; and consequently, second, for the precision of ethical, social and legal discourse. It is therefore

---

[52] Cf. J.S. Robert. Regulating the Creation of Novel Beings. *Health Law Review* 2002; 11: 14–19; R. Bolli. Regeneration of the Human Heart — No Chimera? *The New England Journal of Medicine* 2002; 346: 55–56; J.S. Robert & F. Baylis. Crossing Species Boundaries. *The American Journal of Bioethics* 2003; 3: 1–13; N.J. Jones & W.P. Cheshire. Can Artificial Techniques Supply Morally Neutral Human Embryos for Research? Creating Novel Categories of Human Embryos. *Journal of Medical Ethics* 2005; 21: 29–40.

[53] For instance in the Japanese language the term 'chimera' does not exist; there is no Japanese equivalent for the term 'chimera'. In the context of biomedical research, the term 'chimera' is borrowed and transcripted as 'kimera' by means of Japanese katakana character which only expresses the sound of the word 'chimera' without any semantic denotation to the Japanese lexicology. However there are similar terms which refer to the 'chimera' such as *youkai* (specter) or *kaibutsu* (monster), both of them written in kanji character. But it would be meaningless to use them for the biotechnological chimera. (I am thankful to Prof. Motomu Shimoda of Osaka University for this clarification.)

[54] M. Bader, R. Schreiner & E. Wolf. 2009. Scientific Background. In *Chimbrids. Chimeras and Hybrids in Comparative European and International Research — Scientific, Ethical, Philosophical and Legal Aspects.* J. Taupitz & M. Weschka, eds. Berlin: Springer: 5.

necessary to clarify the semantic differentiation of these concepts in biological use.

Hybrids

A *hybrid* is an entity (a mixture) consisting of a single cell population derived from one zygote, created from two different breeding lines, races or species (including intra-specific and inter-specific hybrid). All of the cells of a hybrid have the same genome — unlike a chimera, in which different genotypes co-exist. Furthermore, there are cases, such as somatic cell nuclear transfer (SCNT), in which the applicability of these proposed definitions is problematic.

Semantically, the term hybrid signifies an entity (usually plant or animal) produced from parents of different breeds or types. Generally, it is something that consists of two or more things or what comes from a mixture of two or more other things. This definition does not express the difference between hybrid and chimera, the way these terms are used in the scientific language. Either the exact and precise scientific description of these two (or more) entities which are being combined into a new one is used (including the type of mixture, developmental stage of the entities involved, etc.); or the word hybrid/chimera is used as a *terminus technicus* (*a* specialised word associated with and rarely known outside a specific industry or discipline). But since there are many possible chimeras and hybrids, the metaphorical language within, otherwise precise, scientific language remains questionable and scientifically inappropriate.

Etymologically, the term hybrid comes from the Greek word *hybris* (hubris) which signifies a series of exclusively negative meanings.[55] Hubris, which means 'vainglory', 'pride' or 'abuse', appears to contradict what scientists would normally want to characterise as a biotechnological hybrid — if an 'act of hubris' denotes an outrageous act, exhibition of pride, or disregard for ethical principles, then this kind of research is something that probably

[55] In Classic Greek, the word *hybris* (υβρις) means vainglory, pride, boast, superciliousness, arrogance, profanation, maltreatment, high-handedness, degrade, and abuse; other negative moral connotations of the word *hybris* are: debauchery, revelry, offence, malefaction, injustice and crime.

should be avoided! Apart of its negative etymological roots, the term hybrid is used in many different disciplines as a *terminus technicus,* but in a very specific and clearly defined sense. For instance, the term hybrid is used in logic, analytical philosophy, linguistics, technology, chemistry (hybridisation), and biology. Intra-specific and inter-specific hybrids are very common in plant and animal breeding. Many agricultural plants grow as hybrids; in plant breeding, hybridisation is an effective means of propagating plant varieties. The term hybrid can be used and understood univocally, if used within a clearly defined semantic framework (as biology provides different and clear definitions of the term hybrid).[56]

Chimeras

A *chimera* can be defined as an entity (a mixture) which contains two or more genetically different type of cells (cell populations) coming from different zygotes of the same, or different, species. If these different cell populations are derived from one species, we speak about *intra-species chimerism*; if the mixed entity is derived from two different species, it belongs to *inter-species chimerism.*

The term chimera denotes various entities that apparently have diverse ontological status and therefore different moral and ethical relevance. Providing some basic differentiation of chimerism, we can distinguish the following types of chimeras:

a) plant chimera: in laboratory;
in nature (e.g. agriculture);
b) animal chimera (experimental);

---

[56] In biology, the term hybrid has various meanings:

a) the offspring of different species
b) the offspring of different genera
c) crosses between different species within the same genus (inter-specific hybrids)
d) crosses between different subspecies within the same species (intra-specific hybrids)
e) crosses between different genera (inter-generic hybrids)
f) crosses between different populations, breeds or cultivars of a single species (principally in plant breeding)
g) in molecular biology, hybrid refers to hybridisation.

c) human-animal chimera;
d) plant-animal-human chimera;
e) human–non-human chimera;
f) embryonic chimera: animal-animal chimera;
human-animal chimera.

Furthermore within human–non-human embryonic chimeras, three different levels can be distinguished: genetic, cellular (tissue), and organ level.

Another distinction regarding chimeras should be made in basic and clinical research. It is obvious that the above mentioned examples of chimeras have different moral relevance, because they have primarily a diverse ontological status, and they *are* different kinds of chimeras. One may not have many objections for the transfer of a limited number of adult human stem cells into an animal embryo, in order to learn how they proliferate and grow during the prenatal period; but one may have very certain opposition to the creation of a human-animal chimeric independent living creature. While the latter may appear to some as morally abhorrent, the main concern regarding animal-human chimeras in the first case is related to the concern as to whether or not such embryonic chimeras will be put to a use that is ethically and/or medically problematic, risky, or dangerous.

Getting the Terminology Right

Based on previous comments and distinctions on hybrids and chimeras, it will be useful to specify some definitions for human–non-human chimeras and hybrids. In general, it is accepted that a hybrid contains chromosomes from different species (or subspecies) together in the same nucleus, where they are free to recombine if possible. On the other hand, genetic recombination would not occur in a chimera, which contains distinct cell populations possessing genetic material from different sources. However, if cell fusion occurs, then this distinction may be blurred.[57] Due

[57] BioCentre: The Centre for Bioethics and Public Policy. 2007. *The New Inter-Species Future? An Ethical Discussion of Embryonic, Fetal and Post-Natal Human–Non-Human Combinations*. Available at: http://www.bioethics.ac.uk/index.php?id=23 [Accessed 2 February 2009].

to the lack of specific definitions regarding the different combinations of human and non-human entities, including gametes and pluripotent stem cells,[58] for the purposes of this chapter, the following definitions, proposed by *The Centre for Bioethics and Public Policy* (UK),[59] will be used:

A) Human–non-human chimera
A biological organism made up of genetically distinct population of human and non-human cells.

Aa) Embryonic or foetal human–non-human chimera
A human embryo or foetus into which at least one cell of a non-human life form has been introduced; or a non-human embryo or foetus into which at least one cell of a human life form has been introduced.

Ab) Post-natal human–non-human chimera
A human person in which non-human animal cells, tissue or organs have been transplanted; or a non-human animal in which human cells, tissue or organs have been transplanted.

B) Human–non-human hybrid
A biological organism created through the use of cells of different human and non-human origins:

— a human ovum that has been fertilised by sperm of a non-human life form;
— an ovum of a non-human life form that has been fertilised by human sperm;
— a human ovum into which the nucleus of a cell of a non-human life form has been introduced;

[58] Cf. R.A. Ankeny. No Real Categories, Only Chimeras and Illusions: The Interplay Between Morality and Science in Debates Over Embryonic Chimeras. *American Journal of Bioethics* 2003; 3: 31–33; H.T. Greely. Defining Chimeras... and Chimeric Concerns. *The American Journal of Bioethics* 2003; 3: 17–20.
[59] BioCentre: The Centre for Bioethics and Public Policy. 2007. *The New Inter-Species Future? An Ethical Discussion of Embryonic, Fetal and Post-Natal Human–Non-Human Combinations.* Available at: http://www.bioethics.ac.uk/index.php?id=23 [Accessed 2 February 2009].

— an ovum of a non-human life form into which the nucleus of a human cell has been introduced;
— a human ovum or an ovum of a non-human life form that otherwise contains chromosomes from both a human being and a non-human life form.

From the proposed scope of these definitions, only the variant *embryonic or foetal human–non-human chimera (Aa)* is of specific interest for the purposes of this chapter. I will not address the issues with respect to the variant *post-natal human–non-human chimera (Ab),* because a regular framework of clinical and research ethics would normally apply due to the participation of a human agent. I will also not consider variant *human–non-human hybrids (B)* in the sense that the 'terrifying' humanised animals or animalised 'walking and talking' humans, and whose creation is normally beyond generally acceptable moral boundaries, are confined to an interesting topic of the popular media, rather than a serious concern to scientists.

Apart of the ambiguity of the definitions of chimera and hybrid, another unclear definition concerns the terms '*embryo*' and '*foetus*'. While it is determined for clinical purposes that the product of fertilisation (before implantation into a uterus) is an embryo (and the trimester system is employed to determine the subsequent foetal stages), the terms embryo and foetus are not clearly defined in ethical discourse. The term '*functional embryo*', which has been introduced (where cloned embryos are concerned) in order to distinguish an embryo able to develop to term when implanted into a uterus, brings even more problems than clarity. Since the functionality of a human embryo cannot be tested without serious ethical concerns, it is problematic to apply the term 'functional embryo' to human embryos.[60]

We are witnessing rapid progress in the development of cloning techniques; especially in the creation of animal cloned embryos. Many

---

[60] Cf. M. Bader, R. Schreiner & E. Wolf. 2009. Scientific Background. In *Chimbrids. Chimeras and Hybrids in Comparative European and International Research — Scientific, Ethical, Philosophical and Legal Aspects.* J. Taupitz & M. Weschka, eds. Berlin: Springer: 5.

researchers have requested to create and use embryos that contain human nuclear DNA, contained within an animal oocyte. One goal is to produce embryonic stem cells from such entities; the justification is that there is a lack of human oocytes for this research, and animal eggs offer a ready source, which also does not risk exploitation of women. In this context, the term 'specified embryo' has been proposed.[61] The specified embryos are classified as follows:

a) human somatic cloned embryo: an embryo produced by transferring the nucleus of a human somatic cell into a human enucleated egg;
b) human embryonic cloned embryo: an embryo produced by transferring the nucleus of a human embryonic cell into a human enucleated egg;
c) human split embryo: an embryo produced by a split of a human embryo;
d) human-animal hybrid embryo: an embryo produced by having a human gamete and an animal gamete fertilised each other;
e) human-animal fused embryo: an embryo produced by transferring the nucleus of a human cell into an animal enucleated egg;
f) animal-human fused embryo: an embryo produced by transferring the nucleus of an animal cell into a human enucleated egg;
g) human-human chimeric embryo: an embryo produced by unification as a result of aggregation of a human embryo and other human embryo or cells;

---

[61] The classification of specified embryos is gratefully taken from Prof. Motumu Shimoda of Osaka University, who follows the definitions proposed by the Japanese legislator (Law Concerning Regulation Relating to Human Cloning Techniques and Other Similar Techniques, 2001; Guidelines for Handling of a Specified Embryo issued by the Japanese Ministry of Education, Culture, Sports, Science and Technology in 2001 as amended in 2006; The Basic Concepts on Handling of Human Embryo issued by the Council for Science and Technology Policy in 2004) — M. Shimoda. Bioethical Discussions on Specified Embryos in Japan. 2009. Scientific Background. In *Chimbrids. Chimeras and Hybrids in Comparative European and International Research — Scientific, Ethical, Philosophical and Legal Aspects.* J. Taupitz & M. Weschka, eds. Berlin: Springer: 809–816.

h) human-animal chimeric embryo: an embryo produced by unification as a result of aggregation of a human embryo and an animal embryo or cells;
i) animal-human chimeric embryo: an embryo produced by unification as a result of aggregation of an animal embryo and human cells.[62]

Equally problematic is the term '*species*'. A species, one of the basic units of biological classification:

> '[C]onsists of organisms that are very similar in anatomy, physiology and genetics, due to having relatively recent common ancestors. Most textbooks define a species as all the individual organisms of a natural population that generally interbreed at maturity in the wild and whose interbreeding produces fertile offspring. This definition serves quite well when normal breeding mammals are concerned. However, as soon as hybrids or chimeras are considered, the term becomes inadequate'.[63]

When, however, the rare cases of fertile inter-species hybrids are taken into account, and the question is asked about the species a mixed embryo is belonging to, then the traditional terminology of speciesism is useless.[64]

The species of human beings is noteworthy, because so far no natural hybrids with other species have been reported. 'But it is also obviously the most problematic species in ethical terms when mixed creatures,

---

[62] According to the Japanese law (Act Concerning Regulation Relating to Human Cloning Techniques and Other Similar Techniques, 2001), the production of specified embryos is regulated as follows:

— transfer of any specified embryo into uterus is prohibited: a) – i)
— production of specified embryos is conditionally permitted: a) and i)
— production of specified embryos is prohibited for the time being: b) – h).

[63] M. Bader, R. Schreiner & E. Wolf. 2009. Scientific Background. In *Chimbrids. Chimeras and Hybrids in Comparative European and International Research — Scientific, Ethical, Philosophical and Legal Aspects.* J. Taupitz & M. Weschka, eds. Berlin: Springer: 6.
[64] Cf. *ibid.*

chimbrids, are concerned'.[65] Within this analysis, it is essential to specify if human–non-human chimeras and hybrids belong to the human species as well.[66] From the scientific point of view, there is no a clear definition what human being means: what *IS* human.[67] Creation of chimeras and hybrids, while living human and animal biological material is mixed, fundamentally challenges our understanding of humanness: what it *IS* to be a member of the species *human being*.[68]

HUMAN–NON-HUMAN EMBRYONIC CHIMERAS: DEMARCATION OF THE SEMANTIC SCOPE

Chimerism belongs to a challenging field within contemporary biomedical research. Not all forms of chimerism raise the same moral concerns. Some of them fall under the classical framework of the ethics of biomedical research, such as informed consent requirements, or the 'Three Rs' concept in animal research.[69] Since this chapter primarily deals with human–non-human chimeras on the embryonic level, many aspects and

---

[65] *Ibid.*

[66] Anyway there are difficulties in applicability of the terms hybrid and chimera in certain cases. In order to avoid these difficulties, the international research project, dealing with human-animal mixtures, created the word "chimbrid" as a comprehensive term to cover both chimeras and hybrids and also all similar genetic mixtures that are not directly covered by the regular terms such as chimera and hybrid — Cf. Summary, Conclusions and Recommendations. 2009. In *Chimbrids. Chimeras and Hybrids in Comparative European and International Research — Scientific, Ethical, Philosophical and Legal Aspects.* J. Taupitz & M. Weschka, eds. Berlin: Springer: 435.

[67] Cf. M. Bader, R. Schreiner & E. Wolf. 2009. Scientific Background. In *Chimbrids. Chimeras and Hybrids in Comparative European and International Research — Scientific, Ethical, Philosophical and Legal Aspects.* J. Taupitz & M. Weschka, eds. Berlin: Springer: 6.

[68] Humans, similarly to other mammals, have around 25,000 genes; there are only very few differences in each single gene between the different species. Moreover, there are hardly any genes that can be found only in humans and not in animals. Biologically humanity lies in the genome. Anyway the question of which genes (and how) make a particular mammal to human remains unanswered.

[69] On the 'Three Rs' and the ethics of animal suffering, see Yeates, this volume.

areas of chimerism will not be discussed. Those omitted forms of chimerism include: chimerism in transplantation medicine, such as xeno-transplantation; macrochimerism (i.e. mixed allogeneic chimerism that is defined as engraftment of haematopoietic stem cells achieved by bone marrow transplantation);[70] microchimerism (including microchimerism which may occur in somatic cell nuclear transfer); and transgenic animals with human genes (such as double transgenic rats for the human renin angiotensin system, transgenic animals with the human kinin B1 receptor or transgenic mice with a human T-cell receptor).[71] Furthermore the extreme form of chimerism, such as animal-human gestation (placing a human embryo into an animal, placing human sperm into an animal, placing an animal embryo into a human, and placing animal sperm into a woman) is not covered here, although an embryonic stage is involved. Although one might expect that chimeras are always artificially created, natural (spontaneous) chimerism does occur rarely (e.g. haematopoietic chimerism). Regardless, only the artificial chimerism remains within the scope of this essay on the specific clarification of ontological status.[72]

Various Types of Ontological Status of Human–Non-Human Embryonic Chimeras

Ontological Priority

Biomedical research using chimeras oscillates between ideas of the 'humanisation' of animals, and the 'animalisation' of humans. This means that the ontological status of human–non-human chimeras will similarly shift between humanness and animalness, and between the status of a

---

[70] B.G. Exner *et al.* Mixed Allogeneic Chimerism to Induce Tolerance to Solid Organ and Cellular Grafts. *Acta Haematologica* 1999; 101: 78–81.

[71] Cf. M. Weschka. 2009. Transgenic Animals Carrying Human Genes. In *Chimbrids. Chimeras and Hybrids in Comparative European and International Research — Scientific, Ethical, Philosophical and Legal Aspects.* J. Taupitz & M. Weschka, eds. Berlin: Springer: 39–43.

[72] Cf. Summary, Conclusions and Recommendations. 2009. In *Chimbrids. Chimeras and Hybrids in Comparative European and International Research — Scientific, Ethical, Philosophical and Legal Aspects.* J. Taupitz & M. Weschka, eds. Berlin: Springer: 457.

human and status of an animal. The ontological status of the entities produced by incorporation of animal and human biological material will also reflect the degree of such alteration. For ethical assessment, the degree to which such alteration might have effects on the features of existing or future *persons* (and animals, with capacities of agency) concerned will be determinative in ethical deliberations.[73] In these deliberations, one might focus on physical appearance, cognition, intellect, sense, behaviour, emotion, and ability. The ontological status of entities produced by incorporation of human biological material into an existing animal will depend on the degree of possible 'humanisation' of the existing or future animal (the greater probability of 'humanisation' of animals and 'animalisation' of humans, the stronger the need for regulation and restrictions).[74] It is obvious that there is a need for appropriate tools to determine the ontological degrees of 'humanisation' in respect to 'animalisation'. This would make it possible to distinguish between various chimeras: not all chimeras have the same ethical implications, since they have diverse ontological status.

This approach will prevent simplification or reaching hurried conclusions;[75] likewise it will give us the necessary (and diverse) ontological ground for questions in respect to the troublesome concept of human (and animal) 'dignity': We need to be prepared to ask, 'How can we preserve our human rights and dignity despite the fact that our "humanness" may no longer be the exclusive possession of *Homo Sapiens*?'[76] Not all chimeras interfere with (human and/or animal) 'dignity' in the same way — beside the fact of the equivocal hermeneutics of 'dignity'. Chimeras may be used as a by-pass strategy — for example, stem cell researchers have highlighted the shortage of human oocytes as a barrier to future advances; so, to avoid using human oocytes, and thereby the gender issues this inevitably raises, animal oocytes have been proposed. But this raises the question of the ontological status of animals, and not only

[73] Cf. *ibid.*

[74] *Ibid*: 456.

[75] Cf. J. Fletcher. 1988. *The Ethics of Genetic Control. Ending Reproductive Roulette.* Buffalo: Prometheus Books: 172.

[76] L.M. Glenn. When Pigs Fly? Legal and Ethical Issues in Transgenics and the Creation of Chimeras. *Physiologis* 2003; 46: 254.

the question of the ontological status of humans.[77] One does not necessarily require a Levinasian notion of ethics in order to prioritise ontological status, *before* specification of moral duties to others (moral status).[78] Finally, the production of animal-human chimeras challenges our notion of human being;[79] in other words the fact that the human being, in different ways and levels mixed with animal, leads to the pre-eminently ontological question 'What *is* a human being?'

Crossing Species Boundaries as an Ontological Issue

In the contemporary discussion on the ethics of human-animal chimeras, the issue of crossing species boundaries is predominantly taken as an issue as to whether we ought to transgress these limits existing between different species. On the one hand, the biological category of 'species' serves as a definition of what a species is (what it is not, and what another species is). Without an idea of species boundary, the standard biological system of classification and categorisation would lose its meaning. But, on the other hand, it is difficult to apply our classification and categories for novel beings or 'in-between' species, that do not occur in nature, and which do not fall under the (well) defined categories used in biology.[80]

Species, as basic units of biological classification, determines all the individual organisms of a natural population. However, the term '*species*'

[77] For instance to use animal eggs/embryos instead of human eggs/embryos for creation of chimeras.

[78] Cf. M.A. Warren. 1997. *Moral Status: Obligations to Persons and Other Living Things.* Oxford: Clarendon Press, New York: Oxford University Press. Authors who deal with the personhood of embryos usually distinguish embryos as persons, non-persons, and potential persons (cf. A. Campbell, G. Gillett & G. Jones. 2005. *Medical Ethics.* New York: Oxford University Press: 4th edition: 101–106.

[79] Cf. R. Streffer. At the Edge of Humanity: Human Stem Cells, Chimeras, and Moral Status. *Kennedy Institute of Ethics Journal* 2005; 15: 347–370.

[80] For instance a chimera combined of 99% of animal cells and of 1% of human cells is probably still an animal (and it would be difficult to call this animal a "humanised animal"). Perhaps such term could be used in the case when 99% of neuronal cells of human-animal chimera are human ones. Cf. H.T. Greely *et al.* Thinking About the Human Neuron Mouse. *American Journal of Bioethics* 2007; 7: 27–40.

is not unproblematic in the context of chimeras, because the traditional terminology of speciesism is inadequate: while it is obvious that the attempt to create a human-animal entity by gestation would mean to cross species boundaries, is it less evident that all chimeras created by various combinations of human and non-human cells would cross species boundaries. 'Species boundaries between humans and animals may be crossed in a number of ways'.[81] It is difficult to discuss the question if we should/can/shall cross the species boundaries,[82] since it is tough to set the determinative species lines for chimeras.

Therefore some people argue that, for human–non-human chimeras, the species categorisation is pointless (at least biologically), and therefore morally irrelevant.[83] From another point of view, it would not be helpful to reject our developed biological classification based on species definitions and their boundaries. For example, it would be expected that society would attempt to quantify the different moral significance between creating a 'humanzee',[84] a mouse with 100% of human embryonic neural cells, or to transplant few human cells into a mouse embryo. Therefore it is still ethically relevant to distinguish between species because species boundaries do have moral relevance.[85] Some people, admitting the moral relevance of species boundaries, would argue that interspecies boundaries can be crossed in certain cases, and such experiments may be conducted ethically.[86] From

[81] J. Harris. 1992. *Wonderwoman and Superman. The Ethics of Human Biotechnology*. Oxford, New York: Oxford University Press: 148.

[82] Cf. J.S. Robert & F. Baylis. Crossing Species Boundaries. *The American Journal of Bioethics* 2003; 3: 1–13.

[83] Cf. A.W. Siegel. The Moral Insignificance of Crossing Species Boundaries. *The American Journal of Bioethics* 2003; 3: 33–34.

[84] For instance to create a chimpanzee with a human brain. Cf. J.D. Loike & M. Tendler. Reconstituting a Human Brain in Animals: A Jewish Perspective of Human Sanctity. *Kennedy Institute of Ethics Journal* 2008; 18: 347–367; R.J. White. Chimeric Monkeys With Human Brains: A New Bioethical Black Hole. *Artificial Organs* 2007; 31: 423–424.

[85] Cf. R. Streiffer. In Defence of the Moral Relevance of Species Boundaries. *The American Journal of Bioethics* 2003; 3: 37–38.

[86] Cf. P. Karpowicz, C.B. Cohen & D. van der Kooy. Developing Human–Non-Human Chimeras in Human Stem Cells Research: Ethical Issues and Boundaries. *Kennedy Institute of Ethics Journal* 2005; 15: 104–134.

the statement of moral significance of species boundaries, it does not necessarily follow that crossing species boundaries *ipso facto* interferes with an idea of moral rightness. Crossing species boundaries is very common in contemporary biology and in biomedical research. Various levels and forms of crossing species should be distinguished, because many forms of it may be identified, and it is not obvious that all boundary crossings are transgressions of moral boundaries. Furthermore, we have to distinguish on which level the crossing of species boundaries occurs — on genomic, cellular, tissue, organ, organism, or embryonic level. In this context, we finally have to address the question of identity. How is the biological identity of humans as a species related to personal identity? To what extent, would human identity be affected by creation of human-animal chimeras? The question arises when one considers the meaning of 'not-fully-human', and the (philosophical) anthropological status of chimeric being and its legal implications;[87] similarly, the clarification of the ontological status of human–non-human chimeras is a precondition for the discussion on human dignity and chimerism.[88] Can, for example, a human–non-human chimera have dignity, since it is not fully human, and therefore lacks a prerequisite, on some understandings, for such a property?

(Or from another perspective, what does it mean to be an enhanced human? If we understand the human-animal chimerism as a form of extension of our humanity to which we are even obliged, then we have to enhance ourselves by means of biotechnology including human-animal transgenetic chimerism as for instance transhumanists suggest.)[89]

We need to have some ontologically specified framework of these novel entities called 'human–non-human chimeras'. These mixtured entities transcend our traditional categories; or more precisely, our traditional

---

[87] Cf. J.T. Eberl. Creating Non-Human Persons: Might It Be Worth the Risk? *American Journal of Bioethics* 2007; 7: 52–54; L.M. Glenn. A Legal Perspective on Humanity, Personhood, and Species Boundaries. *American Journal of Bioethics* 2003; 3: 27–28; S. John *et al.* Law Should Recognize Value of Interspecies Embryos. *Nature* 2008; 451: 627.

[88] Cf. I. de Melo-Martín. Chimeras and Human Dignity. *Kennedy Institute of Ethics Journal* 2008; 18: 331–346.

[89] Cf. J. Savulescu. Human-Animal Transgenesis and Chimeras Might Be an Expression of Our Humanity. *The American Journal of Bioethics* 2003; 3: 22–25.

categories and classifications are neither pertinent nor applicable. The main problem in clarifying this framework consists in a broad spectrum of combinations and possibilities regarding human–non-human chimeras. Beside some specific situations such as human-animal gestation (which, belonging rather to curiosities, are not of a real scientific interest or of clinical application), we are of need for some tools which could help us to clarify the ontological status of individual human–non-human chimerical combinations.

A Suggested Matrix as a Framework for Ontological Status of Human–Non-Human Mixtures

Individual types of human–non-human chimerical mixtures raise, not only a wide range of ethical and legal problems, but first of all they raise a conceptual problem: what they are (the ontological level), and in which terms they are described (semantic level)? It seems that the appropriate approach to the complex phenomenon of 'chimeras' would be to develop a matrix of these variations, which could be used as a framework into which individual combinations could be located. This could specify the ontological status of these individual combinations, serving to help us understand and assess such entities in normative enquiries.

Table 1 is a modified table from the published results of the *Chimbrids project.*[90] I have also incorporated the matrix proposed by Bernhard and Schweitzer.[91] It summarises the currently possible procedures to mix human and animal material. Not all of these possibilities and combinations

[90] Table C.1. in: Summary, Conclusions and Recommendations. 2009. In *Chimbrids. Chimeras and Hybrids in Comparative European and International Research — Scientific, Ethical, Philosophical and Legal Aspects.* J. Taupitz & M. Weschka, eds. Berlin: Springer: 439–440.

[91] Cf. H.P. Bernhard & R.J. Schweizer. 2009. Chimeras and Other Human-Animal Mixtures in Relation to the Swiss Constitution and Swiss Laws: A Case for Regulatory Action. In *Chimbrids. Chimeras and Hybrids in Comparative European and International Research — Scientific, Ethical, Philosophical and Legal Aspects.* J. Taupitz & M. Weschka, eds. Berlin: Springer: 706–715, here 713.

Table 1: Human-Animal Embryonic Chimeras

Procedure	Source (Donor)	Recipient (Stage)	Result (Organism)	Application (Examples)
Stem cell (SC) transplantation	Human: embryonic SC, adult SC, neural SC	Animal: blastocyst, post-gastrulation embryo	Chimeric organism donor/recipient ratio depending on developmental stage and evolutionary relationship ('humanised' animals)	Research on human development, pluripotency[92] and SC differentiation[93]
Embryo transfer	Human embryo	Animal foster mother	Parent and offspring exhibiting microchimerism	No apparent scientific interest
Embryo mixing	Human embryo	Animal embryo	Chimera	No apparent scientific interest
Gamete fusion	Human sperm	Animal oocyte	Activated animal oocyte	Clinical fertility testing (historic: human/ape hybrid generation)[94]

[92] J.P. Lee *et al.* Stem Cells Act Through Multiple Mechanisms to Benefit Mice with Neurodegenerative Metabolic Disease. *Nature Medicine* 2007; 13: 439–447.

[93] J.D. Flax *et al.* Engraftable Human Neural Stem Cells Respond to Development Cues, Replace Neurons and Express Foreign Genes. *Nature Biotechnology* 1998; 16: 1033–1039.

[94] K. Rossiianov. Beyond Species: Il'ya Ivanov and His Experiments on Cross-Breeding Humans and Anthropoid Apes. *Science in Context* 2002; 15: 277–316; N. Patterson *et al.* Genetic Evidence for Complex Speciation of Humans and Chimpanzees. *Nature* 2006; 441: 1103–1108.

are currently performed, and not all possible combinations are included into the table.[95] Its limitation is given by embryo involvement in these mixtures. The categorisation is based on the terms 'source' (which seems to be more appropriate than the term 'donor') and 'recipient'; although both terms are, to a degree, inappropriate. While the term 'source' is a rather neutral and nonpersonal description, the term 'recipient' refers to the activity of someone who is accepting something. The classification of various mixtures (chimeras) takes into account the combinations of specific cell types, tissues and organs, diverse procedures and products resulting from the mixtures created.

For ontological status assessment of individual combinations, the consideration of diverse procedures and resulting organisms is of crucial significance. Similarly relevant is the respective stage of development of used and created mixtures and properties of both entities source and recipient. Developmental stage and properties of entities involved and procedures used are important because, in many cases, biological entities are recovered from persons, human foetuses or embryos, in the context of reproductive medicine, being therefore subject to specific ethical assessment (and legal provisions). The emphasis is given on interspecies human-animal combinations on embryonic level.[96] Further examples of procedures with already established or intended applications are given in the *Chimbrids report*.[97]

---

[95] More remote and rather theoretical options and applications such as animal-human combinations (beside xenografts for medical treatment which are still under moratorium) make the chimerism rather more difficult. Animal-human combinations are not covered in the table since they are currently of no apparent scientific interest. Which do not mean that these theoretical experiments, undertaken for other than scientific reasons, may challenge the ontological status of such combinations and exhort for appropriate regulatory action preventing intentional misuse.

[96] In difference to the Table C.1. from the Chimbrid project report (see above), SNCT, chromosome transfer (human somatic cell info animal embryonic stem cell), and gene transfer (human cDNA library into animal embryonic stem cell) are not covered.

[97] Summary, Conclusions and Recommendations. 2009. In *Chimbrids. Chimeras and Hybrids in Comparative European and International Research — Scientific, Ethical, Philosophical and Legal Aspects*. J. Taupitz & M. Weschka, eds. Berlin: Springer: 437–440.

Embryo Ontological Status

Since the human embryo or human embryonic stem cells (hESCs) can be involved in chimeras' production, it is of relevance to specify the ontological status of the human embryo. No particular framework for the ontological status of hESCs will be proposed, provided that the human embryo as a source for hESCs is a necessary condition. The by-pass strategy to avoid the ethical constraints of embryonic research, through the reprogramming or inducement of somatic SCs [so-called induced pluripotent stem cells (iPS cells)], is scientifically questionable, because it is not evident that the alternatives from non-embryonic sources do have the same differentiation potential as embryonic SCs.

There are several approaches to the ontological status of embryos; some of them under the following distinct titles.[98] I have chosen the systematic classification provided by Knoepffler[99] who, specifying the ontological status of embryo, distinguishes preformistic positions (classic dualistic theory, programme theory, potentiality theory and genealogic theory) and epigenetic positions (individualisation theory, cell theory, organism theory).

A) *Preformistic Positions*

The ontological status of human embryos cannot be answered scientifically on an empirical basis solely. For this clarification, a meta-empirical level of argumentation is needed. Various preformistic positions come out of the presumption that, from the moment of the fusion of gametes (fertilisation), a human person exists; or that, within further prenatal development, the human body (foetus) serves as a medium in which the human person, existing from the moment of fertilisation, appears.

---

[98] For example Bonnie Steinbock distinguishes in this context biological humanity view, person view, and interest view. See B. Steinbock. 2007. Moral Status, Moral Value, and Human Embryos. In *The Oxford Handbook of Bioethics*. B. Steinbock, ed. Oxford, New York: Oxford University Press: 416–440.

[99] N. Knoepffler. 1999. *Forschung an Menschlichen Embryonen. Was ist Verantwortbar?* Stuttgart, Leipzig: Hirzel Verlag: 59–116.

Aa) Classic dualistic theory

The core of the *dualistic theory* consists in the thesis that an embryo is a 'human person' because of the defining presence of a 'soul'. The background of this theory is the dualistic doctrine of two substances (soul, body), according to which the human being is a 'person' because of the moral-essentiality to be found in the (ever-present) soul. In this theory, 'person' denotes the presence of a soul; or, the soul is the bedrock for the 'personness'. Having a very long history in some religious thought, this theory tends to be considered as incompatible with modern scientific observations.

Ab) Programme theory

The foundation of the *programme theory* is the conviction that an embryo contains a unique programme for its actual 'personness'. Fertilisation is considered as a starting point for presence of the 'human person', because the genetic information already present (as a unique programme) represents an existing unique human being, qua 'person'. This means that the genome is the basis of the uniqueness and personness of the human being. Therefore it can be called also the 'genetic school of person', since the genome is what creates a human person. This theory raises a number of anomalies. For example, the existence of monovular twins (in spite of the fact that they share the same genome, they are distinct persons). Furthermore, the development of a teratoma from the genome (embryo) will be another chasm for genetic-centric theories, which, in addition, are contradictory to scientific 'facts'.

Ac) Potentiality theory

The main postulate of this theory is the following one: the human embryo is a 'person' because it has an active potentiality to manifest (later) its 'personness'. Based on this *active* potentiality (it will, all things being equal, attain this status; unlike an entity which has passive potentially, and therefore requires another event to occur for it to be actualised), a human embryo is a human person from the fusion of gametes. Given the right conditions (and nothing is done to stop it) the human person will be manifested later. The essential moment for the process of further active potentiality is fertilisation (thus, sperm and oocyte have passive potentialities). Apparently, the Aristotelian doctrine of active and passive potency is beyond this theory based on the paradigm of substance ontology. The development of personal features (activisation of potencies) is the goal of this substance (active potency).

From empirical observations gained through IVF, the majority of active potentialities who are ontologically 'human persons' *disappear* before they are able to manifest their 'personness'. Regarding embryonic chimeras, it is not clear if such entity (human person) has an active potency to manifest its personness. The potentially argument is often dismissed because an actuality of personhood is not the same as the potential for personhood: in the former case, the person exists, and therefore has moral standing. By definition, the latter does not exist in person form (and may never do so).

Ad) Genealogic theory

The *genealogic theory* lies in the thesis that a human embryo is a person due to its affinity to persons. According to this theory, there is only one criterion for the ontological status of the human embryo: namely the biological affiliation of embryo to the human species. Therefore the beginning and the end of the human person cannot be separated from the beginning and the end of human life. So the human embryo is 'someone', not 'something', because there is no transition from 'something' to 'someone', and he/she (embryo) has to be handled as human person (having moral status of a person). Both terms 'something' and 'someone' are semantically not irreducible, i.e. we cannot reduce 'someone' to 'something' and vice versa. Regardless, semantically, the embryo can be understood as 'something' or as 'someone'. Zygote, embryoblast, and trophoblast can be understood as 'someone', but can also develop into a teratoma as well (then, if the argument follows, a teratoma is 'someone' as well). Although some people call a zygote a human person, the same zygote is understood as 'something' by other people.

B) *Epigenetic Positions*

All introduced preformistic theories are not adopted universally, and they are not, without problematic inferences, compatible with our scientific knowledge; though some of them, the programme theory as an example, seem to be closer to the scientific observations. The diverse difficulties evident in many preformistic theories lead to a search for alternatives which interpret the embryo as *becoming a person*.

Ba) Individualisation theory

According to the *individualisation theory*, an embryo is a human person after implantation. This theory could come both from the Aristotelian substance ontology, and the classic dualism theory. It holds that human nature (embodied in an individualised human being) is the decisive characteristic for ontological status of an embryo. Biologically, the precondition for individuum is the primitive streak, which develops after nidation. The difference to the preformistic position of substance ontology is the premise regarding the timing. The human embryo is not a 'human person' from the moment of fertilisation, but from the moment of nidation when it is an individual, that is cannot divide into one or more 'persons'.

Consequently, there is no problem with ontological status of twins, teratomas, and chimeras (at least with chimeras for research, i.e. *in vitro*) and as such, they cannot be persons since they did not pass the stage of implantation and individualisation).

Bb) Cell theory

The *cell theory* holds that an embryo is a cluster of cells, and no more, and therefore that it does not have a moral standing as a person. 'Embryo' is therefore understood as a delineated event or process: the former stages do not exist (i.e. they have passed and are no longer relevant), and the future stages do not exist yet (and therefore are not relevant at this time). The strength of this position lies in its compatibility with the scientific knowledge. It is not the potentiality, but the time continuum what is of significance. The stages of a developing human being consist of certain time periods, and which build the time continuity. The language of substances is losing its meaning — in the same sense that a larva is not (yet) a butterfly, and which therefore means that the two stages have different and incomparable values. The cell theory is based on process ontology (or the German term 'Ereignisontologie'). The consequence is that a 'larva' cannot be interpreted ontologically as a 'butterfly', and accordingly, an 'embryo' is not a 'human person' (although it may be a human being). The anthropological presupposition of this theory is that *persons* are living being with rationality and self-consciousness (comparable with the 'being with a will' discussed by Kant, and whose capacity for 'self-law' makes it part of the moral world). In contrast to that, human embryos are neither rational nor self-conscious; they are 'things': a cluster of human cells with which agents can make use of.

Bc) Organism theory

The basic form of the *organism theory* is the notion of embryo as the beginning of one or more human beings which gradually become human persons.

From scientific point of view, 'human beings' can be understood as open, biological systems. Ontologically this means that these open systems are organisms with a beginning and end; and with their own story (narrative) and history (process/event). Human embryos are human organisms which occur/happen and, normally and given the right conditions, become human persons. This ontological hermeutics includes time (continuity), process (contemporaneity), and dialogic relationship (persons are relational beings). In this light, the development of a human being is a gradual process in which a human being is developing into a human person.

Summary

Each of the above theories has its strong and weak aspects. For instance classic dualistic theory does not justify the simultaneous spiritualisation which comes under fertilisation; programme theory tends to underplay necessary conclusions from scientific findings; the potentiality theory does not explain why fertilisation produces a person *in actu*; the genealogic theory does not give reasons for embryo's affinity to persons; the individualisation theory does not explain why the primitive streak is the decisive criterion for personness; and the cell theory keeps open the question of time as the decisive moment (why exactly in this moment and not in that moment).

CHIMERA ONTOLOGICAL STATUS

What needs specific attention is the ontological status of the chimera. The ontological status of the ancient chimeras was mythological, while the ontological status of the research chimeras is real and new in addition. The main difficulties consist in the fact that we do not have an appropriate ontological category for the chimera which is both *real* and *mixtured entity* of two (or more) species. Chimerism within contemporary biomedical research is a specific challenge to philosophy to provide the needed reflection for these real chimeras from ontological point of view.[100] On the level of human-animal embryonic chimeras, basically two approaches can be taken: either to consider the ontological status of human and animal species concurrently, or to propose a new and specific category for human-animal embryonic chimeras as novel entities (and this new category could serve as the base for chimeras' ontological status discussion.

Embryonic Chimeras' Ontological Status

In human-animal embryonic chimera research, not only (human) embryos, but chimeras as specific novel entities are affected. Two types of embryonic chimeras should be distinguished: a) chimeras where an animal embryo is involved and b) chimeras where a human embryo is involved.

For the first type, the decisive criterion is the ontological status of an animal embryo. Here at least three different interpretations of an animal embryo's ontological status may be given: an animal embryo is an entity substantially distinct from the human embryo (strong anthropocentrism) on the ontological level; an animal embryo has the same ontological status as a human embryo (vitalism, some forms of utilitarianism); the animal embryo's ontological status comes from the fact that animal embryo is a living being, developmentally close to the human embryo and as such is worth of a specific protection (animal protection).

So the respective understandings of animal embryo ontological status will be taken into the account.

---

[100] It would exceed the scope of this article to provide such comprehensive philosophical reflection on the chimeras' ontological status.

For chimeras where human embryo is involved, the respective understanding of human embryo ontological status (as discussed above) has to be taken into the account.

CONCLUSIONS

In order to answer the simple ontological question what chimera is, or better what human-animal embryonic chimeras are, several aspects and levels have to be taken into account. For the determination of the ontological status of a specific human-animal mixture, an explicit framework is needed so as to characterise and explain the kinds of mixtures involved. Any combination of human and animal materials is not simply human or not entirely animal, because the kinds of entities one is normally taking about share features and properties of both of animal and human; the relevant ontological features are therefore dependent upon the ratio of the original source and the recipient (whether human or animal), and on the developmental stage and evolutionary relationship of both of them. Understanding the state of the art science, and the appropriate semantics, are preconditions for clarification of chimeras' ontological status. Various matrices can be of help while providing a framework into which individual combinations (chimeras) can be located, and by which ontological status of these individual combinations could be specified and understood. Depending on the ontological status of both human and animal embryo, the ontological status of human-animal embryonic chimeras reaches from the ontological status of a human person (preformistic positions) to various forms of gradualist argument (epigenetic positions).

Only one ontological position has a clear and unequivocal answer to the question what human-animal embryonic chimera is, namely the position 'all-or-nothing', according to which a human embryo has the full ontological status of a human being ('all') and to use the human embryo to create a human-animal chimera would be a crime synonymous with killing or murder, beside the immoral trespassing of species boundaries and brutal dehumanisation (animalisation) of humans. This would be an impassable ontological (and consequently moral) barrier for usage of animal (or animal embryos) in chimerism, due to violation of human dignity.

For all other positions the clarification of the ontological status of the relevant chimera is needed. To clarify the ontological status of human-animal embryonic chimeras means to differentiate carefully. The proposed categorisation of both human and animal embryo ontological status together with the matrix can be of help. They are important tools for the ethics of creating human–animal chimeras. What needs a specific consideration is the human-animal chimera as an ontological category.

10

RELIGION, CIVIC VIRTUE AND THE STEM CELL DEBATE

Teoh Chin Leong

INTRODUCTION

This chapter argues for a set of normative standards that ought to exist in public debates on ethical issues that can have an effect on the direction of public policy. In particular, it examines the role that religion can play in public discourse. It is implicit that religion has a positive role to play given any society that cherishes freedom of religion and expression and which believes in according equal respect to all its citizens. Religious considerations, hence, need not be 'privatised' or kept out of public policy debates. However, there are limitations on how religious discourse ought to be presented in the public sphere. These restrictions or qualifications apply equally to all public discourse in pluralistic, multicultural democracies regardless of their initial starting points.

In particular, I will examine in some depth Robert Audi's plausible account of how religion ought to be incorporated into public policy debates.[1] I will also argue for the need to instill an overlapping consensus of procedural discourse virtues integral to ethical rationality in public debates involving contentious matters of morality. This will lay the conceptual ground needed for the final section where I take up two case studies involving religious and secular speech related to the moral permissibility of embryonic stem cell research.

[1] R. Audi. 2000. *Religious Commitment and Secular Reason*. Cambridge, UK; New York: Cambridge University Press.

SETTING THE CONTEXT: SUBSTANTIVE AND PROCEDURAL ETHICS

In deciding how one ought to proceed with ethical deliberation, the issue is often framed in terms of a choice to be made between *substantive* ethical argumentation and *procedural* accounts of decision-making. There is disagreement about which form of decision-making settles the question of the legitimacy of decisions so made. Substantive moral reasoning is argued to confer legitimacy because decisions made on the basis of such reasoning directly address the issues at stake in the debate. Furthermore, to the extent that the better argument wins the day, moral argumentation may also be considered epistemically superior to procedural accounts of decision making. Critics, however, argue that pluralistic societies can never hope to adjudicate between competing moral claims by pronouncing one to be uncontroversially 'better' in some sense than another. There is a plurality of incommensurable moral claims and value systems, and this diversity needs to be respected, or at least accepted. Pronouncing one view 'better' than another and making that the basis of law is coercive to minority views.

A procedural account, on the other hand, focuses on the *process* of decision making. When decisions are made according to accepted processes, the decision is considered (morally, legally or politically) legitimate because the requirement of procedural justice (variously defined) has been met. Depending on the context, such processes can take the form of procedurally fair or representative public consultations, subject or patient selection in medical research, resource allocation and other policy making processes, to cite just a few examples. There is, therefore, no direct need to address substantive ethical issues as long as decisions are made on the basis of fair procedures. Critics, such as Ashcroft, argue that this approach begins with an unwarranted 'presumption of undecidability' or intractability about the moral issues under consideration.[2] As a result, political consultation and consensus-making inappropriately take the place of agreement on the basis of rational moral argumentation on

---

[2] R. Ashcroft. Fair Process and the Redundancy of Bioethics: A Polemic. *Public Health Ethics* 2008; 1: 3–9: 3.

core substantive issues. In addition, Ashcroft questions whether political consensus-making, which need not be based on rigorous ethical deliberation and consideration of evidence, is enough to make policy decisions legitimate.[3]

This basic line of argumentation has also been extended to cases where the 'procedure' in question requires appeal to a country's constitution. In such a case, policy is considered legitimate as long as it is consistent with the country's constitution, as opposed to merits-based legal or political legitimacy conferred on the basis of an 'all-things-considered', 'full merits' deliberation of the case at hand.[4] Michelman argues that process-based appeal to the constitution will not suffice, since citizens still need to assess the constitution itself on its ethical merits applied to the case at hand. There is thus no escape from substantive moral deliberation. Complex socio-ethical problems cannot be legitimately solved by simply running them by the constitution as if there are no interpretative or ethical challenges with such a procedural approach.[5] Other thinkers, like Habermas and Rawls, have been accused of proposing evaluative strategies in public policy that redefine or skirt the main moral issues (of abortion or euthanasia) altogether.[6]

This debate sets the context for my paper. I want to argue that the contrast between substantive and procedural accounts of ethical decision

---

[3] *Ibid.*, 5–6.

[4] Rawls, for instance, argues that '...in considering whether to make homosexual relations between citizens criminal offenses, the question is not whether those relations are precluded by a worthy idea of full human good as characterised by a sound philosophical and nonreligious view, nor whether those of religious faith regard it as sin, but primarily whether legislative statutes forbidding those relations infringe the civil rights of free and equal democratic citizens. This question calls for a reasonable political conception of justice specifying those civil rights, which are always a matter of constitutional essentials'. See: J. Rawls. The Idea of Public Reason Revisited. *The University of Chicago Law Review* 1997; 64: 765–807: 780.

[5] F.I. Michelman. Constitutional Legitimation for Political Acts. *The Modern Law Review* 2003; 66: 1–15.

[6] J. Finnis. Natural Law and the Ethics of Discourse. *Ratio Juris* 1999; 12: 354–373: 367–370.

making presents us with a false dilemma. There are procedural or process-based elements even within substantive moral argumentation. However, the role of these procedural virtues is limited to providing normative guidance on the *conduct* of ethical deliberation and the nature of public discourse. There is, thus, a different, and more fruitful, way of thinking about 'procedures' in the context of ethical deliberation, and which is often left out of consideration when we talk about the standards that ought to apply in public policy debate. I want to consider especially how religion can be incorporated into public debate from a procedural perspective. I begin with an account of Audi's position on this issue before supplementing it with my own position.

THE CULTIVATION OF AN ETHIC OF CITIZENSHIP

Audi argues that the purpose of any state is to provide conditions for the flourishing of its citizens. While the concept of 'human flourishing' can be difficult to define, we need just a brief sense of what it entails for the purposes of this paper. In the most general sense, 'human flourishing' is concerned with living well together in a community. In a liberal, pluralistic democracy, 'flourishing' involves ensuring that values such as freedom and equality are respected. However, given the fact of pluralism, there also exists an 'ethics of citizenship', of which the cultivation of civic virtue is an essential part. It is important that in order to live well together in a diverse, pluralistic society, the conditions for reducing resentment, alienation and divisiveness, and increasing cooperation, harmony and respect, are met. I refer to this set of goals, and others that can be derived from them, as our 'flourishing goals'.

Audi explicitly contrasts his 'ethic of citizenship' position with an 'ethic of rights'. In his view, 'we can act wrongly... even when we are within our rights'.[7] It is thus unhelpful to jostle for air time in the public arena based purely on one's right to do so. While Audi allows for one's right to the freedom of expression, he also argues that we need a higher

[7] Audi, *op. cit.* note 1, p. 207.

standard of discourse if we are establishing public policies which are inevitably coercive in nature. We need to argue from civic virtue and with a considered civic voice; a concept I will explore in the next section. This applies to both individuals and institutions, whether religious or secular. What seems to motivate Audi's appeal to an ethic of citizenship is the fact that living in a pluralistic community requires us to moderate our intentions, speech and actions in a way that promotes our collective flourishing goals. It is an approach that proceeds from the 'outside-in': from the reality of diversity and our communal goals to its effect on individual conduct. According to Audi, rights talk, proceeding from the 'inside-out', can be divisive and alienating. We need a different way of speaking and relating to each other, even if this will not guarantee resolution to the most troubling ethical issues of our time.

It is important to note that our flourishing goals are goals that any reasonable citizen can agree on and adopt. They are not values that are completely foreign to us, and thus they can constitute a common starting point for regulating public debate. As will be shown, these values do not trump substantive values that are brought to bear in ethical debates (say for instance, 'the sanctity of life'). Instead, they are meant to moderate the *process* of ethical deliberation, not its eventual outcome. The question: 'What are we aiming for in public discourse on policy matters?' can thus be answered by saying that *public debate should procedurally exemplify our flourishing goals*.

THREE PRINCIPLES OF CIVIC VIRTUE

When one engages in advocacy in relation to changing the law or influencing public policy, there are at least three principles that must be observed if one is to act from civic virtue. These principles do not apply to someone who is simply expressing herself freely on a subject since she has a right to do so. According to Audi, the principles are: (i) the principle of secular rationale; (ii) the principle of secular motivation; and (iii) the principle of theo-ethical equilibrium. When we internalize these principles, we tend to speak with what Audi considers to be a *laudatory civic voice*. I take these principles in turn.

The Principle of Secular Rationale

This principle states that 'citizens have a prima facie obligation to have, and to be willing to offer, an (evidentially) adequate secular reason'[8] in advocacy for or support of a particular public policy that may restrict human conduct. To have a secular reason means that the reason has an:

> '...evidential [or normative] force, that is, ability to justify, [that] does not depend on — but also does not deny — the existence of God and, more broadly, does not depend on theological considerations (or on the pronouncements of a person or institution *as* a religious authority)'.[9]

The implication is that reasons perceived to be religious justifications for instituting a law or changing a policy are (generally) inadmissible from the point of view of civic virtue, not because they are bad reasons, *qua* reasons, but because they do not promote our flourishing goals. In particular, a religious reason for a change in law can be resented by those of differing faiths and those without a faith who do not share the religious reason in question. It would appear as an imposition of values or standards that they cannot accept, made worse by the fact that they have been institutionalized into policies or laws that they must now abide by.

By contrast, adequate secular reason, it is alleged, provides the common ground and voice that is acceptable to the diversity of faiths and beliefs that inhabit any pluralistic, multicultural community, precisely because it is neutral with respect to religious considerations. In addition, having secular justification as the grounds for coercive laws 'tends to reduce the chance that a majority representing one religion or denomination will abridge the rights — including the religious liberties — of another religion or denomination'.[10] What operates quite forcefully behind the scenes in such reasoning is the 'do-unto-others' principle. Hence, if a religious community objects to the principle of secular rationale in public

---

[8] *Ibid.*, 212.

[9] R. Audi. 2007. *Moral Value and Human Diversity*. Oxford: Oxford University Press: 97. See also: *Ibid.*, 89.

[10] Audi, *op. cit.* note 1, p. 212.

discourse, Audi would remind them 'how they themselves [would] wish to be treated by those who disagree with them for religious reasons, particularly where their religious conduct might be restricted'.[11] The use of adequate secular rationale thus carves out a common justificatory space that can be offered for analysis in a way that promotes our flourishing goals. The latter includes preventing a sense of alienation and promoting fairness and reciprocity in our treatment of each other when it comes to coercive laws or policies.

Despite the importance of this principle, Audi insists that it does not relegate religious considerations into oblivion. It does not lead to the privatization of religion, or the absurd scenario of people internally divided between their secular and religious selves.[12] Indeed, Audi argues that the principle also rules out many 'secular' arguments, including reasons based on atheistic or anti-religious considerations, if they do not meet the standards set out above.[13] Audi includes considerations of 'public health, public safety...educational need, or national defense',[14] amongst adequate secular reasons.

Some points of clarification are in order. To say that we employ secular reason means that this rationale can be taken to be independent of, though it may run parallel to (and from the point of view of the devout may even arise from), any religious commitment or reason we may hold. In addition, the latter may not, in normal circumstances, replace the former in the justificatory space, if we are being civically virtuous. Evidential or justificatory independence from God in the form of a secular basis or grounding for a proposition or moral principle 'does not imply independence of God in general. Nor does it imply that the "faculty" of reason is secular, in the sense that it is not capable of reaching religious knowledge'.[15] Audi argues that religious and secular considerations are often in harmony with each other, so that the Ten Commandments, for instance, have justificatory appeal to both the religious and non-religious.

---

[11] *Ibid.*, 203.
[12] *Ibid.*, 214.
[13] *Ibid.*, 87. See also: Audi, *op. cit.* note 9, p. 137.
[14] Audi, *op. cit.* note 1, pp. 86–87.
[15] *Ibid.*, 89.

A secular reason given in such a context will thus also be acceptable to the religious, even if there is disagreement about the ultimate source of value. It is in this way that Audi claims his position does not unduly hamper the possibility or proper exercise of religious discourse.

Audi also distinguishes 'public' reasons or justifications from secular ones. The former is sometimes interpreted to imply that a justification has to be intelligible, acceptable or in some sense familiar to the general public for it to count as an adequate public reason. Audi argues that his secular reasons cannot be reduced to mere public justifications of the kinds outlined above because 'a public could be ill educated or blinded by prejudice'.[16] Hence, 'intelligibility', 'acceptability' and 'familiarity' cannot be appropriate or sufficient criteria for the adequacy of secular reasons.[17]

Instead, if:

> '...a reason is secular, no special religious qualifications are needed to understand it; if it is adequate, any appropriately educated person can understand it; and if it is an adequate reason for a law or public policy, then either it or something it clearly implies will at least normally be intelligible to a normal adult with a good high school education'.[18]

But secular understanding and basic intelligibility are not sufficient defining features of adequate secular rationality. For Audi, 'an adequate reason provides enough justification to make it at least minimally reasonable to do (or believe) the thing in question',[19] regardless of its actual acceptability or familiarity to the general public. Furthermore, to qualify

---

[16] *Ibid.*, 90.

[17] In addition, Finnis criticises Rawls for his distinction between 'comprehensive doctrines' and 'public reasons', where the latter cannot be based on the former. This allows Rawls to simply assert that arguments against abortion made on the basis of comprehensive religious or philosophical doctrines are not part of an 'overlapping consensus' of perspectives that everyone can agree on, and also not 'reasonable'. See: Finnis, *op. cit.* note 6, p. 367. If inclusivity of perspectives is a valuable social good, then this is one reason to prefer Audi's conception of 'secular reasons' to Rawls' use of 'public reasons'.

[18] Audi, *op. cit.* note 1, p. 90.

[19] *Ibid.*, 90.

as actually possessing or *having* an adequate reason, one must go beyond mere acceptability of reasons for a position or course of action because the reasons could be accepted unreflectively; say because one already wants to believe the conclusion and is looking for *any* reasons whatsoever that could play a justificatory role. Audi argues that we also need to examine the rationality or credibility of the reasons given and whether they are indeed plausibly connected or relevant to the proposed action or position.[20]

Unlike Rawls, who (in his earlier work) forbids the use of 'comprehensive doctrines' in public debate, Audi believes his approach is preferable because it allows for the use of comprehensive views in the moral space that exists between one's right to free speech and our obligations towards the principles of civic virtue.[21] However, a religious citizen may wish to ensure public comprehensibility or accessibility of her own reasons even when derived from her comprehensive views since communicability is key to 'avoiding alienation and civil strife'.[22] This appears to rule out esoteric reasons such as those based on mystical perception of what God wants in the relevant situation and cases where no explanation is offered for one's position at all.

Finally, our prima facie obligation to give adequate secular reasons varies with one's role in society and the context of our speech. In general, people in positions of social responsibility and influence, such as government officials or clergy, have a stronger obligation to adhere to the principle of secular rationale. This obligation is also greater if we find ourselves in certain circumstances, such as appearing on public television to make a speech. Again, the ultimate purpose of the principle is that it is a constitutive part of an ethic of citizenship which aims at promoting our flourishing goals.

---

[20] *Ibid.*, 91.

[21] For criticisms of Rawl's later views when he *does* allow for the use of comprehensive doctrines, see: *Ibid.*, 159–160. See also: C.B. Cohen. 2006. Religion, Public Reason, and Embryonic Stem Cell Research. In *Handbook of Bioethics and Religion*. D.E. Guinn, ed. New York: Oxford University Press: 138.

[22] Audi, *op. cit.* note 1, p. 159. For further public discourse standards that can help ensure a moderate civic voice in the public arena, see: *Ibid.*, 172–176.

The Principle of Secular Motivation

This second principle of civic virtue states that:

> '...one has a (prima facie) obligation to abstain from advocacy or support of a law or public policy that restricts human conduct, unless in advocating or supporting it one is sufficiently *motivated* by (normatively) adequate secular reason'.[23]

To be 'sufficiently motivated' means that the reason is enough to explain one's actions and would motivate us to act even in the absence of other reasons (including religious ones) that could play a motivating role. Hence, even if a religious reason was sufficiently motivating, we could still consider a secular reason sufficiently motivating if it was important enough to move us to act and if we can act from (or because of) that secular reason apart from any religious reasons we may have.

According to Audi, the principle of secular rationale is more basic and important than the principle of secular motivation. The importance accorded to the latter principle appears to be motivated by a concern that if it were not met, the equalitarian or neutrality principles (or both) would be breached as well. The equalitarian principle calls for neutrality amongst different religions in public affairs.[24] The neutrality principle states that in the public sphere, one should be neutral towards religion as such.[25] This would rule out anti-religious sentiments as appropriate grounds for a particular coercive law or policy (for example, disallowing discussions of creationism in the school curriculum because one thinks the idea of God is absurd). But it would also rule out policies preferring the religious (in general) to the non-religious (for example, mandating prayer sessions in schools because it is thought that one ought to be in touch with one's spiritual side). The flourishing goals that are important here, concern avoiding a sense of coercion and alienation that can arise from the

---

[23] *Ibid.*, 96.

[24] *Ibid.*, 35–37.

[25] *Ibid.*, 37–41.

domination or favouring of either the religious (or a particular religion) or the anti-religious.

There is a concern that secular reasons offered may only be a (conscious or unconscious) rationalisation of religious considerations and hence may not be sufficiently motivating as reasons. However, if the secular reasons really do motivate, then even though those reasons were sought from initially religious motivations, one would have satisfied the principle of secular motivation. Audi believes that the *manner* in which we present our case is important and that it is civically virtuous to be clear and transparent in the motivations that actually move us because such a way of relating reveals to others who we really are. It is thus an essential part of an ethic of citizenship that promotes our flourishing goals when *trust* can be cultivated amongst discoursing parties who know where we are really (motivationally) coming from.

The Principle of Theo-Ethical Equilibrium

The third principle of civic virtue — that of 'theo-ethical equilibrium' — is meant to help facilitate the realisation of the first two principles discussed. It states that:

> '...where religious considerations appropriately bear on matters of public morality or of political choice, religious people have a prima facie obligation...to seek an equilibrium between those considerations and relevant secular standards of ethics and political responsibility'.[26]

The purpose of this endeavour is to reach a state of integration, where one's religious and secular beliefs, attitudes and desires, align with each other in a mutually consistent and supportive way.[27] This can help in the practice of civic virtue when a conscientious and rational citizen can present secular justifications for public policy that are sufficiently motivating and which reflect one's religious convictions as well. Audi argues that

[26] *Ibid.*, 136.
[27] *Ibid.*, 121.

there is much overlap between religious and secular moral grounds, motives, concepts, principles and obligations, especially in the Hebraic-Christian tradition, to believe that equilibrium is possible. He notes, however, that there are better and worse states of equilibria (including better and worse ways of attaining equilibria) and these states can be fragile when it comes to complex matters of morality.

The application of this principle requires both a sense of fallibilism and the openness to reconsider both religious and secular justifications for an action or belief when disequilibrium occurs. Hence:

> '...a seemingly sound moral conclusion that goes against one's scriptures or one's well-established religious tradition should be scrutinised for error; a religious demand that appears to abridge moral rights should be studied for such mistakes as misinterpretation of what it requires, errors in a translation of some supporting text, and distortion of a religious experience apparently revealing the demand; a major moral principle derived from only one of the five sources of religious obligation[28] should...be tested against one or more of the other four and perhaps also against some secular source'.[29]

Furthermore,

> 'Given the conception of God as omniscient, omnipotent, and omnibenevolent, the possibility of theo-ethical equilibrium is to be expected; and a mature, conscientious theist who cannot reach it should be reluctant or unwilling to support coercive laws or public policies on a religious basis that cannot be brought into that equilibrium'.[30]

An important outcome of this principle is that the integration of religious and secular elements, for instance through consensus, compromise or

---

[28] The five sources Audi refers to are scripture, non-scriptural religious authority or community, tradition, religious experience and natural theology. *Ibid.*, 116–117.
[29] *Ibid.*, 130.
[30] *Ibid.*, 130.

reconciliation, can now be accomplished on principled grounds, as opposed to merely instrumental, pragmatic or prudential grounds.

AN INSTITUTIONAL ETHICS OF CITIZENSHIP

It is significant that the three principles of civic virtue outlined above also apply to institutions in contexts of advocacy for coercive laws and policies. So, for instance, institutional citizenship requires the willingness to adopt and practice an institutional principle of theo-ethical equilibrium. But, while religious institutions should also attempt to meet their obligations of citizenship, they should do so, under normal circumstances, whilst observing (the institutional principle of) ecclesiastical political neutrality; and at the individual level, clerical political neutrality. Audi argues that, just as governments should not interfere with religions,[31] religions too should not interfere with governments. If we are to attain our flourishing goals and avoid socio-political polarizations, governmental neutrality with respect to different religious organisations is paramount. Political action by religious institutions or their representatives,[32] however, makes such governmental neutrality difficult, since politicians may then feel compelled to favour one religious organization or discriminate against another in an effort to garner votes.

While understanding the importance of allowing religious institutions to exercise moral leadership in addressing important issues of the day, Audi cautions against sliding into overtly political action which could also erode the moral authority of institutions mired in politics. In addition, religious institutions may be concerned about preserving in their congregation (and also in public officials and ordinary citizens) a measure of autonomy in making political judgments and decisions. A lot has to do

---

[31] In discussing the importance of separating the church from the state, Audi talks about the need to adhere to three separation principles. He refers to the first principle as the 'libertarian principle' of church-state separation, which allows for freedom of religion. See: *ibid.*, 33–35.

[32] For example, when religious representatives publicly support or endorse political candidates and parties, or openly pressure lawmakers into instituting coercive laws and policies.

with the context and voice with which clerical deliverances are made, and how these can be perceived by the public. Putting a distance between religious views and politics, however, will do much to encourage 'the exercise of reflective and independent citizenship'.[33]

A lack of political neutrality can also lead to religious organisations disintegrating into discord and conflict where unity, harmony and the promotion of spiritual goodness amongst their followers is a key, perhaps primary, goal. Corruption of various kinds can also creep in if political advocacy by clerical elements is too strong.

Individuals and institutions (including secular ones like educational institutions) that are able to appreciate and practice these three principles of civic virtue are more likely to be able to speak with others, including those whom we deeply disagree with, with the appropriate *civic voice* and hence collectively promote our flourishing goals.

FIVE OBJECTIONS

There are some objections that can be leveled against Audi's theory of an ethic of citizenship. I examine five principal objections that, by addressing, will set the stage for a fuller conception of the procedural virtues needed in public discourse which I develop in the next section.

Objection 1

Firstly, while Audi tries to preserve an arena of free speech for religious citizens, he clearly believes that rights are not enough for one to act in a morally praiseworthy way. We need, in addition and at a higher normative standard: an ethic of citizenship incorporating certain civic virtues, especially when there is advocacy for coercive laws and policies. To act rightly (as opposed to acting within our rights), civic virtue would thus trump our rights, at least in certain circumstances.

But it is not clear how this distinction between rights and virtue is to be maintained and respected in practice. At least in terms of public

[33] *Ibid.*, 47.

discourse, as it is usually understood and conceived by the citizenry, it is not clear what free speech is *for* if it was not thought to be able to influence policy. It would instill the feeling that one would only be taken seriously if one spoke only with a civic voice. While there may be good reasons for speaking with a civic voice, the realization of this by those who want to be taken seriously (and who wouldn't?) would 'trickle down' all the way, as it were, to the level of speech rights. Hence, what began as respecting one's right to free speech over and above the need for civic virtue, has now turned into a kind of dominance of civic virtue in the public arena. To be sure, one would still have the right to speak in civically unvirtuous ways, given one's right to free speech. But whenever one does that, it would be as if one were asking to be ignored since, on Audi's account, such views are civically inadmissible in public policy debates if they are not presented with the requisite civic voice. I believe that the obligation to always speak with a civic voice is not necessarily a bad thing, and would argue that one should welcome the implication that higher standards of discourse ought to prevail in the public space. In the next section, I will outline further aspects of civic virtue that ought to apply in public speech in the hope that they will address the weaknesses in Audi's account.

Objection 2

Apart from the challenge of actually communicating the complexity of Audi's theory of ethical citizenship and civic virtue to those who matter most, viz. ordinary citizens themselves, there is a second objection that can be made. While the justificatory and motivational principles are meant to avoid a feeling of alienation and resentment amongst citizens who may feel that one party is being favoured or else dominating public discourse, it is possible that our flourishing goals will fail to be met even where the principles are consciously adopted.

One reason for this is that the feeling of being 'dominated' or 'out of favour' is not simply tied to believing that one's interlocutor has inadequate secular reasons or is inappropriately motivated in the ways Audi has described. Oftentimes, suspicion that someone doesn't have the 'right' motives comes from observing one's manner of dialoguing or even simply from finding out that someone is in fact religious, and so assumes that every position henceforth will be a concealed religious argument meant to foist her values on the unsuspecting. To address this misconception in motives (if there indeed is one) would require a change in relational manner and comportment such that it reflects a genuine sense of fallibility. But if *this* is needed in order not to come across as dogmatic or wanting to dominate the other with one's values, then it is the civic virtue of fallibility, not Audi's principle of secular motivation, that does the conciliatory work.

In addition, given the adequacy requirement of a reason (that it 'provides enough justification to make it at least minimally reasonable to do (or believe) the thing in question'),[34] discord can arise when policies are consistently adopted on the basis of such minimal reasonableness (which remains for now ill-defined). One could hope that the better argument will prevail in public discourse, but nothing in Audi's principles seems to indicate that that is even a desirable goal, unlike accounts of political legitimacy that stress the importance of substantive argumentation. There are also questions of the priority or weighting that can be given to different values that may provide a different assessment of what is minimally reasonable to do or believe given a certain circumstance. Hence, 'domination', 'alienation' and 'dogmatism' can still enter by the back door having satisfied Audi's principles, especially if one is on the receiving end of a coercive law or policy so justified.

Objection 3

A third objection is that it is conceptually possible but psychologically and practically difficult, if not impossible, to determine whether one is sufficiently motivated by secular as opposed to religious reasons. Rationalisation in human beings is a complex knot; difficult to tease apart in terms of whether one reason is 'truly' behind or motivating or causing our belief in something else. It would seem better, especially in light of Audi's positive valuation of transparency and openness to reveal who we really are, to have a religious citizen admitting her religious motivations but yet being able to offer secular reasons that may be sufficiently motivating to her interlocutors though not necessarily to her. Audi rejects this as desirable only to

[34] *Ibid.*, 90.

the extent that the religious person does not declare that the secular reasons she offers are non-motivating, since those reasons would then be assumed to be motivating and that would be insincere and manipulative, or at best conceals how she really feels.[35] However, if the goal is to increase trust, surely an open-minded interlocutor could accept that there are different paths to the same conclusion? And as long as he finds the secular reason sufficiently motivating, we can perhaps agree that we can be appropriately, though differently, moved to the same conclusion in the spirit of achieving a measure of consensus. There need be no insincerity or manipulation going on, and certainly no sense of being 'dominated' coercively, if one freely accepts a secular reason that is offered as both adequate and sufficiently motivating, irrespective of the motivational state of one's interlocutor.

Objection 4

A fourth objection stems from the fact that the principle of theo-ethical equilibrium appears to be primarily a way for facilitating the alignment or integration of religious and secular reasons and motivations. The objective is to maintain secular justifications and motivations at the level of public discourse aimed at influencing law and public policy. However, if the goal is to prevent a sense of alienation in citizens (in this case alienating religious citizens), then it would surely be a principle of civic virtue that non-religious citizens go through a similar process of reflective equilibrium themselves. In particular, it can be just as alienating for religious citizens when moral conclusions based on religious considerations have to find a secular basis in civic speech, while there is no such constraint on the quality of secular considerations, for instance, by non-religious citizens, towards their own preferred policy ends. I am thinking here about secular considerations for advancing certain scientific or medical ends based purely on scientific or economic reasoning, which would appear to pass the test of adequate secular reason and motivation, but not necessarily adequate *moral* reasons and motivations.

For instance, a scientist may value a kind of technological determinism, where as long as the technology allows for something to be accomplished,

---

[35] *Ibid.*, 99.

then he would argue that it should be done, say in relation to human cloning or genetic enhancement. One way of criticising such a scientist would be to argue that perhaps he hasn't sufficiently examined or appreciated the moral dimensions of the issue at hand and ought to engage in a wider process of reflective equilibrium before making a final judgment. Oftentimes, what leads to discord and alienation in heated moral debates is not the fact that there are competing views per se, but the narrowness of certain positions adopted that are then foisted on others, as if no other value positions exist or could be taken to be morally central or even reasonable. If our flourishing goals are important then some additional procedural virtues are needed in public discourse beyond Audi's three principles of civic virtue.

Of course, one could argue that as long as the technologically deterministic scientist in my example does not push for the adoption of coercive policies, no real damage is done even if he reasons from a narrow set of presuppositions. However, just as Audi believes that we can act wrongly even when we are within our rights, so too can we act wrongly even if liberties or freedoms are not directly compromised. Liberty need not be the only or even the key value in deciding on the morally appropriate course of action. Considerations of social justice, say in the case of a policy on genetic enhancement, may be more decisive.

Objection 5

A final objection is that Audi hints at how religious considerations can be incorporated into the public space, but does not describe the normative force that permissible religious involvement can have in enriching our moral understanding and improving our civic lives. Audi can perhaps be accused of looking too much at the appropriate form that religious discourse should take when it accords with civic virtue, without appreciating the positive substantive role religion can have on virtue formation and ethical deliberation.[36] Audi's principle of theo-ethical equilibrium

[36] Though admittedly, Audi mentions the heuristic role of religious arguments and sacred texts as 'inexhaustible sources of ideas, standards, and practical wisdom'. *Ibid.*, 77. What he does not fully bring out, however, is how this heuristic role can actually *constitute* civic virtue rather than being merely consistent with it.

certainly allows for such a substantive role to be more fully reflected, and it is to this task of elaborating on certain key procedural elements of ethical rationality that we now turn.

PROCEDURAL VIRTUES IN PUBLIC ETHICAL DISCOURSE

So far, there has been an underlying assumption in this paper that ethics or political morality will be decisive in public policy making. The truth is that policy can arise from a multitude of factors, including considerations tied to amassing or maintaining political power, winning party votes, appeasing the masses, furthering non-moral economic ends or simply feeling compelled to follow international treaties for economic or political reasons. However, to the extent that moral considerations are over-riding in public policy or legal decisions, there are normative standards that can be properly applied to its practice. I argue, therefore, that we do better in facilitating Audi's 'flourishing goals' if certain *procedural* principles are added or emphasised in the cultivation of our civic voice, particularly in complex issues of morality.

The principles or virtues I have in mind are not esoteric: they are simply the virtues that constitute *good form* or practice when one engages in ethical discourse. It is important to note that 'procedural' here does not mean 'mechanical' or imply that it is unthinking in some way. In a procedural account of ethical citizenship, it is the principles, values, virtues, attitudes and dispositions that accompany civic engagement that are important. In ethical deliberation, important procedural elements include:

- an exploratory openness to the issue at hand;
- a sense of fallibility in one's reasoning;
- empathy in understanding and considering differing perspectives;
- reflection on how one's emotions affect one's reasoning and conclusions;
- consistency in the use of moral principles or reasons across different contexts; and
- universality, fairness and sincerity in the application of these normative discourse standards amongst discoursing parties.

The appeal is to an overlapping consensus of procedural ethical rationality already familiar in academic circles.[37] These are certainly elements that can be thought of as constitutive of the practice of reflective equilibrium but it pays to be able to separate the individual virtue-based elements that could make such a practice not just workable but also worthwhile.[38]

What are the affective, normative and epistemic presuppositions of the method of reflective equilibrium? Amongst the virtues required would surely be (and I repeat some of the virtues already mentioned): openness, honesty, sincerity in the pursuit of consensus or truth, self-knowledge, striving for authenticity in our feelings and beliefs, understanding our own motivations and emotions, fallibility and openness to external criticism, empathy, understanding, the principle of charity, fairness, striving to be inclusive of member concerns in discourse, relinquishing self-righteousness or arrogance, guarding against rationalisation and the preparedness to change or revise one's reasons, beliefs and conclusions.[39] These are largely moral traits of character. If the concept of reflective equilibrium is thought to be important, then the traits of character which it presupposes must also be developed. A proper functioning of the method of reflective equilibrium thus requires a proper functioning of elements of ethical being or character on which it depends. Once these traits or

---

[37] I mean the term 'overlapping consensus' in the Rawlsian sense of a consensus that can be affirmed by people holding diverse religious, moral or philosophical positions. See: J. Rawls. The Idea of an Overlapping Consensus. *Oxford Journal of Legal Studies* 1987; 7: 1–25. In this paper, I make the argument that the procedural virtues, principles, attitudes and dispositions that are constitutive of ethical rationality are those that people of different intellectual or moral orientations can accept when they engage in ethical discourse.

[38] Again, the influence here is Rawlsian. In 'reflective equilibrium' we are looking at achieving a considered position which reflects a measure of settled consistency in our principles as they are applied to concrete cases after due reflection.

[39] This goes beyond what Finnis attributes to Socrates and Plato as ideal discourse standards or conditions, viz. 'knowledge, goodwill, and frankness'. Finnis elaborates on them thus: '...(i) a sound, wide-ranging education, (ii) goodwill towards the other parties to the discourse/discussion (indeed, the kind regard one has towards one's friends), and (iii) willingness to speak frankly (even when that involves admitting one's mistakes, self-contradictions, and self-refutation), and not to feign agreement'. See: Finnis, *op. cit.* note 6, p. 355.

virtues are in place, the *character* of ethical discourse changes; they help to (procedurally) guide and facilitate fruitful dialogue amongst discoursing parties in an open, civil and respectful manner. This goes beyond merely considering whether ethical deliberation should proceed substantively or if a politically fair process is enough. Moral legitimacy seems to imply a *virtue-based process legitimacy* whenever we engage in moral reasoning. It involves the mutual cultivation of ethical being in the very act of public deliberation and engagement.

Without an appreciation and conscientious application of these process-related, virtue-based standards of thought, speech and conduct, the manner in which ethical discussion ought to take place in any rational or deliberative democracy could deviate far from what is civically virtuous. It is not just what is said that is important, but also *how* and *why* it is said. It is perhaps surprising that such procedural virtues readily meet with acceptance when presented to rational people (both religious and non-religious) in regulating the conduct of genuine ethical inquiry (hence constituting an overlapping consensus). Yet the signs of such virtue on display in the public arena are nearly always absent, whether in the newspapers, public talks, letters to the forum, on the internet or in public and interest group debates. Part of the problem is precisely that ethical discourse is seen as *debate* rather than as a *dialogue*. Morality is thought to be a mere expression of emotions or subjective preference or dogma, not open to reasonable criticism or reformulation. But if we expand the scope of civic virtue to include the procedural virtues just stated, we can further enrich and promote our flourishing goals in the process. This emphasis on the desirability of procedural discourse virtues collapses the distinction between the right to free speech and speech that is civically virtuous that was the basis of our first objection above.

RELIGION AND THE CULTIVATION OF EXPLORATORY OPENNESS

Before we proceed to consider how this (and Audi's) framework of civic virtue may be applied to the current controversy on stem cells, let me outline the positive substantive role religion can have on ethical deliberation situated within one of our procedural virtues — that of *exploratory openness*. This will help us to see how religion can have a greater role to play in public discourse than Audi seems to allow. On the basis of the virtue of exploratory openness, religious involvement can be seen as a *constitutive* part of civic virtue. This goes beyond Audi's account, where religious concerns are only seen as civically virtuous if they can be conveyed with secular rationale and motivation, and in line with theo-ethical equilibrium.

As citizens who are constituted, within our very persons, by diverse communal and role-based influences, values and affiliations, the need to seek a distinctive and authentic voice that defines our being is a challenging one. If we grant, as I think is reasonable, that we cannot know from the outset how we feel or ought to feel about complex matters of morality that concern contemporary society, it seems to follow that the path to self-discovery and self-making consists in an exploratory openness to different thoughts, ideas and experiences. These can provide us with the raw material with which we can work to eventually find ourselves. One aspect of this search for a settled sense of our moral identity consists in broadening our ethical or moral consciousness. We need to cultivate a richer, deeper sense of moral awareness.

Yet (and this is important) in relatively *new* and complex issues of bioethics, for instance, public debate proceeds from settled (and sometimes unchallengeable) convictions based on scenarios and background assumptions that may or may not hold when applied to a different situation. How can we expand our moral horizons and imagination? As Murdoch argues, 'I can only choose within the world I can *see*'.[40] We have to be sensitised to the diversity of the values-laden landscape before us; we have to be able to see potentially morally problematic aspects of that landscape and how our actions (and inaction) can change the ethical meaning of that landscape. The cultivation of moral perception and moral imagination, through an *affective* (and not merely intellectual) engagement of the heart and mind, is a way of combating moral blindness.

If this is correct, then religious contributions to (what the Catholic Church refers to as) 'the formation of conscience' or the shaping and

---

[40] I. Murdoch. 2001. *The Sovereignty of Good*. Routledge: 35–36.

testing of our basic moral intuitions can be crucial. This doesn't mean we have to fully accept what religious authorities tell us; but it also means there is no reason to dismiss those considerations out of hand, especially if we believe that religions contain a repository of not just divine but also humane and compassionate wisdom that we can learn from. Developing on the ideas of James Gustafson, Cahill suggests that:

> 'Theological language, and religious stories and images, can sometimes effectively move into public settings — not to dominate, alienate, or condemn, but to stimulate the emotions and imaginations of discussion partners, as they seek to move together toward better understanding of the human condition and more humane, just, and beneficent practices and policies of biomedicine'.[41]

Religious discourse can preserve its distinctiveness even when it is found in public discourse when the purpose is to educate our emotions, expand our moral consciousness or reaffirm a spirit of solidarity through reflection on common elements in our humanity. According to Cahill:

> 'To the degree that any one image, story, moral principle, or concrete moral analysis can appeal to a variety of values and commitments, it can have a chance to influence public life by raising the profile of one pattern of associational behaviour over another'.[42]

Religious symbols and stories can, for instance, highlight and help us reconsider contexts related to:

> '...the universal human need for health and vulnerability to illness; the inevitability of death; the reality of social exploitation; democratic political traditions of equality, respect, and fairness; and multiple other religious and moral traditions of other-concern and altruism'.[43]

---

[41] L.S. Cahill. 2006. Theology's Role in Public Bioethics. In *Handbook of Bioethics and Religion*. D.E. Guinn, ed. New York: Oxford University Press: 45.
[42] *Ibid.*, 44.
[43] *Ibid.*, 44.

The key point here, as shown in objection five above, is that Audi needlessly restricts the positive civic role of religion. The cultivation of civic virtue, through the principle or virtue of exploratory openness, can itself require a greater openness to religious considerations than Audi's three principles of secular rationale, secular motivation and theo-ethical equilibrium seem to allow. While Audi permits the use of religious language and reasons in the public arena on the basis of one's rights, he does not consider this use by itself as *constitutive* of civic virtue. The importance of exploratory openness also highlights the fact that the narrow-minded technologically deterministic scientist we encountered (the basis of objection four) is not being civically virtuous if he lacks a basic moral awareness of the relevant issues and why they may be important to a variety of people. Increasing one's moral consciousness has an educative effect and can help us imaginatively extend and empathically cast our minds towards, for instance, possible harms caused, injustices committed or obligations that remain unfulfilled within the ethical domain. A morally attuned citizenry could then better act on this consciousness after due deliberation, leading to reduced alienation and increased harmony in line with our civically-based flourishing goals.

CIVIC VIRTUE AND THE STEM CELL DEBATE

While a procedural account of ethical rationality and civic virtue may not give definitive answers on substantive matters of moral controversy, such as those surrounding the ethical permissibility of embryonic stem cell research, it can outline some possible approaches to considering the issue and rule out as civically inadmissible other lines of reasoning. The ideals of citizenship I have discussed, if seen as reasonable, should take our level of reasoning beyond mere personal preference (or prejudice) for a candidate or policy choice, to something that can be defended on the grounds of civic responsibility. For the purposes of partially illustrating how such a procedural approach might work, I will examine two different instances of public speech: one religiously-based, and the other a secular perspective on stem cell research.

Does the *Donum Vitae* Constitute Civically Virtuous Speech?

To begin, I examine how an emphasis on procedural virtue can be used to assess the Catholic Church's official position on embryonic stem cell research. This position finds its basis in the original debate on abortion where the central issue was also the moral status of the embryo. I will limit my discussion to only the following statements from the *Donum Vitae*[44] and it would be worth quoting this at some length:

> 'This Congregation is aware of the current debates concerning the beginning of human life, concerning the individuality of the human being and concerning the identity of the human person. The Congregation recalls the teachings found in the *Declaration on Procured Abortion*: "From the time that the ovum is fertilised, a new life is begun which is neither that of the father nor of the mother; it is rather the life of a new human being with his own growth. It would never be made human if it were not human already. To this perpetual evidence... modern genetic science brings valuable confirmation. It has demonstrated that, from the first instant, the programme is fixed as to what this living being will be: a man, this individual-man with his characteristic aspects already well determined. Right from fertilisation is begun the adventure of a human life, and each of its great capacities requires time...to find its place and to be in a position to act". This teaching remains valid and is further confirmed...by recent findings of human biological science which recognise that in the zygote resulting from fertilisation the biological identity of a new human individual is already constituted...
>
> Thus the fruit of human generation, from the first moment of its existence, that is to say from the moment the zygote has formed, demands the unconditional respect that is morally due to the human being in his

[44] The concern here is with the *use* of speech as exemplified in these statements. Hence if these statements are used, say by an interest group, with the intent of advocacy for restrictive laws or public policies, then the statements can be evaluated on the basis of its civic virtuousness. I am not claiming that, as the document stands, it is in fact being used with such intent.

> bodily and spiritual totality. The human being is to be respected and treated as a person from the moment of conception; and therefore from that same moment his rights as a person must be recognised, among which in the first place is the inviolable right of every innocent human being to life'.[45]

What resources do we have to assess the civic virtuousness of these statements?

To begin, let us take a slight detour to consider if one may have justification in the public funding of stem cell research irrespective of the statements above. We will have to distinguish between two levels of coercion here.

Arguably, public funding of stem cell research involves what Audi refers to as secondary as opposed to primary coercion.[46] An example of primary coercion, the kind that requires adequate secular justification, is taxation. Given that taxation is justified, the subsequent use of taxes in ways which may be against the will or desires of some citizens is a secondary form of coercion less in need of justification according to the principle of secular rationale. This is because the purpose of the primary form of coercion (taxation in this case) was, presumably, justified in the first place. For instance, primary coercion in the form of taxation for the purpose of enhancing scientific and medical research can be justified on the secular basis of improving public health when promising drugs, therapies or treatments are developed for eliminating disease and reducing suffering. Hence it is assumed that any subsequent use of taxes (within the limits of the original justification) is permissible, including the funding of research on stem cells. In any pluralistic democracy, there are bound to be secondary uses of taxation to which individuals disagree. Consensus is not the justificatory ground here. Rather it is whether there was adequate

---

[45] Congregation for the Doctrine of the Faith. 1987. *Instruction on Respect for Human Life in Its Origin and on the Dignity of Procreation: Replies to Certain Questions of the Day.* Available at: http://www.vatican.va/roman_curia/congregations/cfaith/documents/rc_con_cfaith_doc_19870222_respect-for-human-life_en.html [Accessed 30 Jul 2009]. Henceforth, we shall refer to this document as the *Donum Vitae*.

[46] Audi, *op. cit.* note 1, p. 88.

justification of taxation at the primary level to begin with. It is not, of course, that secondary coercion requires no justificatory reasons at all. However, to the extent that it does, the principle of secular rationale still applies. And if we accept Audi's distinction that primary coercion requires more secular justification than secondary forms of coercion, then public funding of stem cell research appears in less need of justification provided they are consistent with our primary ends.

One objection to this line of reasoning, and one that a Catholic convinced of the statements given in the *Donum Vitae* may give, is that I may agree with a primary form of coercion, without agreeing that it is justified in every application at a secondary level of coercion even when the goals are consistent at both levels. In the case of stem cell research, one may object on moral grounds that not all means are morally permissible even for the good secular ends of reducing suffering and disease. The destruction of embryos in stem cell research is one means that is ethically impermissible in scientific research because it involves the killing of human life.

Let us consider this objection at the secondary level in light of the principle of secular rationale and motivation. According to Audi, a religious argument for personhood at the moment of conception can be transformed into a secular argument:

> 'Think of the genetic argument for the personhood of the zygote: roughly, the argument that since all the genetic information needed for its development into a person is present at conception, the zygote *is* a person at that point'.[47]

This certainly seems to be, at first look, an adequate secular rationale; and appears to be the basis of the Catholic Church's position. The latter is shown to be the case when the *Donum Vitae* argues that 'modern genetic science' has shown that 'from the first instant, the programme is fixed as to what this living being will be'. It is hence admissible as civically responsible speech. In addition, the statements show an awareness of competing arguments that have been given in the debate. They also

---

[47] *Ibid.*, 97.

attempt to engage in wide reflective equilibrium by bringing in considerations from modern science.

However, Audi's approach may suggest that to the extent that a Catholic who is offering this argument is not sufficiently motivated by the secular considerations just offered, he is not being civically virtuous. In particular, Audi's project shows that it may be hard to hold this secular line of reasoning as being adequate without smuggling in certain religious presuppositions that actually motivate it. For instance, because the religious 'think of the zygote as ensouled by God at the moment of its formation or...simply have been brought up to think of all human life as sacred'.[48]

The procedural virtue here that might be absent is the virtue of *sincerity* in offering secular reasons that one would believe to be adequate apart from one's religious commitments.[49] Given our earlier criticism that it may be difficult to discover if one is merely rationalising an argument in favour of a conclusion that is already antecedently held by us or whether we are genuinely moved or motivated by it, the conscientious citizen may wish to consider if he would deem his secular arguments fallible or open to criticism. The latter, if we recall, are part of the procedural virtues of ethical rationality we all agree on. To the extent that he believes, prior to examination, that his arguments are infallible, he is not being civically virtuous.

There is a complication here. If one believed that God is an inerrant source of ethical wisdom, then the religious citizen would be *rationally committed* to a position of infallibility based on her prior set of religious beliefs.[50] However, this doesn't allow the religious citizen to reject the principle of fallibility. This is because it is entirely consistent to believe

---

[48] *Ibid.*, 97.

[49] Audi suggests some questions a conscientious citizen might want to ask themselves to determine 'motivational weight', including: 'How persuasive does a consideration seem to us? Are we influenced by it through commitment to some authority backing it or by its content...? How concerned or upset would we feel if it were challenged or could not be realized in action? How did we acquire it, and does this show anything about the strength of its grip on us?' *Ibid.*, 106.

[50] C.J. Eberle. 2002. *Religious Conviction in Liberal Politics*. Cambridge, U.K.; New York: Cambridge University Press: 264.

in biblical inerrancy whilst allowing for the possibility that our limited reasoning capacities have led us to error in our interpretation of inerrant biblical sources. As noted above, 'a major moral principle derived from only one of the five sources of religious obligation should...be tested against one or more of the other four and perhaps also against some secular source'.[51] We should thus at least test the statements in the *Donum Vitae* against other Catholic sources, and be open to criticism and the prospect that the argument is wrong. Indeed, as we shall see below, there are Catholic theologians with differing views about the status of the embryo who have arrived at these conclusions through a process of rational inquiry. These are elements that any religious protagonist would have to be open to (re)considering as well, and to understand why they would conclude in the way that they do when opinions differ.

In so far as adopting an attitude of fallibility and openness to criticism, as well as the virtue of consistency, is considered civically virtuous, the following lines of thinking may also be of concern to the conscientious Catholic thinker. Robert P. George has made the following observation:

> 'It is worth pointing out that contrary to a common misunderstanding, the Catholic Church does not try to draw *scientific* inferences about the humanity or distinctness of the human embryo from *theological* propositions about ensoulment. It works the other way around. The theological conclusion that an embryo is "ensouled" would have to be drawn on the basis of (among other things) scientific findings about the self-integration, distinctness, unity, determinateness, etc., of the developing embryo'.[52]

If this is true, and the statements in the *Donum Vitae* above appear to support the eagerness of the Catholic Church to support scientific reflection, then the following statements are puzzling:

> 'At the Second Vatican Council, the Church for her part presented once again to modern man her constant and certain doctrine according to

[51] Audi, *op. cit.* note 1, p. 130.
[52] R.P. George. Embryo Ethics. *Dædalus* 2008; 137: 23–35: 24.

which: "Life once conceived, must be protected with the utmost care; abortion and infanticide are abominable crimes". More recently, the Charter of the Rights of the Family, published by the Holy See, confirmed that "Human life must be absolutely respected and protected from the moment of conception".... Certainly no experimental datum can be in itself sufficient to bring us to the recognition of a spiritual soul; nevertheless, the conclusions of science regarding the human embryo provide a valuable indication for discerning by the use of reason a personal presence at the moment of this first appearance of a human life: how could a human individual not be a human person? The Magisterium has not expressly committed itself to an affirmation of a philosophical nature, but it constantly reaffirms the moral condemnation of any kind of procured abortion. This teaching has not been changed and is unchangeable'.[53]

Two points bear pointing out. Firstly, the scientific arguments mentioned above do not cohere with a more detailed look at the scientific evidence since the publication of the *Donum Vitae* in 1987. In seeking to 'gain a greater coherence between moral theology and modern embryology', Shannon & Wolter (describing their position as Catholic) conclude after surveying the relevant biological data:

'Given the findings of modern biology, there is no evidence for the presence of a separate ontological individual until the completion of either restriction or gastrulation, which occurs around three weeks after fertilisation. Therefore, there is no reasonable basis for arguing that the pre-embryo is morally equivalent to a person or is a person as a basis for prohibiting abortion'.[54]

Of course, there is some room for debate here, with others arguing that it is only at around the 14-day mark when the primitive streak is formed that

---

[53] Congregation for the Doctrine of the Faith, *op. cit.* note 45.

[54] T.A. Shannon & A.B. Wolter. 2005. Reflections on the Moral Status of the Pre-embryo. In *Contemporary Issues in Bioethics: A Catholic Perspective*. Lanham, MD.: Rowman & Littlefield Publishers: 85.

'the embryo can no longer split into several individuals'.[55] The point here is that the basis for this disagreement is scientifically grounded on identifying the point of individuation as being morally relevant, and there appears to be nothing that indicates the presence of a distinct individual at the moment of conception. It is worth noting that Shannon & Wolter's arguments were made while aware that they had to be 'reasonable' and capable of being 'reasonably defended in the public sector'.[56] Hence, using the empirical criterion the Catholic Church itself employs, embryonic stem cell research would be permissible up to 14 days from the time of fertilisation even on the strictest scientific view.[57]

Secondly, even if we are to challenge the exact moment that individuation occurs, it is because science conceives of itself as a fallibilistic enterprise that such a challenge would be deemed permissible, subject to the best evidence of human biology. It would hence be inconsistent to declare, given this dependence on the fallibility of science, that abortion is a 'teaching [that] has not been changed and is unchangeable' since the sanctity of human life at the point of conception is a 'constant and certain doctrine'. This resolute 'certainty' and spirit of absolutism would seem to go against the possession of an open attitude and disposition which may be considered a precondition of genuine moral engagement.

Therefore, one may conclude that anyone who publicly argues on the basis of the statements given in the *Donum Vitae* for a restrictive law or public policy on embryonic stem cell research would not be adopting *adequate* secular justification (since the best science appears not to support statements about personhood 'occurring' at the point of conception)[58] and

---

[55] Cohen, *op. cit.* note 21, p. 131.

[56] Shannon & Wolter, *op. cit.* note 54, p. 86.

[57] This is not to suggest that there is no controversy about the 14-day limit, since the primitive streak could develop over a period of time and not necessarily emerge on day 14 itself. But this criterion wouldn't push the point of impermissibility to the moment of conception.

[58] But see George, *op. cit.* note 52, pp. 34–35, where he sketches evidence that 'the human embryo, from the zygote stage forward, is a unitary human organism'. He seems to agree though that 'the issue is not definitively settled'. And that is precisely the point from the point of view of maintaining a spirit of fallibility and openness to critique that is central to the scientific enterprise.

would at the same time also be arguing inconsistently and without due openness to critique and fallibility. As a consequence, he would not be arguing in a civically virtuous manner.

The case study on a particular use of the *Donum Vitae* outlined above is not meant to be a definitive refutation of the moral impermissibility of embryonic stem cell research. That was not the original intention, and there are bound to be counter-arguments to the views expressed here. Instead, I am highlighting the ways one could assess whether the relevant speech, if given in the context of advocacy in prohibiting stem cell research or other coercive laws and public policies, could be considered civically virtuous. If one agrees with the basic procedural elements of civically responsible speech as discussed in this paper, then in their public speech they would do well to take into account virtuous attitudes, dispositions and actions that can better lead to the attainment of our collective flourishing goals.

The Stem Cell Debate in the Media

Of course, non-religious speech made in the public arena should also be subject to the same procedural standards of civic virtue. We will conclude by examining an example of this in the media in relation to the stem cell debate. While this is not the place to explore the role of the media and its relation to the ideals of citizenship, it should go without saying that the media can have a profound effect in shaping the hearts and minds of its viewers or readers. As such, one can argue that it ought to be evaluated according to the use of its civic voice. For the purposes of illustration, I will limit my evaluation to an article which appeared in the *Los Angeles Times* in 2005. While that article was meant to be an opinion piece, my analysis so far should have cautioned us against making too stark a distinction between the right to free speech and speech that is consistent with civic virtue.

In his article, 'Bioethicists Fiddle as Patients Die', Michael Kinsley seems to have little patience for the importance of careful moral argumentation on the ethics of stem cell research, although ironically he employs some argumentation himself in other parts of his opinion piece.

Hence, he states that 'arguments against therapeutic cloning (cloning for medical purposes) tend to be abstract and poetic... But on the subject of stem cells, I am not in the mood for poetry'.[59] He also seems to endorse a version of scientific or technological determinism, where it is thought that science ought to trump any consideration of ethics. He believes, for instance, that:

> 'Scientists look for solutions. Although there are no guarantees, when you put more scientists onto a problem, you increase your chance of solving it. By contrast, professional ethicists tend to look for problems. When you put more ethicists onto a problem, you can end up with more problems. Cad that I am, for example, it never occurred to me to worry that cloning embryos for stem cells "exploits women as egg donors not for their benefit". But it occurred to [Leon] Kass...'[60]

This deterministic tendency to unquestioningly prioritise science over ethics was noted above and is an attitude that can be potentially alienating to citizens genuinely concerned about difficult issues of practical ethics, regardless of their religious affiliations. In addition, Kinsley sees no place for religion in the stem cell debate: '...I have no trouble feeling that the government should value my life more than the lives of these clumps. God may disagree. But the government reports to me and to other adult Americans, not to God'.[61] With respect to treating religious citizens as equal and inclusive partners in public conversation, this line of reasoning would not be civically virtuous, for it prohibits religious involvement in public debate.

When he does take the ethics seriously, Kinsley understates the complexity of the issues that can be at stake. His solution to the concern about the exploitation of women for their eggs, for instance, is to have 'a

---

[59] M. Kinsley. 2005. Bioethicists Fiddle as Patients Die. *Los Angeles Times* 22 May. Available at: http://articles.latimes.com/2005/may/22/opinion/oe-kinsley22: 2. [Accessed 21 Aug 2009].

[60] *Ibid.*, 2.

[61] *Ibid.*, 1.

simple release form' so that women who have undergone IVF can give up their unwanted eggs having provided informed consent.[62] Indeed, part of the procedural virtues of exploratory openness, adequate moral perception and the respectful consideration of competing viewpoints seem to be absent in the statements already quoted; and also when he concludes that '[i]t's amusing in a way to think of scientific breakthroughs sitting on hold while someone noodles his way through arcane ethical mazes of his own devising'.[63]

Kinsley appears to be questioning the point of ethical deliberation altogether in scientific research.[64] It may thus be worth bearing in mind that it is both the right and the responsibility of the public, *qua* citizens, to make explicit their concerns with respect to major medical or scientific research, advancements or technologies. The professional ethicist, and the public when they speak about ethics, is merely reminding us of

---

[62] *Ibid.*, 2. The concern about the exploitation of women in this context can take several forms. See: F. Baylis and C. McLeod. The Stem Cell Debate Continues: The Buying and Selling of Eggs for Research. *Journal of Medical Ethics* 2007; 33: 726–731, for more detailed discussion of the ethical tensions in egg procurement, including whether to reimburse egg donors (those who donate leftover eggs after IVF for reproduction) as opposed to egg providers (non-IVF women who provide their eggs purely for research). In addition, there is the challenge of regulating the supply of eggs from economically disadvantaged women both within a country and across borders so that they are not disproportionately represented, thus increasing the potential harm that they may face.

[63] Kinsley, *op. cit.* note 59, p. 2.

[64] A charitable interpretation of Kinsley would be that he believes that there are just three important arguments against stem cell research and he finds them all wanting (in the ways he specifies in his article). However, a procedural account of the principles and virtues important to public discussion clearly goes beyond the for-and-against thrust of argumentation Kinsley believes to be the sum total of ethical discourse. It is the *manner* in which this public discourse takes place that is important, especially when there can be repercussions on our flourishing goals. It is a strength of a virtue-based procedural account of ethical deliberation that it can temper a purely substantive approach to argumentation. It should also be noted that without the supplementary process virtues discussed above, Kinsley's speech would have been considered civically permissible if assessed according to Audi's three principles of civic virtue alone. I am skeptical, however, that such speech would pose no problems to the promotion of our flourishing goals.

the range of values that inhabit our world. Because he is sensitive to the world of values and the different perspectives before him, the ethicist isn't, as Kinsley suggests, muddling through 'ethical mazes of his own devising'.[65] He doesn't simply conjure up issues out of thin air, unconnected and irrelevant to the real world. Instead, he gives us reason to pause and think, not rush unreflectively forward, oblivious to some other set of values we may be trampling all over. Seen in this light, public debate does not necessarily aim only at the 'moral breakthrough' Kinsley suggests will never come because all the considerations are already, and have always been, before us.[66] Instead, civically-conscious public engagement ensures due consideration of and respect for the values of others.

Of course, some ethical positions may be mistaken. They may be based on shaky premises, or the inference to a particular conclusion may be unwarranted. It is the task of ethicists to help formulate and evaluate arguments to clear such misconceptions and pave the way for a better understanding of the issues at hand. Yet, Kinsley impatiently dismisses this important work as 'abstract and poetic, concerned with the nature of humanity and stuff'.[67] One wonders which area of pursuit would be worth the effort put into it if indeed it wasn't concerned with the 'nature of humanity'? To this end, the goal of open and mature public debate is to, amongst other things, help uncover the complexities, conflicts and nuances of a central aspect of our humanity — that of the values we cherish and why they matter so much to us, including values inspired by religion. It is a requirement of civic virtue that this exercise in the consideration of values is undertaken seriously and sincerely (not perfunctorily), that it continues to engage the minds of future generations and to challenge and shape their consciences, even after a law has been passed on a particular issue. In the process, it is the procedural virtues of civic discourse outlined in this paper that are crucial and which ought to guide the *spirit* of public debate and inquiry.

---

[65] *Ibid.*, 2.

[66] *Ibid.*, 1.

[67] *Ibid.*, 2.

CONCLUSION

In the context of public policy debate on complex issues of morality, I have argued for the need to go beyond a consideration of ethical legitimacy in terms of fair-process or substantive argumentation. The latter requires the cultivation of character-based process virtues central to ethical rationality and reflective equilibrium. In considering the place of religion in public debate, Audi's three principles of secular rationale, secular motivation and theo-ethical equilibrium can serve as procedurally valid starting points for civically-conscious discourse. However, they can be supplemented and strengthened by the account that has been given of character-based discourse virtues. I have shown how these procedural virtues, attitudes and dispositions can be applied to the current stem cell debate. More importantly, I have shown how these virtues can help shape the nature and character of public ethical deliberation, including the kinds of reasoning and ways of relating to one another that would be considered civically virtuous. An ethic of citizenship that aims to promote our flourishing goals whilst ensuring the moral legitimacy of ethical debate and public policy decisions cannot afford to neglect these character-based process virtues.

ACKNOWLEDGEMENTS

I am grateful to Benjamin Capps for helpful comments and discussion of various drafts of this chapter, without which my ideas would have been less developed.

Part Two

GLOBAL PERSPECTIVES

11

REJUVENATED FEDERALISM: STATE-BASED STEM CELL RESEARCH POLICY

Geoffrey Lomax

INTRODUCTION

National policy regarding the funding of stem cell science occupies an exceptional space in the United States. August 2001 marked the first time a US president had ever taken up a matter of bioethical import as the sole subject of a major national policy address in announcing sharp restrictions on research eligible for federal funding.[1] The stem cell field was subsequently described by commentators as an 'extraordinary tapestry', in which scientific and political threads are delicately intertwined.[2]

The restrictive federal context from 2001–2009 served as a catalyst for the emergence of state-based research programmes in the US. By 2006, eight states had developed policies and/or programmes expressly to support research not eligible for federal funding. Five jurisdictions initiated state-administered funding programmes designed to advance research and economic development.

Public-sector programme development within this 'extraordinary tapestry' presents challenges for public administration. Challenges arise because stem cell science touches a series of controversial issues for which

---

[1] O.C. Snead. The Pedagogical Significance of the Bush Stem Cell Policy: A Window into Bioethical Regulation in the U.S. *Yale Journal of Health Policy, Law, and Ethics* 2005; 5: 491–504.

[2] D. Kennedy. Stem Cells: Still Here, Still Waiting. *Science* 2003; 300(5621): 865.

there is intractable disagreement. Under conditions of socio-political controversy, particularly involving issues of science and technology, it is essential that public agencies strive for administrative legitimacy.[3] Such legitimacy is generally pursued through procedural mechanisms that promote pluralistic decision-making in a manner that accords with our image of a just and effective government.

This chapter explores how states have addressed administrative challenges encountered in stem cell research programmes. This story is told from my vantage point as an administrator with the California stem cell agency with responsibility for facilitating the development and implementation of normative ethical standards for research conduct. Observations from this experience correspond to issues of democratic governance and the role of state-state interactions in public policy development. These observations may serve to elucidate theoretical work suggesting proceduralism remains a valuable facilitator for democratic policy-making particularly with regard to controversial technologies.[4]

In addition, the stem cell experience continues to raise questions about the distribution of authority between federal and state governments — the concept of federalism. This chapter provides an opportunity to highlight the role of state-state interactions in the development of a common regulatory-policy framework to advance the scientific enterprise. My thesis is that the collective application of procedural mechanisms by states for policy development, combined with the formation of inter-jurisdictional networks within the sphere of publically funded stem cell science programming, has served to enhance legitimacy and advance effective governance. The stem cell experience may provide a useful model for responsible governance of controversies involving science and technology through state action — a *rejuvenated federalism*.

---

[3] L.J. Virelli III. *'Political' Science: Peer Reviewers as Agents of Administrative Legitimacy*. SSRN 2008. Revised (and published) as: 'Training the Elephant in the Room: Scientific Peer Review and Administrative Legitimacy'; last revised March 24, 2009; *Administrative Law Review*, Fall 2009; Available at: http://papers.ssrn.com/sol3/papers.cfm?abstract_id=1259801.

[4] B. Capps. Authoritative Regulation and the Stem Cell Debate. *Bioethics* 2008; 22(1): 43–55.

SOVEREIGN ACTION AND SOCIAL CONTROVERSY

The imposition of restrictions on the conduct of federally funded research in the US through 2009 served as impetus for sovereign action by individual states. State actions, relating to stem cell research policy, have generally followed a three-stage trajectory: (1) programme initiation, (2) administrative development and implementation, and (3) creation of interstate support networks. Programme initiation has occurred through a variety of constitutional mechanisms — executive orders, legislative statutes, citizens' initiatives and regulation. Some policies served to expressly permit activities not eligible for federal funding while others authorised funding to specifically promote research and economic development.[5]

Efforts to initiate state-based research programmes were, and continue to be, marked by social controversy rooted in historic debates over the fate of the human embryo — 'embryo politics'.[6] For example, the *California Stem Cell Research and Cures Initiative* received over seven million votes, but programme funding was delayed due to a series of legal challenges by 'pro-life' organisations. Legislative and administrative efforts continue to be marked by contentious debate and political polarisation.[7] To the extent stem cell research involves the destruction of human embryos; it will remain a symbol for larger intractable values conflicts driven by powerful social, cultural and political forces.[8] Further, the association of stem cell science with biotechnical innovation — therapeutic cloning, chimeras, gene modification among other methods — and commercial enterprise is a source of antagonism from the 'secular left'.[9]

---

[5] A.D. Levine. Policy Considerations for States Supporting Stem Cell Research: Evidence from a Survey of Stem Cell Scientists. *Public Administration Review* 2008; 68(4): 681–694.

[6] D.C. Wertz. Embryo and Stem Cell Research in the United States: History and Politics. *Gene Therapy* 2002; 9(11): 674–678.

[7] R. Korobkin & S.R. Munzer. 2007. *Stem Cell Century: Law and Policy for a Breakthrough Technology*. New Haven: Yale University Press: xiii, 322.

[8] R.M. Green. Embryo as Epiphenomenon: Some Cultural, Social and Economic Forces Driving the Stem Cell Debate. *Journal of Medical Ethics* 2008; 34(12): 840–844.

[9] V. Postrell. 2005. Criminalizing Science. *Forbes*.

SOCIAL CONTROVERSY AND ADMINISTRATIVE LEGITIMACY

It is against this backdrop of deep-rooted societal controversy across the political spectrum that public agencies have been charged with the development and implementation of research-enabling programmes and policies. Under such conditions it is of paramount importance that agencies strive for administrative legitimacy through accountability, procedural integrity and transparency in decision-making.[10] Societal controversy can actually advance this task by serving as a lens to focus or frame critical issues and advance public understanding and participation in agency decision-making.

The pursuit of administrative legitimacy has been characterised as a 'duty of official life by establishing the sanctity of public office as a public trust'.[11] Early models for public administration involved value-neutral and technically schooled functionaries applying the 'bureaucratic apparatus of authority' to direct the 'business' of government.[12] Such models have given way to the expectation for public deliberation and direct citizen participation. In the US and elsewhere, the later half of the 20th century brought suspicion of the growing size and reach of government, the power of experts and the effects of technology. Activists of all persuasions reacted by demanding more direct control in decisions that affected them.[13] Today there is an expectation that mechanisms will exist for citizens to be engaged in more direct democracy including opportunities to influence the formulation of public programmes. In light of these expectations, public agencies are not only viewed as programme administrators, but facilitators of processes designed to support democratic governance.

---

[10] Virelli, *op. cit.* note 3.

[11] W. Wilson. 1886. *The Study of Administration.*

[12] M. Weber, H.H. Gerth & C.W. Mills. 1946. *From Max Weber: Essays in Sociology*. NY: Oxford University Press: xi, 490.

[13] N. Roberts. Public Deliberation in an Age of Direct Citizen Participation. *The American Review of Public Administration* 2004; 34(4): 315–353.

PROCEDURAL FRAMEWORKS AND LEGITIMACY

Procedural frameworks for participatory democracy have been the subjects of considerable scholarly attention both conceptually and empirically. For matters of health-science and technology policy, there is an emphasis on process transparency and evidence based adjudicative decision-making.[14] This discourse echoes themes from the broader literature over the governance of technologies with documented or perceived risks to the environment.[15] Historic debates emphasise the value of a 'discursive community' to foster collaboration and constructive deliberations in the policy development process.[16] The stem cell debate has added a degree of specificity by fostering consideration of how ethics may be incorporated into science policy and regulation.[17]

Empirical work suggests deliberative approaches among 'configurations of actors' provide ongoing feedback to support evidence-based and socially responsive policy development.[18] 'Policy oriented (loop) learning' is viewed as a mechanism through which actors can contribute to building a body of evidence to support the attainment of superior outcomes.[19] For

---

[14] Virelli, *op. cit.* note 3; J. Frenk. Balancing Relevance and Excellence: Organizational Responses to Link Research with Decision Making. *Social Science and Medicine* 1992; 35(11): 1397–1404; and J.F. Pfaff & C.P. Guzelian. Evidence Based Policy. *Fordham Law Legal Studies Research Paper 976376.* 2007.

[15] G.P. Lomax. From Breeder Reactors to Butterflies: Risk, Culture, and Biotechnology. *Risk Analysis* 2000; 20(5): 747–753.

[16] R.F. Heller, T.D. Heller & S. Pattison. Putting the Public Back into Public Health. Part II. How Can Public Health be Accountable to the Public? *Public Health* 2003; 117(1): 66–71; and T. Meppem. The Discursive Community: Evolving Institutional Structures for Planning Sustainability. *Ecological Economics* 2000; 34(1): 47–61.

[17] B. Capps. 2006. Procedural Ethics and the European Stem Cell Debate. In *Jahrbuch für Wissenschaft und Ethik*, P. Ameriks & J. Stolzenberg, eds. Berlin: Walter de Gruyter.

[18] A. Iannantuono & J. Eyles. Environmental Health Policy: Analytic 'Framing' of the Great Lakes Picture. *Environmental Management* 2000; 26(4): 385–392; J. Schmandt. Civic Science. *Science Communication* 1998; 20(1): 62–69; and S. Tsuchiya & T. Tsuchiya. A Review of Policy Exercise Interactive Learning Environments. *Simulation Gaming* 2000; 31(4): 509–527.

[19] P. Van der Knaap. Policy Evaluation and Learning: Feedback, Enlightenment or Argumentation? *Evaluation* 1995; 1(2): 189–216.

public agencies charged with facilitating the development of stem cell research programmes these models and experience provide direction for programme development.

In fact, state-based stem cell research programmes have adopted, or in some cases applied existing frameworks, designed to ensure process transparency, weight of evidence decision-making and ongoing opportunities for stakeholder review and comment. Established administrative procedures in states serve as the foundation for a baseline level of public participation in the context of formal rule-making proceedings. State-based stem cell programmes have gone beyond traditional review and comment, proceeding to expand participation. For example, the California Institute's strategic planning process, a non-regulatory agency-initiated initiative, included an advisory committee that convened in public and involved interviews with over 70 scientists, clinicians, patient advocates and others; held three scientific conferences; and conducted two focused planning meetings.[20]

DEVELOPING NORMATIVE ETHICAL STANDARDS FOR RESEARCH

The California Institute utilised a deliberative approach for the development of standards governing sponsored research. The substance of these policies has been described previously, so this description emphasises process.[21] Policies were first conceptualised at public meetings through give-and-take discussions involving an institute advisory committee and the public. Deliberations were iterative. Institute staff was charged with developing specific options to address particular policy aspirations. Participants had access to supporting materials; such as briefing papers, expert presentations and model guidelines, and they were invited to submit their own ideas and comment on each specific proposal. Vigorous give-and-take discussions involving both advisory committee members and the public often ensued. In addition to direct policy deliberations, the

[20] CIRM. 2006. *CIRM Scientific Strategic Plan*. San Francisco, CA: CIRM.

[21] G.P. Lomax, Z.W. Hall & B. Lo. Responsible Oversight of Human Stem Cell Research: The California Institute for Regenerative Medicine's Medical and Ethical Standards. *PLoS Medicine* 2007; 4(5): e114.

institute held a series of statewide meetings to assess needs and gather additional comments on ethical issues related to stem cell research.

This deliberative process preceded the initiation of administrative (e.g. public notice and comment) procedures required by state law for regulatory rule-making. While this approach is not unprecedented — it is increasingly common for public agencies to have public deliberations in advance of new regulation — the institute's commitment represented an exceptional resource commitment and level of due diligence. Nine public meetings were held over an eight-month period prior to initiation of the formal notice-and-comment administrative proceedings. Subsequently two additional rounds of deliberations between agency staff, the advisory committee and the public were conducted. The process culminated with a public record providing response to over 100 specific comments.[22] The institute maintains a standing advisory committee to evaluate the need to amend existing or develop new research standards. This committee is convened on an ongoing basis and individual committee members interact with diverse constituencies supporting a plurality of viewpoints on policy considerations.

The California Institute has employed similar processes for the development of policies governing intellectual property, research administration and institute governance. The final adoption of any policy is at the discretion of the institute's governing board. Deliberations at the board-level offer additional opportunity for public participation and comments. In addition, there is a series of external checks to support legitimacy and transparent governance. For example, the financial practices and policies of the institute and the governing board are the subject of review and audit by the California Controller.[23] In addition, the institute benefited from an audit by the state auditor and a review by a state commission concerned with effective governance.[24] Similar processes have been mirrored in

[22] CIRM. 2006. *Summary and Response to Public Comment for the Proposed CIRM MES Regulations*. San Francisco, CA: CIRM.

[23] CIRM. 2007. *CIRM Annual Report 2007*. San Francisco, CA: CIRM: 48.

[24] BSA. 2007. *California Institute for Regenerative Medicine*, B.o.S. Audits, ed. Sacramento: California State Auditor: 97; and Little Hoover Commission. 2008. *Public Hearing on the California Institute for Regenerative Medicine*. Available from: http://www.lhc.ca.gov/studies/agendas/Nov08.html.

other US states. For example, in New York State an ethics committee, operating in public, advises the Empire State Stem Cell Board on research standards.[25]

STATE-STATE INTERACTIONS IN POLICY DEVELOPMENT

A number of state-based research programmes were initiated between 2004 and 2006. States developed a range of policies, alluded to previously, to support programme implementation including ethical standards, procedures for scientific peer review and grants administration and intellectual property policies.[26] Federal laws and guidelines provided some guidance — notably the *National Academies Guidelines for Stem Cell Research*, the *Common Rule*[27] and *National Institutes of Health* administrative policies. Frequently, however, federal policies had to be adapted in a manner appropriate to the legal peculiarities of the respective states. For example, a number of states had new or existing laws governing transfer of human biological materials or donation of gametes and embryos for research.[28] This policy interaction introduced complexity into programme implementation.

Simultaneously, there was recognition of the need for regulatory compatibility among jurisdictions to advance development of the broader field. For example, the California *Stem Cell Research and Cures Initiative* charges the institute with advancing stem cell research and other vital medical technologies, for the development of life-saving treatments and cures. Other states are charged with similar mandates to balance programmatic goals with the needs for effective review and oversight. In attempting to fulfill these mandates, states have come to recognise that

---

[25] NYSTEM. 2008. *Empire State Stem Cell Board Strategic Plan.*

[26] S. Stayn. A Guide to State Laws on hESC Research and a Call for Interstate Dialogue. *BNA Medical Research Law and Policy* 2006; 5(21): 718–724.

[27] The Common Rule is a rule of medical ethics in the United States. These regulations governing Institutional Review Boards for oversight of human research came into effect in 1981 following the 1975 revision of the Declaration of Helsinki.

[28] G.P. Lomax & S. Stayn. Similarities and Differences Among Stem Cell Research Policies: Opportunities for Policymakers, Patients, and Researchers. *BNA Medical Research Law and Policy* 2008; 7(21): 695–698.

'border issues' or policy variation could potentially become a barrier to collaboration and exchange that is vital for advancing their common mission.[29]

Recognising the technical challenges posed by policy interaction and potential for 'border issues' to create unintended barriers to research, the state of Connecticut convened a multi-jurisdictional workshop in 2007 to consider opportunities for interstate collaboration.[30] This workshop resulted in the formation of the *Interstate Alliance on Stem Cell Research* (IASCR). The alliance is dedicated to fostering effective interstate collaboration, by assisting states in developing research programmes and by promoting efficient and responsible use of public funds.[31]

IASCR participants include representatives from state and national jurisdictions responsible for facilitating policy development and programme implementation. The alliance has spent considerable time evaluating inter-jurisdictional variance in state policy. In addition, participants have developed informal networks to address specific policy areas — intellectual property, research standards, grants administration and banking of research materials. The networks often concentrate on developing options to address complexities arising from state-state and state-federal policy interaction. Collectively, these research activities and inter-jurisdictional networks serve to enhance the evidentiary basis for programme implementation within member states. For example, IASCR members have developed proposals for reciprocal policy agreements between state and international jurisdictions to support the efficient exchange of research materials.[32] The California Institute revised its ethical standards to be more consistent with federal guidelines and other state regulations based on evidence derived from IASCR policy research.

---

[29] H.T. Greely. Moving Human Embryonic Stem Cells from Legislature to Lab: Remaining Legal and Ethical Questions. *PLoS Medicine* 2006; 3(5): e143.

[30] StemConn. 2007. Interstate Collaboration on Stem Cell Research. In *Connectitut's Stem Cell Research International Symposium*.

[31] IASCR. 2009. *The Interstate Alliance on Stem Cell Research*. Available from: http://www.iascr.org/ [Accessed 1 Feb 2009].

[32] G. Lomax & A. McNab. Harmonizing Standards and Coding for hESC Research. *Cell Stem Cell* 2008; 2(3): 201–202.

In addition, states have been restrained in the development of unique intellectual property requirements based on analysis that underscores the pre-eminence of federal law and the role of patents in encouraging socially valuable innovation.[33]

STEM CELL SCIENCE AND FEDERALISM

Federalism is a fundamental concept in US government referring to the boundaries between federal and state authority. From a descriptive perspective, federalism is a shorthand moniker for a complex set of political, legal, and economic relationships within a system of divided sovereignty.[34] Stem cell research has served to catalyse dialogue concerning federalism and bioethics policy development.[35] D'Andrea suggests a framework for evaluating the efficacy of centralised (federal) vs. decentralised (state or local) approaches to policy development with regard to issues of efficiency, social capital and justice. This framework may be applied to consider the effectiveness of state stem cell programme development.

With regard to programme efficiency it is suggested that a centralised federal approach may be more efficient by virtue of creating uniform standards. The obvious problem in the stem cell case is that states were responding to a restrictive federal policy, so the only alternative was a decentralised approach. There is merit to the assertion that a uniform approach supports efficiency through economies of scale and reduces the potential for inefficiencies created by border issue regulatory friction. In fact, during the development of the California Institute's ethical standards, numerous commentators suggested regulations should be based on national models for informed consent and oversight to provide consistency.[36] Issues of efficiency and uniformity were a particular imperative during public workshops over intellectual property policy. Commentators emphasised

[33] R.B. Korobkin & S.R. Munzer. Stem Cell Research and the Law. *UCLA School of Law Research Paper 06-05*. 2006.

[34] A. Erbsen. Horizontal Federalism. *Minnesota Law Review* 2008; 93(2).

[35] A. D'Andrea. Federalizing Bioethics. *Texas Law Review* 2005; 83: 1663–1715.

[36] CIRM. 2006. *Summary and Response to Public Comment for the Proposed CIRM MES Regulations*. San Francisco, CA: CIRM.

that institute regulations need to be consistent with national policy governing patenting and licensing regimes.[37] The same themes have been echoed in other states. States appear to have achieved an optimal resolution by taking a decentralised approach to research authorisation — allowing experiments not eligible for federal funding — but adopting oversight, intellectual property and administrative policies generally consistent with centralised federal guidelines and regulations.

The issues of social capital and justice relate to pluralism, democratic participation and fairness in policy-making. Mazzone suggests the deliberative approach taken by state stem cell programmes is important because it provides important opportunities for citizens to meet, work out differences, and participate in self-governance. The process in turn builds social networks and trust that can ultimately inform enlightened federal policy-making.[38] Siegel asserts that pluralism is promoted when state policies differ along various dimensions on controversial issues in American culture.[39] Stem cell science is a model for such differences. In addition to programmes designed to advance research not eligible for federal funding, a number of states have imposed restrictions, including criminalisation, which exceeds federal policy.[40] Thus, a decentralised approach has resulted in a highly pluralistic approach to research regulation.

Justice in policy-making tends to be concerned with the prevention of harm and distribution of public goods. One advantage of decentralisation is that it allows states to serve as laboratories for democracy and consider the distributional effects of polices. Indeed, with regard to justice-related concerns, state stem cell programmes have been a source of policy innovation. The California Institute's research standards contain novel provisions requiring free treatment to research donors for direct and proximate

[37] CIRM. 2008. *Intellectual Property Regulations Consolidation Project*. San Francisco, CA: CIRM.

[38] J. Mazzone. The Social Capital Argument for Federalism. *Southern California Interdisciplinary Law Journal* 2001; 11(27): 27–62.

[39] N. Siegel. International Delegations and the Values of Federalism. *Law and Contemporary Problems* 2008; 71: 93–113.

[40] National Conference of State Legislation. 2008. *Stem Cell Research*. Available from: http://www.ncsl.org/programs/health/Genetics/embfet.htm [Accessed 1 Feb 2009].

medical complications.[41] Such requirements do not exist in federal policy. The institute's intellectual property policy constrains certain types of exclusive patent licenses to promote the sharing of research materials and requires 25 per cent of certain royalty streams to be returned to the state.[42] Consistent with approaches taken elsewhere, vital research materials such as cell line and cell-derived products must be made available for basic research.[43] In addition, there are requirements for the development of affordable access plans for the eventual distribution of cell therapies. These specific examples are indicator policies that reflect the ongoing desire to ensure broad health and economic benefit from stem cell research.[44]

Given state stem cell programs are in relatively early stages of development, indicators of the efficacy of these policies are just emerging. As theory would suggest, a decentralized approach has advanced policy innovation designed to promote equity and fairness.[45] For example, a recent study funded by the National Science Foundation, describes the involvement of multiple stakeholders and concludes that California has established itself as a major center for stem cell research effecting both the distribution biotechnological infrastructure, start up firms and investment of venture capital in the United States.[46] Now that the federal government has lifted the 2001 funding restrictions and targeted biomedical research for economic stimulus funding, there may be opportunities to learn from the experience of states to further advance the field — a rejuvenated federalism.

---

[41] G.P. Lomax, Z.W. Hall & B. Lo. Responsible Oversight of Human Stem Cell Research: The California Institute for Regenerative Medicine's Medical and Ethical Standards. *PLoS Medicine* 2007; 4(5): e114.

[42] D.E. Winickoff. Governing Stem Cell Research in California and the USA: Towards a Social Infrastructure. *Trends Biotechnology* 2006; 24(9): 390–394.

[43] R. Brownsword. Stem Cells, Superman, and the Report of the Select Committee. *Modern Law Review* 2002; 65(4): 568–587.

[44] M.T. Longaker, L.C. Baker & H.T. Greely. Proposition 71 and CIRM — Assessing the Return on Investment. *Nature Biotechnology* 2007; 25(5): 513–521.

[45] A. D'Andrea. Federalizing Bioethics. *Texas Law Review* 2005; 83: 1663–1715.

[46] Adelson, J. The California stem cell initiative: Persuasion, politics, and public science. *American Journal of Public Health* 2010: published online ahead of print.

CRITIQUES OF A STATE-BASED APPROACH

Some commentators have questioned the efficacy of state-based approaches for the regulation of biotechnology.[47] These critiques tend to converge around limitations in agency authority or the reach of policies enabling programme initiation. With regard to stem cell science, they advocate centralised approaches with authority emanating from a federal commission.[48] These approaches emphasise public consultation and democratic decision-making, but the specific mechanisms advocated are substantially similar to existing state-level deliberative processes. Given the paucity of evidence to support the efficacy of any particular deliberative approach or mechanism, the advantage of this configuration is not immediately evident. As Pieterse has suggested there is no case, example or validated model of participatory democracy on a major scale.[49] Further, centralised approaches amplify potential risk associated with creating a 'fifth arm of government' outside the networks of democratic control.[50] Such risks could be associated with any advisory body, but centralised ones appear less likely to support pluralism and self-governance by virtue of their national scale. As Siegel has highlighted, it is uncontroversial descriptively that federal rules have prevented different parts of the US from governing themselves in ways that accommodate variance in normative values.[51]

PLURALITY AND LEVELS OF ENGAGEMENT

Concerns over the efficacy of state-based approaches may emanate from the fact that the configurations of actors engaged in deliberations concerning programme implementation do not necessarily reflect a plurality

---

[47] F. Fukuyama. How to Regulate Science. *Public Interest* 2002; Winter (146): 3–23.

[48] F. Fukuyama & F. Furger. 2009. *Beyond Bioethics. A Proposal for Modernizing the Regulation of Human Biotechnologies*. Washington DC: The Paul H. Nitze School of Advanced International Studies: 471.

[49] J.N. Pieterse. Participatory Democratization Reconceived. *Futures* 2001; 33(5): 407–422.

[50] S. Jasanoff. 1990. *The Fifth Branch: Science Advisers as Policymakers*. Cambridge, MA.: Harvard University Press: xiii, 302.

[51] N. Siegel. International Delegations and the Values of Federalism. *Law and Contemporary Problems* 2008; 71: 93–113.

of society overall. This tendency should be anticipated; because, once stem cell research is constitutionally sanctioned, an incompatible position is created for those who oppose embryo destruction on moral grounds.[52] This incompatibility explains why adherents to a 'pro-life' position have engaged in legal and policy actions intended to prevent programme initiation. The legal challenges in California sought to block programme implementation by overturning the constitutional amendments of the *Stem Cell Research and Cures Initiative*. 'Pro-life' constituencies have successfully advocated for laws that restrict and even criminalise research involving embryo destruction in some states.[53] At the federal level, the 'pro-life' focus is on ongoing enactment and expansions of policy that prohibits the use of embryos in research. Given this incompatibility, there is no perceived advantage and potentially great risk — though perceived tacit acceptance of an illegitimate endeavor — of participating in downstream programme development. In California, 'pro-life' organisations have not been openly present at public deliberations convened pursuant to programme development, and other states report a similar experience.

It should be expected that deliberations concerning programme development and implementation involve a narrower set of interests, as compared to society as a whole. Experience suggests that deliberations attract a configuration of actors that (1) aspire to programme benefits — researcher institutions, patients, industry among others — or (2) activists concerned with issues of governance, social justice and participatory democracy in general. This point does not imply that administrators should not be sensitive to the range of societal concerns. Rather it explains why deliberations over operational priorities may be somewhat narrowed in relation to broader societal debates. Administrators are generally charged with a duty to address a defined set of issues and needs. Consequently, the public record will tend to reflect agency responsiveness to a self-selected group of participants engaged in these deliberations.

---

[52] B.M. Dickens & R.J. Cook. Acquiring Human Embryos for Stem-Cell Research. *International Journal of Gynecology and Obstetrics* 2007; 96(1): 67–71.

[53] National Conference of State Legislation. 2008. *Stem Cell Research*. Available from: http://www.ncsl.org/programs/health/Genetics/embfet.htm [Accessed 1 Feb 2009].

This self-selection process should not be viewed as a threat to plurality or democratic decision-making. There is ample opportunity for advocates of a more restricted approach to stem cell research to influence policy at the level of programme initiation. In the US, policy initiation, and by extension administrative agency charge; is determined by the will of the people either through elected representatives or, in some jurisdictions, through voter referendum. This point is evidenced by enactment of restrictive state and federal laws. Plurality is maintained because the democratic system offers levels of engagement commensurate with an actor's core interests. In the long run, no consensus may ever be achieved regarding the moral status of the embryo, suggesting internal and external discord will reign freely at multiple levels.[54]

THE EMERGENCE OF FEDERAL STEM CELL POLICY

The year 2009 brought a change in the US presidency and national stem cell policy. After taking office, President Obama directed the US National Institutes of Health (NIH) to develop guidelines to support *responsible, scientifically worthy human stem cell research, including human embryonic stem cell research, to the extent permitted by law.*[55] The process, which resulted in the release of final guidelines in July 2009, mirrored states' experience and supports the premise that principles of federalism serves to advance effective governance of stem cell science.

Specifically, the NIH introduced a draft policy, and then initiated a process of public review and comment. The draft policy catalysed state-state interactions and broader 'networking' among the stem cell research community. US state members of the *Interstate Alliance on Stem Cell Research* engaged NIH and articulated a number of considerations for aligning the guidelines with existing policy.[56] These considerations, based

[54] L.M. Solomon & S.A. Brockman-Lee. Embryonic Stem Cells in Science and Medicine, Part II: Law, Ethics, and the Continuing Need for Dialogue. *Gender Medicine* 2008; 5(1): 3–9.

[55] F. Register. 2009. Draft National Institutes of Health Guidelines for Human Stem Cell Research Notice. G.P. Office, ed. Government Printing Office: 18578–18580.

[56] IASCR. 2009. *IASCR Notes from Discussion of the Draft NIH Guidelines.*

on states' experience with research programme administration, emerged as formal recommendations to NIH. A remarkable consensus emerged among states, research institutions and patient organisations over how the guidelines could be optimally aligned with established research practice.[57] The final NIH Guidelines incorporated the major recommendations of the broader research community.

THE PATHWAY TOWARDS CLINICAL APPLICATION

This volume emphasises ethical challenges relating to medical applications of stem cell therapies. This chapter has focused on procedural mechanisms that have served to advance effective policy governing basic research; suggesting they have been efficacious in advancing responsible science in a pluralistic environment. A major goal of stem cell science is to translate this basic research into therapeutic products. There are clear indications that the primary federal authority, the US Food and Drug Administration (FDA), will be assertive in evaluating clinical applications. For example, the FDA approved the first clinical trial involving human embryonic stem cell-derived therapeutics in January 2009, and numerous studies involving investigational stem cell-based products have been submitted.[58]

Perhaps more importantly the FDA has initiated efforts to promote communication and exchange between the agency and its stakeholders with the goal of facilitating development of safe and effective therapeutic products. Specifically, the FDA has supported the development of collaborative partnerships, including state-based programmes, to consider risk management and related issues for clinical trials. The timing of this effort is exquisite because the regulations of clinical trials must be achieved through a national authority. However, this collaborative approach suggests the FDA seeks to draw on the collective experience of the research community. While it is premature to forecast specific issues requiring

[57] IASCR. 2009. *Advancing the Promise: Leading Research Institutions, Patients and Scholars Comment on the Draft NIH Guidelines for Human Stem Cell Research.*
[58] D.W. Fink Jr. FDA Regulation of Stem Cell-Based Products. *Science* 2009; 324(5935): 1662–1663.

resolution, indicators suggest a credible process will be in place to address them as they emerge.

CONCLUSION

Stem cell science has become embroiled in intractable value conflicts driven by powerful social, cultural and political forces. Against this backdrop US states have been charged with the development of programmes designed to promote research, advance cell therapies and stimulate economic development. States have responded by employing procedural mechanisms designed to ensure transparency, consistency and due process in policy development. As the intrinsic technical challenges posed by this mandate became apparent, state, national and international networks emerged to address nuanced policy considerations and support the evidentiary basis for policy development. Consistent with the principles of federalism, a new federal policy has emerged that incorporates states' experience with stem cell policy development. This chapter has highlighted numerous public policy innovations that have emerged to support ethically and socially responsible stem cell science. At the current time, it is critical to maintain this interaction between state and federal jurisdictions to support the development of responsible clinical application of stem cell science — a rejuvenated federalism.

12

HYBRID EMBRYOS — ETHICS, LAW AND RHETORIC IN THE UNITED KINGDOM'S STEM CELL POLICY

Natasha Hammond-Browning and Søren Holm

It is a trite platitude that scientific progress is fast and unpredictable, and the stem cell area is one area where this platitude has been verified several times. When we began to write this paper in early autumn 2008, hybrid embryos were the best thing after 'sliced bread'. They were going to solve the so-called 'egg supply' problem in stem cell research; and great political energy had just been expended on legalising their creation in a number of countries. During the debate in the United Kingdom parliament it was, for instance, claimed that:

> '...there is not a great deal of scientific pressure at the moment to do research on true hybrids, but there is a lot of such pressure to do research on cytoplasmic hybrids. The reason is clear: there is a great shortage of human eggs. If it were possible to do this research using animal eggs, there would be a virtually unlimited supply. I remind your Lordships that we are talking about research that is essential for the future'.[1]

In March 2009, when we were finalising the paper, hybrid embryos had appeared to have fallen from this position of prominence, and been overtaken by induced Pluripotent Stem (iPS) cells as the next big thing.

[1] Lord Harris of Pentregarth 3 Dec 2007. *House of Lords Hansard (Debates)*. Vol 696, Col 1522–1523 HL.

In this chapter we will therefore first describe and analyse the development of UK policy in relation to hybrid embryos. We will then briefly describe recent developments concerning iPS cells, and analyse some common challenges faced by hybrid and iPS cells in the transition from basic to clinical research.

The UK has consistently been at the forefront of regulating developments in human fertilisation and embryology; it was the first country to formally regulate fertility treatments in the 1990s, further expanding this regulation to encompass, for example, embryos created specifically through somatic cell nuclear transfer and human embryonic stem cell research, and now it is leading the way in regulating experimentation upon hybrid embryos.[2]

As will be seen, the legislation of the UK refers to hybrid embryos as 'human admixed embryos', however for the purposes of this paper the authors will refer to such embryos as hybrids. These embryos are often referred to by scientists as cytoplasmic hybrid embryos to indicate the mix of animal cytoplasm and the human nuclear DNA. The term 'true hybrids' will be used to refer to embryos created with human and animal gametes.

Hybrid embryos have three possible uses: for use in general stem cell research (i.e. solving the general 'egg supply' problem); to derive stem cells from people with specific diseases for research; and finally, as the basis for personalised stem cell treatments (so-called 'therapeutic cloning'). It could be argued that there is now no scientific reason to use hybrid embryos to derive stem cells from people with specific diseases, due to the advent of iPS cells (thus bypassing the cloning process); and that the same holds with regard to personalised treatments, because it can be pursued more effectively by iPS cell technology. However, it could, on the other hand, be argued that the use of hybrid embryos for general stem cell research is still valid, although developments in iPS cell methods may also make this use obsolete.

[2] The 1990 Act has now been replaced by the Human Fertilisation and Embryology Act 2008, which incorporates various amendments, added since inception, and adapted to keep pace with scientific developments.

HYBRIDS AND THE HFEA

Hybrid embryos first came to the attention of the UK's embryology regulator, the Human Fertilisation and Embryology Authority (hereafter referred to as the HFEA) in November 2006 when it:

> '…received applications from two different research teams for a licence to derive stem cells from human embryos. However, in order to overcome the shortage of egg donors, the researchers proposed using animal eggs instead of human eggs to create the embryos'.[3]

As these applications raised for the first time significant social and ethical implications, the HFEA decided to postpone a decision upon the licence applications until after a public consultation on this matter. The HFEA consultation, *Hybrids and Chimeras,* ran for three months from April to July 2007, and set out the legal, scientific and ethical background to the creation of hybrid embryos clearly, before seeking public opinion.

Following the public consultation, the HFEA considered how it should approach the licensing of hybrid research. They concluded that not only did such research fall legally within the HFEA's remit, there was also *'…no fundamental reason to prevent cytoplasmic hybrid research'.*[4] As such, if an individual research team can prove that hybrid embryo research is 'necessary and desirable' as required by the legislation, then a licence could be granted.

The two original separate licence applications, from King's College London and the University of Newcastle-upon-Tyne, were approved by the HFEA and granted in January 2008.[5] A third research licence application from the University of Warwick has since been approved.[6]

---

[3] HFEA. 2007. *Hybrids and Chimeras: A Consultation on the Ethical and Social Implications of Creating Human/Animal Embryos in Research*: para 1.3.

[4] HFEA. 2007. *Hybrids and Chimeras: A Report on the Findings of the Consultation*: para 7.2.

[5] HFEA. 2008. *HFEA Statement on Licensing of Applications to Carry Out Research using Human-Animal Cytoplasmic Hybrid Embryos.* 17th January. Available at: http://www.hfea.gov.uk/418.html [Accessed 22 Feb 2009].

[6] HFEA. *University of Warwick* HFEA Current Research Projects. Available at: http://www.hfea.gov.uk/en/1699.html [Accessed 22 Feb 2009].

The legislative requirement that the use of embryos is 'necessary and desirable' for the research will, in the future, be far harder to prove since the rapid developments involving iPS cells raise questions as to the grounds of 'necessity' (conversely, no such grounds exist for iPS cell research). The Act will not justify the issuing of licences for hybrid embryo research where a viable alternative exists, and which does not require the use of embryos.

Since human iPS cells where first derived in 2007, the methods for induction has developed very rapidly, and iPS cells can now be derived without any permanent change of the genome.[7] This means that iPS cells are quickly becoming a scientifically valid alternative to hybrid embryos for many research purposes since the newer techniques are likely to make them more like 'standard' embryonic stem cells than the techniques first described in 2007.

Interestingly, the projects related to the first two licences to be granted by the HFEA have recently been refused funding by the Medical Research Council (hereafter referred to as the MRC). Accusations of the funding refusal occurring due to ethical objections have been rejected by the MRC who claimed that the applications were rejected following rigorous peer review which does not allow for moral objections to influence the outcome.[8] There has also been a general shift in funding towards adult stem cells, principally due to the advent of iPS cells, with the MRC last year increasing funding of adult stem cells from 46% to 61.3% of its overall funding for stem cell research.[9] This is not a deliberate change in overall policy, but merely a shift in the split of the overall allocation to stem cell

[7] K. Takahashi *et al.* Induction of Pluripotent Stem Cells from Adult Human Fibroblasts by Defined Factors. *Cell* 2007; 131: 1–12; J. Yu *et al.* Induced Pluripotent Stem Cell Lines Derived from Human Somatic Cells. *Science* 2007; 318: 1917–1920; K. Kaji *et al.* Virus-Free Induction of Pluripotency and Subsequent Excision of Reprogramming Factors. *Nature* 2009; 458: 771–775; and K. Woltjen *et al.* PiggyBac Transposition Reprograms Fibroblasts to Induced Pluripotent Stem Cells. *Nature* 2009; 458: 766–770.

[8] S. Connor. 2009. Funding Halted for Stem Cell Research. *The Independent* 13 Jan. Available at: http://www.independent.co.uk/news/science/funding-halted-for-stem-cell-research-1332000.html [Accessed 19 Jan 2009]; and MRC. 2009. *MRC Defends Position on Stem Cell Research Funding*. Available at: http://www.mrc.ac.uk/consumption/groups/public/documents/content/mrc005376.pdf [Accessed 19 Jan 2009].

[9] I. Sample. 2009. Rival Stem Cell Technique Takes Heat Out of Hybrid Embryo Debate. *The Guardian* 13 Jan. Available at: http://www.guardian.co.uk/science/2009/jan/13/hybrid-embryos-stem-cells/print [Accessed 19 Jan 2009].

research as a result of the peer review and grant panel processes. In spite of the fact that there are currently three research teams with licences to undertake hybrid embryo research within the UK, and are still legally able to do so, two have no funding for such work and are likely to stop work as soon as the money that they do have runs out whilst the third, Warwick, is yet to start whilst a grant proposal is completed.[10]

The HFEA claim that hybrid embryo research was within its legal remit has also been challenged. The HFEA took this view based upon the previous House of Lords decision in *Quintavalle.*[11] The case was brought by Bruno Quintavalle on behalf of the Pro-Life Alliance, who challenged the view that embryos created by somatic cell nuclear transfer fell within the remit of the HFEA. The House of Lords held that embryos created by somatic cell nuclear transfer did fall within the legal definition contained within the *Human Fertilisation and Embryology Act 1990* (the 1990 Act), if given a *purposive reading* — as they were 'live human embryos'.[12] The Courts have taken a liberal interpretation of the 1990 Act, as it would not be desirable to leave such embryos outside of the statutory regulation when Parliament had clearly intended embryo research to be carefully regulated. Although it was a purposive interpretation which was taken towards section 1 of the 1990 Act, this was still a liberal approach to take in the sense that the Court could have given a literal interpretation as they did with s3(3)(d). So by taking this liberal approach they included embryos not specifically referred to in the Act. It could be argued that hybrid embryos were also not desired when the 1990 Act was brought in and so the HFEA would need the Court to again take a purposive, liberal interpretation.

The HFEA would understandably be hopeful that, should the regulation of hybrid embryos be challenged in the Courts under the 1990 Act, then a purposive interpretation would again be made. The concern of a court challenge arising was played out when the Christian Legal Centre and Comment on Reproductive Ethics (a second 'Pro-life' group) sought a

---

[10] S. Connor. 2009. Funding Halted for Stem Cell Work. *The Independent* 13 Jan. Available at: http://www.independent.co.uk/news/science/funding-halted-for-stem-cell-research-1332000.html [Accessed 19 Jan 2009].

[11] *R (on the application of Quintavalle) v Secretary of State for Health* [2001] 4 All ER 1013, [2002] 2 All ER 625, [2002] 2 All ER 113.

[12] N. Hammond. Revisiting Quintavalle — Knee Jerk Reactions and Illogical Judgments. *Medical Law Monitor* 2006; 13 (6): 7–12 and 13 (7): 7–8.

judicial review of the HFEA decision claiming that '…the HFEA had exceeded its jurisdiction in licensing the conduct of human/animal hybrid research because it was only empowered to license research using human embryos'.[13] Although the application for judicial review was refused by the High Court in December 2008,[14] such matters, at that time, were covered by the 1990 Act, pending the implementation of the 2008 revision (which came into force in October 2009). It is now completely clear, from the legal perspective, that hybrid embryos (so defined) fall within the remit of the HFEA, and that research upon such embryos is legally permitted. The enactment of the *Human Fertilisation and Embryology Act 2008* (the 2008 Act) was a long time coming into being, and the debate surrounding hybrid embryos was some of the fiercest. It is to this that we turn to now.

DEBATE

The UK Government has not always been supportive of allowing the creation of hybrid embryos for research purposes. Back in 2000, the then Government agreed with a recommendation made in the Report: *Stem Cell Research: Medical Progress with Responsibility* (the 'Donaldson Report'), that the creation of cytoplasmic hybrid embryos should be prohibited, and additionally called upon the relevant funding bodies not to support this type of research.[15]

---

[13] M. Allyse. 2008. Legal Challenge Over 'Hybrid Embryo' Research. *BioNews* 28 November. Available at: http://www.bionews.org.uk/new.lasso?storyid=4092 [Accessed 1 December 2008].

[14] M. Allyse. 2008. Legal Challenge over 'Hybrid Embryo' Research Fails. *BioNews* 16 November. Available at: http://www.bionews.org.uk/new.lasso?storyid=4127 [Accessed 19 December 2008].

[15] Department of Health. 2000. *Stem Cell Research: Medical Progress with Responsibility. A Report from the Chief Medical Officer's Expert Group Reviewing the Potential of Developments in Stem Cell Research and Cell Nuclear Replacement to Benefit Human Health.* London: Department of Health: para 2.62 and recommendation 6. Available at: http://www.dh.gov.uk/en/Publicationsandstatistics/Publications/PublicationsPolicyAnd Guidance/DH_4065084 [Accessed 15 Aug 2008]. Department of Health. 2000. *Government Response to the Recommendations Made in the Chief Medical Officer's Expert Group Report 'Stem Cell Research: Medical Progress with Responsibility'*. London: Department of Health: para 8. Available at: http://www.dh.gov.uk/en/Publicationsandstatistics/Publications/ PublicationsPolicyAndGuidance/DH_4123598 [Accessed 22 Feb 009].

The prohibition on the creation of true hybrids and chimeras can also be seen in the Consultation on the 1990 Act, although the Government did open up the discussion to consider the creation of cytoplasmic hybrid embryos.[16] In the proposals for revised legislation, the prohibition of creating true hybrid embryos is continued, although a regulation-making power is suggested so as to permit some research under the new Act should the need arise for hybrid embryo research to be undertaken in the future.[17]

Following a subsequent report from the House of Commons Science and Technology Select Committee, which considered the Government proposals concerning the use of hybrid and chimera embryos in embryo research, the Government altered the stance which it had previously taken.[18] This about turn by the Government on hybrid embryos can be seen in the Draft Bill.

It is in the Draft Bill that we first see definitions of hybrid embryos and the proposal to allow the creation of such embryos for research purposes. At this point hybrid embryos are referred to as 'inter-species embryos' and are defined as:

(a) *an embryo created by using human gametes and the gametes of an animal,*
(b) *an embryo created by replacing the nucleus of an animal egg or a cell derived from an animal embryo with a human cell or the nucleus of a human cell,*
(c) *a human embryo that has been altered by the introduction of any sequence of nuclear or mitochondrial DNA of an animal,*

---

[16] Department of Health. 2005. *Review of the Human Fertilisation and Embryology Act: Consultation*. London: Department of Health: Section 9.29–9.35. Available at: http://www.dh.gov.uk/en/Consultations/Closedconsultations/DH_4123863 [Accessed 22 February 2009].

[17] Department of Health. 2006. *Review of the Human Fertilisation and Embryology Act: Proposals for Revised Legislation*. London: Department of Health: Section 2.85. Available at: http://www.dh.gov.uk/en/Publicationsandstatistics/Publications/PublicationsPolicyAndGuidance/DH_073098 [Accessed 22 February 2009].

[18] House of Commons, Science and Technology Committee. 2007. *Government Proposals for the Regulation of Hybrid and Chimera Embryos: Fifth Report of Session 2006–2007*. London: The Stationery Office Limited. Available at: http://www.publications.parliament.uk/pa/cm200607/cmselect/cmsctech/272/272i.pdf [Accessed 22 February 2009].

(d) *a human embryo that has been altered by the introduction of one or more animal cells, or*
(e) *any other embryo that contains both —*

  (i) *any haploid set of human chromosomes, and*
  (ii) *any haploid set of animal chromosomes or any other sequence of nuclear or mitochondrial DNA of an animal.*[19]

Part (e) of this section was designed as a 'catch-all' provision, so that any future methods for creating hybrid embryos which are discovered are also encompassed by the Act; and thus designed to avoid the type of challenge previously made by Quintavalle and CORE. However, this section was difficult, and in fact impossible, to explain even by the scientists involved in the field![20] The Joint Committee which reported upon the Draft Bill also criticised the Government approach to defining inter-species embryos. A general definition was suggested which would have been in line with the approach taken in defining entirely genetically-human embryos.[21] Whilst this approach was rejected by the Government, the inexplicable Part (e) was removed from the Bill when it was published on the 8th of November 2007.

The Bill went through numerous amendments before the final version was agreed upon and given Royal Assent on the 13th of November 2008. Provisions relating to parenthood (Part 2 of the Act) have been introduced in April 2009. The remainder of the legislation including regulating the creation of human embryos outside the body, banning sex selection for non-medical reasons, provisions clarifying the scope of embryo research and making it easier to do follow up research using HFEA data will be introduced in October 2009. During the passage through Parliament, the issues of hybrid embryos and abortion became central to the debate and other issues fell by the wayside. Debate concerning hybrid embryos took

[19] Department of Health. *Human Tissue and Embryos (Draft) Bill* (2007) CM7087. London: The Stationery Office: Part 2, Clause 17, sub clause 2(5).
[20] *Joint Committee on the Human Tissue and Embryos (Draft) Bill Volume I: Report* HL Paper 169-I, HC Paper 630-I, refer to paragraphs 162 and 173.
[21] *Joint Committee on the Human Tissue and Embryos (Draft) Bill Volume I: Report* HL Paper 169-I, HC Paper 630-I, refer to paragraph 178.

up a vast amount of parliamentary time; whilst necessary it was also perhaps repetitive since a large amount of the discussion was about the general issue of the moral status of the embryo, discussions which had also played a large role during the debate of the 1990 Act. It is after the first set of amendments that the term 'inter-species embryo' is lost, and replaced with 'human admixed embryo'. The change in terminology occurred due to the debate in the House of Lords, where it was argued that 'human admixed embryo' was a better reflection of what these embryos are, from a scientific point of view:

> '"[H]uman admixed embryo" has been suggested as a more accurate collective term to describe those entities that the Bill seeks to bring clearly within its regulation. The new term is more suitable because it specifies what we debated in Committee: the human admix is nearer to the human end as opposed to the animal admixed embryos'.[22]

The Act defines it as:

> 'For the purposes of this Act a human admixed embryo is —
>
> (a) an embryo created by replacing the nucleus of an animal egg or of an animal cell, or two animal pronuclei with —
>
> (i) two human pronuclei,
> (ii) one nucleus of a human gamete or of any other human cell, or
> (iii) one human gamete or other human cell.
>
> (b) any other embryo created using —
>
> (i) human gametes and animal gametes, or
> (ii) one human pronucleus and one animal pronucleus,
>
> (c) a human embryo that has been altered by the introduction of any sequence of nuclear or mitochondrial DNA of an animal into one or more cells of the embryo,

---

[22] Lord Darzi of Denham 15 Jan 2008. House of Lords Hansard (Debates) Vol 697, Col 1195 HL.

(d) a human embryo that has been altered by the introduction of one or more animal cells, or

(e) any embryo not falling within paragraphs (a) to (d) which contains both nuclear or mitochondrial DNA of a human and nuclear or mitochondrial DNA of an animal ("animal DNA") but in which the animal DNA is not predominant'.

Although not all members of Parliament were happy with this new legal name:

> '…after helpful explication of the language of the "human admixed embryo", is left thinking that the previous phrase, "interspecies embryo", was clearer for the man or woman in the street, the church or the mosque, than what we now offer'.[23]

It could be argued that the term 'human admixed embryo' is in fact misleading to the general public, who find this area of science difficult enough to follow as it is. It could be argued that by including the word 'human' it is suggesting that these are completely or essentially *human* embryos, something which it is acknowledged is difficult to debate and resolve from an ethical and scientific viewpoint. The *legal* name for such embryos does not truly acknowledge the animal contribution, however small that may be, since it does not make it clear what the human is 'admixed' with. While the legal definition of 'human admixed embryos' does clearly acknowledge the animal contribution in the creation of these embryos, most publications (of a non-specialist nature) are likely to exclude such nuances, preferring instead to use the short-hand: 'human admixed embryo'.

The 2008 Act has made it clear that any hybrid embryos created under a licence from the HFEA cannot be placed into a woman.[24] This therefore negates the risk of hybrid embryos being used for fertility treatment.

---

[23] The Lord Bishop of Winchester 15 Jan 2008 Vol 697, Col 1194 HL.

[24] *Human Fertilisation and Embryology Act 2008*:Section 3(2) and Schedule 2, Para 2 (c).

DERIVATION OF STEM CELLS FROM HYBRID EMBRYOS

A question which remains to be resolved is the regulation and permitted uses of any embryonic stem cells which may be obtained from a hybrid embryo. When the HFEA grants a licence for the creation of embryos and the subsequent derivation of stem cells, it also attaches the condition that any resulting stem cell lines must be banked with the UK Stem Cell Bank.[25] The UK Stem Cell Bank then allows other researchers to access those stem cell lines for research. Eventually these stem cell lines may be used in treatments.

The question we ask here is: whether those stem cell lines which are derived from hybrid embryos may be used for treatment? Whilst it is admitted that this possibility is still somewhat in the future for all types of embryonic stem cell lines, it is prudent to consider the issue now.

The HFEA is currently in the pre-implementation stages of its Eighth Code of Practice; and it is expected that further guidance will be contained within the Code of Practice as to who is responsible for the oversight and regulation of the use of hybrid embryonic *stem cells*. The Interim UK Regulatory Route Map for Stem Cell Research and Manufacture also provides some guidance and is discussed further below.

Whilst the HFEA regulates and controls human gametes and human embryos (as well as hybrid embryos), it does not regulate any products derived from those embryos, including stem cells. As previously mentioned, the HFEA makes it a condition of all research licences which have as their purpose the derivation of stem cells from embryos that any resulting stem cell lines must be banked with the UK Stem Cell Bank. Human embryonic stem cells are therefore overseen by the UK Stem Cell Bank. iPS cell-derived cell lines do not involve gametes or embryos in the derivation process, and their derivation is therefore outside of the remit of the HFEA. They can thus be derived without HFEA approval and there is therefore no mechanism for requiring their deposition in the UK Stem Cell Bank or their further research use. The need to regulate iPS cells can be questioned due to their non-controversial sources, although the fact

[25] HFEA. 2008. Appendix A. 7th *Code of Practice*. Available at: http://cop.hfea.gov.uk/cop/pdf/CodeOfPracticeVR_4.pdf [Accessed 22 Feb 2009].

that the Government has taken steps to regulate all other forms of stem cells (embryonic through the HFEA and UK Stem Cell Bank, adult through the Human Tissue Authority) could be one argument for also regulating iPS cells, particularly when they could be used in clinical trials and treatments in the future. It could also be argued that there is a need for regulation or at least oversight in the context of basic research. The EU Tissues Directive regulates clinical research with iPS cells, but not basic research and such research also falls outside the scope of the National Research Ethics Service and of the Human Tissue Authority in the UK. But iPS cells are derived from humans and the donors of the cells from which the iPS cell lines are derived arguably have an interest in their further use being regulated in some way.[26]

The UK Stem Cell Bank controls who accesses the stem cell lines which are banked with it, as well as the permitted research purposes upon those stem cell lines. In deciding what is a permitted research purpose the UK Stem Cell Bank *Code of Practice* reflects the permitted research purposes found in the HFE (Research Purposes) Regulations 2001 (and now incorporated into the 2008 Act), in that it allows access to, and research upon, embryonic stem cell lines only for the following purposes:

(a) research which increases the knowledge about the development of embryos or has the long term goal of helping to increase knowledge about serious diseases and their treatment…
(b) basic cell research which underpins these aims…
(c) development of cell based therapies for clinical trials in respect of serious human diseases.[27]

(It is thought that the UK Stem Cell Bank will also rewrite its Code of Practice so as to reflect the permitted research purposes within the 2008

[26] S. Holm. Who Should Control the Use of Human Embryonic Stem Cell Lines. A Defence of the Donors' Ability to Control. *Journal of Bioethical Inquiry* 2006; 3(1-2): 55–68.

[27] MRC. 2006. *Code of Practice for the Use of Human Stem Cell Lines*: Section 8.1.1, p. 12. Available at: http://www.ukstemcellbank.org.uk/documents/Code%20of%20Practice%20for%20the%20Use%20of%20Human%20Stem%20Cell%20Lines.pdf [Accessed 22 February 009].

Act when it comes into force.) By reflecting the permitted research purposes of the 2001 Regulations, it retains public confidence in the reasons *why* embryos are legally used and destroyed for research.[28] Whilst embryonic stem cells are no longer part of an embryo nor are they classified as an embryo, some people do not distinguish between an embryo and an embryonic stem cell, viewing an embryonic stem cell with the same moral significance as they view an embryo. Others would attach moral significance to these stem cells purely because they are derived from embryos. Due to the controversial source of these stem cells public confidence needs to be retained in the research which is done upon them.

The research licences which have been granted to the three research teams working in London, Newcastle and Warwick also have the condition that any stem cells which are derived from the hybrid embryos must also be banked with the UK Stem Cell Bank.[29] Once banked with the UK Stem Cell Bank they will be subject to the same Code of Practice which controls access to and research upon other embryonic stem cell lines. The foreseeable issue, however, is the UK Stem Cell Bank's last permitted purpose: that of 'developing cell-based therapies for clinical trials in respect of serious human diseases'. This will be an issue as it has been made clear that whilst it may be desirable and necessary to use hybrid embryos for research, it is debatable whether it is desirable to use such embryos for use in *human* clinical trials or treatments.

Using stem cell lines derived from hybrids in clinical trials or treatments may not be desirable due to the lack of knowledge as to what impact the animal mitochondria will play in the development of the hybrid embryo and the derived stem cells. Although such cells are predominantly human in origin (i.e. the nuclear DNA), one cannot assume that the animal component plays no role at all in their function. After all, human mitochondrial diseases are known, and therefore there is reason to believe that animal mitochondria will have a phenotypic effect. One suggestion

---

[28] Refer to Department of Health and Social Security. 1984. *Report of the Committee of Inquiry into Human Fertilisation and Embryology*. London: Her Majesty's Stationery Office: para 11.10 for the limits which were suggested for research involving human embryos.

[29] Confirmed by private correspondence with the HFEA 16 Mar 2009.

for how this problem can be overcome is by performing a second cell nuclear transfer procedure from the hybrid stem cell into a human enucleated cell. This would result in a stem cell with no animal mitochondria.

A similar issue arises in relation to iPS cells. Both types of stem cells are derived through the use of an 'unnatural' technique and it is not possible to foresee and control all the risks associated with these techniques. This presents similar risks to those identified in xenotransplantation. The possible risk of passing infections or diseases from animals to humans, and possibly on into the general population is one that is very clear when dealing with xenotransplantation. Whilst the risk is far less clear with the possible use of hybrid embryo-derived stem cells for treatment, it is still a foreseeable risk. The regulator for xenotransplantation was shut down in December 2006;[30] subsequently the Department of Health has issued guidance for xenotransplantation.[31] Depending upon if the proposed use of xenotransplantation is for research, clinical trials or treatment a scientist will need to approach one or more bodies for approval.

Hybrid embryo-derived stem cells can be compared to xenotransplantation not only for the possible animal/human transmission risks, but also for the bodies which would need to be approached for approval prior to research, clinical trials or treatment. As previously discussed, a researcher who wishes to create hybrid embryos to derive stem cells will require a licence from the HFEA and must have prior approval from a research ethics committee. A researcher wishing to conduct research upon hybrid embryo-derived stem cells would need to approach a research ethics committee for approval, and then the UK Stem Cell Bank for access to the stem cells. A scientist looking to undertake clinical trials and/or treatment involving hybrid embryo-derived stem cells will need to not only receive research ethics committee approval first, but will also need to comply with the EU Tissues Directive and as such would be subject to the controls of the Human Tissue Authority and where appropriate the Medicine and

---

[30] The reasons for the decision to abolish the xenotransplantation regulator are not clear, but it was a part of a general government drive to streamline its regulatory systems. See also S. McLean & L. Williamson. The Demise of UKXIRA and the Regulation of Solid-Organ Xenotransplantation in the UK. *Journal of Medical Ethics* 2007; 33: 373–375.

[31] Department of Health. 2006. *Xenotransplantation Guide*. 12 Dec 2006. Gateway ref. 7345.

Healthcare Products Regulatory Agency.[32] The Interim UK Regulatory Route for Stem Cell Research and Manufacture makes it clear that there are a number of steps and regulatory agencies involved before a hybrid embryo stem cell line would be approved for use in clinical trials and/or treatments. Whilst hybrid embryo-derived stem cell lines are not specifically referred to, the Regulatory Route Map is applicable to all types of stem cell lines.[33]

The EU Tissues Directive, as transposed into UK law by the *Human Tissue (Quality and Safety for Human Application) Regulations 2007* 'sets standards of quality and safety for the donation, procurement, testing, processing, storage and distribution of human tissues and cells'.[34] The high standards which are set may mean that it is sometime before hybrid embryo-derived stem cells can comply and be used in clinical trials and treatments.

THE FUTURE OF HYBRIDS IN CLINICAL MEDICINE

The analysis of the problems associated with clinical use of hybrid stem cells may already be obsolete. It has recently been called into question whether hybrid embryos have any ability to develop to a stage where they can be used to produce pluripotent stem cells. Work undertaken in California with bovine, rabbit and mouse eggs, with comparative work using human eggs, showed that a very low percentage of hybrid embryos

---

[32] HTA, HFEA and MHRA. 2007. *Position Statement on Regulating Human Embryonic Stem Cell Lines for Human Application: Joint Statement from HTA, HFEA and MHRA*: 3 May. Available at: http://www.hta.gov.uk/guidance/licensing_guidance/position_statement_on_regulating_human_embryonic_stem_cell_lines_for_human_application.cfm [Accessed 13 March 2009]. It is assumed that this statement on embryonic stem cells applies to hybrid-derived stem cells as well as those derived from non-hybrid embryos.

[33] Department of Health. 2009. *Interim UK Regulatory Route Map for Stem Cell Research and Manufacture.* Available at: http://www.advisorybodies.doh.gov.uk/genetics/gtac/InterimUKSCroutemap120309.pdf [Accessed 22 March 2009].

[34] The full text of the EU Tissue and Cells Directive can be located on the Department of Health website: Available at: http://www.dh.gov.uk/en/Publichealth/Scientificdevelopmentgeneticsandbioethics/Tissue/Tissuegeneralinformation/DH_4136920 [Accessed 13 March 2009].

developed to the 16-cell stage.[35] Additionally the hybrid embryos failed to produce stem cells that were fully pluripotent. As the authors state,

> 'Our results suggest that bovine and rabbit oocytes do not support appropriate embryonic genome reprogramming of human somatic cell nuclei, and call into question the ability of animal ooplasm to generate patient-specific human stem cells'.[36]

Whilst these initial results are disheartening for those who feel that hybrid embryos are the way forward to stem cell research, others feel that these results do not mean the end of the line for hybrid embryo research:

> 'Understanding what has to be done to overcome these problems would help us understand what reprogramming is all about'.[37]

The fact that the Californian research team has published unfavourable results may also be welcomed, but for different reasons. Scientists are often accused of not publishing 'wrong' or 'poor' results, so this paper should be welcomed for showing the problems which need to be overcome if hybrid embryo research is to continue.

Additionally it needs to be borne in mind that whilst this scientific paper shows that this particular process is difficult, it may still be possible with a different method. However, with the competing technology of induced pluripotent stem cells it may not be economically viable or time worthy to continue with the hybrid embryo route.

Although the UK Government seems to be keen to allow hybrid embryo research and stem cell derivation to occur, but not the use of the

---

[35] Y. Chung *et al.* Reprogramming of Human Somatic Cells Using Human and Animal Oocytes. *Cloning and Stem Cells* 2009; 11(2): 1–11, Table 1.

[36] Ibid., 11.

[37] J. St. John, quoted in: H. Ledford. 2009. Hybrid Embryos Fail to Live Up to Stem-Cell Hopes. *Nature News*: 3 February Available at: http://www.nature.com/news/2009/090204/full/457642b.html [Accessed 9 February 2009].

derived stem cells in clinical trials and therapies, no express prohibition of clinical use can be found in the 2008 Act. From an international perspective it may be very difficult to prevent such stem cells from eventually being used in clinical trials and therapies, if and when the reprogramming issues are overcome.

The International Society for Stem Cell Research (the ISSCR) has recently published guidance for the clinical translation of stem cells.[38] Although the Guidelines refer to the other recent discovery within the field of stem cell research, induced Pluripotent Stem cells (iPS cells), there is no specific mention of stem cells derived from hybrid embryos. The Guidelines are welcome as they lay out clearly the standards which researchers and scientists should be striving for, particularly in countries where regulation is informal or lacking. Acknowledgement of the possible future use of hybrid embryo-derived stem cells would have been of use, the Guidelines may need to be rewritten to take into account such stem cells if and when it becomes apparent that these stem cells could be used in therapies. Whilst the UK Government does not currently want such stem cells to be used in therapies, other countries may not take this stance.

CONCLUSION

The United Kingdom Government was keen to push forward with hybrid embryo research. However, in light of the recent refusals for funding, the development of iPS cells and the problems reported with deriving stem cell lines from hybrid embryos, the usefulness of hybrid embryo research could be far more limited than anticipated when the *Human Fertilisation and Embryology Act 2008* was being debated. This is not to say that hybrid embryo research and stem cell derivation will not serve some purpose; alternative methods for deriving stem cells may successfully be developed and the perfection of techniques to create and derive stem cells are two ways in which hybrid embryos may yet prove to be useful.

---

[38] ISSCR. 2008. *Guidelines for the Clinical Translation of Stem Cells.* Available at: http:www.isscr.org [Accessed 9 February 2009].

13

STEM CELL RESEARCH AND ITS CLINICAL APPLICATION IN CHINA: INTERACTIONS BETWEEN SCIENCE, ETHICS AND SOCIETY

Renzong Qiu and Xiaomei Zhai

INTRODUCTION

Since news of Dolly the sheep was first published in *Nature* in 1997, human cloning and stem cell research have been the topic of ongoing debate in mainland China, both in scientific circles and among the general public. Hundreds of articles on the subject have been published in academic journals, popular magazines, newspapers and websites, and the topic has been featured in a considerable number of television programmes. Decision makers in science and medicine began to address the ethical, legal and social issues involved in biomedicine and biotechnology for the first time in China's history when a meeting of experts was convened to discuss the implications of the *Nature* paper.[1] One can also find evidence of China's willingness to engage with ethical issues at the international level; for example, the Chinese government joined France and Germany in their efforts to persuade the United Nations to endorse a resolution prohibiting human reproductive cloning, despite the fact that some Chinese scientists and philosophers are in favor of it. Ironically, on 8 March 2005, the United Nations Assembly adopted a declaration on human cloning in which member states are required to take *necessary*

[1] I. Wilmut *et al*. Viable Offspring Derived from Fetal and Adult Mammalian Cells. *Nature* 1997; 385 (6619): 810–813.

steps to prohibit all forms of human cloning, because it is incompatible with human dignity and protection of human life. However, this raised many problematic questions, such as: what is included as 'all forms of human cloning'; what is meant by 'human dignity', and why is human cloning incompatible with it; and what is 'human life', and why is it compromised by human cloning? Furthermore, the fact that the world is made up of diverse cultures is not specified in the document.[2] As a result, the Chinese government, together with more than 30 countries, stood against the Declaration. Making sense of China's engagement with bioethics requires an appreciation of the development of biotechnology within the social environment.

STEM CELL RESEARCH IN CHINA'S SOCIAL ENVIRONMENT

The cloning and stem cell debate in China is taking place at a time when the country is in transition from a monolithic society to a more or less pluralistic civil society. The factors influencing the debate are complicated. China's characteristic culture had persisted for thousands of years, and it was built on three teachings: Confucianism, Taoism and Buddhism. Of them, Confucianism is dominant, and is firmly rooted in many Chinese minds and in many social conventions. In the decades after 1949, the chief ideology was a Chinese adaptation of Marxist-Leninist philosophy. Since the new policy in 1987, China has been gradually integrated into the international community, and the influence of Western culture has become increasingly pervasive. Liberalism, feminism and communitarianism became new conceptual resources. With the government's commitment to a market economy and the rule of law, economic and legal factors have also become very important during the last two decades.

After the Western powers knocked open the door to China in 1840, the Chinese people realised there was something lacking in Chinese culture;

---

[2] Fifty-Ninth General Assembly, Plenary, 82nd Meeting (AM). 2005. *Press Release GA/10333: General Assembly Adopts United Nations Declaration on Human Cloning by Vote of 84-34-37.* 8 Mar. Available at http://www.un.org/News/Press/docs/2005/ga10333.doc.htm [Accessed 24 Jun 2009].

but only after half a century of continuing encounters with the Western states, would *Mr. Sai* (science) and *Mr. De* (democracy) be brought into China on 4 May 1910.[3] Even now, the Chinese people commemorate the 4th of May as *Young People Festival* every year; and developing science and technology has now become part of basic state policy for the Chinese government; though the development of democracy lags behind. This state policy has been supported by the Chinese public, and in contrast with science in the West, scientists here still enjoy high regard and trust in the Chinese public. Since 1999, China's spending on research and development (R&D) has increased by more than 20 per cent each year. In December 2006 China had moved ahead of Japan for the first time, to become the world's second highest R&D investor after the US. Spending by central government in 2006 reached RMB71.6 billion, or c£4.7 billion, compared with £3.2 billion by the UK government. A considerable part of this spending is devoted to biotechnology and biomedicine. For example, investment in stem cell science over the five years and up to 2010, is projected to be between RMB500 million (US$63 million) and RMB2 billion (US$250 million).[4] In the *National High-Technology Research and Development Project* (863 Project) and *National Key Basic Research and Development Project* (973 Project) the focus has been on biotechnologies including stem cell research.[5] In recent years the alliance of bio-industry, bio-technology and education has been greatly promoted. It is hoped that the research results of life science and biotechnology will be expediently translated into industry. The development of biotechnology, such as successful cloning of 'Dolly' in 1997, raised a range of ethical issues; so it can be understood that soon after the stem cell *Nature* paper was published, the late Minister of Health, Professor Minzhang Chen,

---

[3] See: W.M. Tu. 1997. Destructive Will and Ideological Holocaust: Maoism as a Source of Social Suffering. In *Social Suffering*. A. Kleinman, V. Das & M.M. Lock, eds. Berkeley: University of California Press: 160.

[4] UK Stem Cell Initiative. 2005. *Report and Recommendations*. Department of Health, London.

[5] See www.863.gov.cn. In 2006 there were 41 projects in stem cell and tissue engineering. Each PI received a grant typically to the amount of millions of Chinese dollars from the government.

unprecedentedly convened a meeting at which scientists, physicians, bioethicists and lawyers were invited to attend to discuss the ethical, legal and social implications of this burgeoning science. The consensus they reached included the need to regulate biomedicine and biotechnology, and the need to set up of some sort of national ethics committee as a policy consulting body. Since 1998, the Chinese government has promulgated a number of regulations to protect the rights and interests of human subjects in research and patients in clinical practice.[6]

STEM CELL RESEARCH AND CHINESE CULTURE

Let us set aside the issue of human reproductive cloning, for there is complete agreement on its prohibition among the member states of United Nations. However, on the issue of human 'therapeutic' or research cloning and human embryonic stem cell research, there is wide disagreement between them. In comparison with Western countries, where there is little agreement between various factions on the issue, Chinese culture provides no barrier to human research cloning and human embryonic stem cell research; and accordingly, there is no disagreement among the

[6] Such as *Law on Practicing Doctors* (National People's Congress, Jun 1998), *Regulation for Protecting Human Genetic Resources* (MOST and MOH, 1998), *Regulation for Drug Clinical Trials* (SFDA, 1999, 2003), *Regulation for Human Assisted Reproductive Technologies* (MOH, 2001, 2003), *Law on Population and Family Planning* (National People's Congress, December 2001), *Ethical Principles and Technical Norms for Human Assisted Reproductive Technologies* (MOH, 2001, revised 2003), *Ethical Guiding Principles for Human Embryonic Stem Cell Research* (MOST/MOH, December 2003), *Regulation for Clinical Application of Human Organ Transplantation Technologies* (MOH, 1 July 2006), *Regulation for Prevention and Treatment of HIV/AIDS* (State Council, 2006), *Regulation for Ethical Review of Biomedical Research Involving Human Subjects* (January 2007, MOH), *Regulation for Human Organ Transplantation* (State Council, 1 May, 2007), etc. The State Council is the Chinese central government and the National People's Congress is the Chinese legislature. MOST, MOH and SFDA are the abbreviations for Ministry of Science and Technology, Ministry of Health and State Commission on Population and Family Planning.

All the laws and regulations can be found at the following websites: www.gov.cn; www.npc.gov.cn; www.most.gov.cn; www.moh.gov.cn; www.pop.gov.cn [Accessed 25th June 2009].

government, scientists, scholars in the humanities and social sciences and the public. This may be due to the unique characteristics of Chinese culture.

Traditional cultural values are likely relevant to the public attitude and opinions and the governmental policy. First, under the influence of Confucian pro-life (referring to personal life rather than *human* life in general) viewpoint, saving persons has always been put as the first priority. Now there are hundreds of millions of people who are suffering from diseases like heart diseases, cancers, Parkinson's disease, Alzheimer's disease, spinal injuries, diabetes, immunodeficiency, genetic haematological diseases, hepatitis, hepatocirrhosis, osteoarthritis, osteoporosis, and muscular dystrophy. Patients with organ failure are in the most desperate situation, and it is estimated that about one million patients need organ transplantation each year, but only 10,000 receive an organ for transplantation. The commitment to promote stem cell research and regenerative medicine as a promising frontier in biotechnology and biomedicine is necessary, especially for a country like China, where the long-term cultural tradition has constituted a barrier for saving millions of patients' lives who could have been saved by transplantation medicine. Patients and the public believe on various grounds, that stem cell research will invent a variety of ways to relieve their sufferings. For the government, the priority is always on the agenda of *minsheng* (people's well-being) under the rubric of scientific view of development (*kexue fazhan guan*), putting people first (*yi ren wei ben*), and creating a well-off (*xiaokang*) and harmonious (*hexie*) society as the country entered the 21st century. The improvement of *minsheng* will provide strong legitimacy to the government, and Confucianism requires that the government should fulfill *renzheng* (humane policy), as Confucius and Mencius taught (*Analects of Confucius*; *Meng Zi*).[7] Both the Chinese public and the government are convinced that stem cell research is not a theoretical scientific endeavour just for curiosity or for the sake of science, but a *public good* which promises to save millions of human lives.

---

[7] The Chinese Classics consulted for this chapter are: *Analects of Confucius*, Shanghai: The Commercial Press, 1926; *Meng Zi,* Shanghai: World Bookstore, 1932; *Xun Zi*, in S.T. Zhang: Commentaries on *Xun Zi*, Shanghai: Shanghai People's Press, p. 95.

Not only is there strong support from the Chinese government, scientists and the public for stem cell research, but also the Chinese culture and ideology do not create a barrier to the more controversial aspects of the research, as was seen in some countries in the West. We turn now to some of the ideologies which underlie this acceptance.

The Confucian Concept of Personhood

The Confucian concept of personhood is a monist, gradualist and relational one. For Confucianism, the universe and all of its inhabitants — including persons — are composed of *qi*: a physico-psychological entity with capacity for creation, change and transformation, and which has two basic forms, *yin* and *yang*. The generation, change and transformation of all things are produced by their interaction. The person is a psychosomatic unity: *xing* or *ti* (body, form) and *shen* (psyche, spirit), both of which come from *qi* and are related to each other. So in contrast with the Cartesian dualism that was promulgated in some early ideas of Western medicine, the division between medicine (the body) and psychiatry (the mind) has *never* existed in traditional Chinese medicine.

For Confucianism, the human embryo is a product of *yin* and *yang*. There are many transformations in the process from embryo to newborn. The transformation from embryo/fetus to newborn is something like from a bud to a flower or from seed to plant. There is a continuum between the bud and flower, but the flower is distinct in kind and in degree. In the same vein, the human embryo will develop or transform into a human 'person', but it is not a human person yet, although it has inherent the teleology or self-actualisation to develop into human person. This gradualist view is in sharp contrast with the instantaneous view in some European countries according to which a human being emerges at the instant of fertilisation.[8]

[8] F.B. Zong *et al.* (eds.). 2003. *Ancient Interpretations of Words.* The Commercial Press, pp. 1853–1857. See, for example, the German Embryo Law 1990 (Gesets zum Schutz von Embryonen [Embryonenschutzgesets]); and the Irish Constitution (1937, 8th amendment 1999), both of which recognise the interests of the embryo from the moment of conception.

The third greatest Confucian in Chinese history, Xun Zi (313–238 BC), said: 'Birth is the beginning of person, and death is the end of person. Human *tao* lies in good beginning and good end'. For the Confucian concept of personhood, 'being' is always in the process of 'becoming'. Even after birth, all three aspects of the person: the psyche (*shen*), the vital force (*qi*), and the physical body (*ti*) are imperfect, and are waiting to be cultivated and perfected. No one is born as a 'person'. The person has to be made with effort: person-making (*zuoren*) is a lifetime process. That is why Confucians emphasise: cultivate life (*yangsheng*), cultivate sentiments (*taoyan qingcao*), and cultivate character (*yangxing*).

Xun Zi also argued that a person is an entity which has capacity for social relationship (*qun*). Confucians do not think of a person in terms of a substance which exists in itself, or as a part of any other being, such as the human genome, soul or rationality. Rather they find human beings as distinguishable from animals because of their relational/social capacity. Humans are not as strong as oxen, nor do they run as fast as horses, yet how is it that oxen and horses are being mastered by human beings? That is because humans are capable of social relationships (*qun*) and animals are not. A person is never seen as an isolated individual, but is always conceived of as a part of a network of relations. The self-cultivation of an individual person to become a real (moral) person is a process that is carried out in and through the social context, and for the purpose of fulfilling social responsibility rather than self-actualisation *per se*.[9]

According to the Confucian gradualist view, a human being or a person begins with his/her birth, not the instant when a sperm fertilises an ovum; and the human embryo or foetus has not become a person until this point. It should enjoy due respect, because it can have a certain moral status which is between full person and non-living things. The human embryo/foetus also has no equivalent, so they should not be treated as personal or family property, and they cannot be traded. But the destruction of a human embryo should not be taken as 'killing a human being/person';

---

[9] E. Hui. 2004. Personhood and Bioethics: Chinese Perspective. In *Bioethics: Asian Perspectives — A Quest for Moral Diversity.* R.Z. Qiu, ed. Dordrecht: Kluwers: Ip, PK; Confucian Personhood and Bioethics: A Critical Appraisal, pp. 49–56.

the human embryo is a human biological life: a precursor of person, and not merely a thing like the placenta. Accordingly, it deserves due respect when used in research and ought to be disposed of with due procedure. Without sufficient reason, the manipulation or destruction of an embryo is not ethically permissible. Saving the lives of millions of human persons could be a sufficient reason; but we must see each kind of research in a hierarchy of justification. For example, if there are alternative sources from which to derive pluripotent stem cells for research, such as the use of primordial germ cells from aborted foetuses, or deriving pluripotent cells from 'adult' somatic cells, researchers have no justification for destroying a human embryo. Furthermore, the use of spare human embryos for research, after successful IVF, would be preferable to creating a human embryo for that purpose. However, where alternatives are not available for research in the near future (e.g. making adult stem cells pluripotent), or for translational therapeutic purposes, the use of nucleus transfer to create an embryo from which to derive stem cells should not be absolutely prohibited. Rather, it should be deemed permissible, or even necessary, but it should be subject to strict regulation. Due respect must be given to the entities which are between persons and which enjoy a higher moral status than those things (e.g. a stone) which have no moral status. A person enjoys full respect; a stone has no moral status. In between are non-human animals, human embryos and foetuses and corpses, and these deserve modest, but not full, respect.

When the Confucianist says that the human embryo should enjoy due respect, it is meant that: the human embryo may be used in research only extracorporeally, and only when it is no more than 14 days old; the human embryo may be used only in cases where the research goal cannot be achieved with other methods; the human embryo should not be treated as a commodity or as property; and scientists should in some way acknowledge the human embryo's contribution to human health and life. Due procedure means that after use, the human embryo should be buried or cremated with a ceremony.[10]

---

[10] See: R.Z. Qiu. Human Cloning: Arguments For and Against. *Journal of Central China University of Science and Technology* 2005; 19(3): 108–118.

Legal and Regulatory Factors

Legal and regulatory factors also play an important role in the debate on cloning and stem cell research issues. In Article 9, Chapter II Citizens (Natural Persons), *General Principles of the Civil Law,* it is stipulated that 'A citizen shall have civil rights from birth to death'. In Article 101, Section 4 Personal Rights, *General Principles of the Civil Law*, it is stipulated that 'The citizen's personal dignity shall be protected by law'. In Article 28, *Law of Succession,* it is stipulated that 'At the time of the partitioning of the estate, reservation shall be made for the share of an unborn child'. And in Article 302, *Criminal Law*, it is stipulated that 'Whoever steals from or insults a corpse shall be sentenced to a fixed-term imprisonment of up to three years'. The implications of these articles are that a natural person comes into being at the moment of birth. A human embryo or foetus is not a person for the purposes of law; and neither is a corpse. However, there is some transitivity: both the human embryo or foetus and the corpse can be seen as having a certain interest. A person enjoys full respect of his or her personal dignity, and a 'pre-person' (embryo or foetus) or 'post-person' (corpse) enjoys due (not full, but modest) respect.

Different social groups in China support stem cell research with various, sometimes conflicting, reasons or motives. Scientists may be motivated by the hope of saving lives, or by the desire to promote their own career, personal fame or interests; biotech companies may see stem cell research and its future clinical application as a promising business that may bring maximum profits to them; patients and the public hope that stem cell research will relieve their suffering; and the government sponsors stem cell research from the perspective of scientific development and progress, and the 'prosperous' and 'harmonious society' programme. Thus, both the cultural and the legal environment in China favour stem cell research; and measures are geared to allow the smooth and regulated realisation of the science. However, in the same period another development is noteworthy and it is relevant to stem cell research.

AWARENESS OF PATIENTS' AND HUMAN SUBJECTS' RIGHTS

In this section, we turn to the noteworthy development is the birth and growth of bioethics in China. The *National Conference on Philosophy of Medicine* held in Guangdong in December 1979 initiated an irreversible process which led to the birth of bioethics in China. The process included a focus on, for example, the ethical issues in life-sustaining technologies, assisted reproductive technologies, organ transplantation, and genetics. The 1979 Guangdong Conference may be seen as a watershed in bioethics development in China. Subsequently:

- In 1980, the journal, *Medicine and Philosophy* was founded, under the sponsorship of the *Chinese Society for Philosophy of Nature, Science and Technology,* affiliated with the *China Association of Science and Technology*;
- A series of bioethics articles in the journal *Philosophical Problems in Natural Sciences* were published under the sponsorship of the *Institute of Philosophy,* affiliated with the *Chinese Academy of Social Sciences*;
- A teaching workshop on bioethics to train graduate students[11] was held in Southeast University, Nanjing in the Summer of 1986, under the sponsorship of the *Ministry of Education*;
- The first book on bioethics[12] in China was published in 1987;
- The first legal case of euthanasia and the first legal case of assisted reproductive technologies were debated around 1988;[13]
- The first *National Conference on Social, Ethical and Legal Issues in Euthanasia* was held in Shanghai in July 1988; and

[11] Some of them have later become the backbone of bioethics in China, such as Xiaomei Zhai who is now the Executive Director of the Center for Bioethics, Chinese Academy of Social Sciences/Peking Union Medical College; Member of Ethics Committee, the MOH; Vice-President of Chinese Society for Bioethics; Member of HUGO Ethics Committee.

[12] R.Z. Qiu. 1987. *Bioethics.* Shanghai: Shanghai People's Press; 1988. *Between Life and Death: Moral Dilemmas and Bioethics.* Hong Kong: Chinese Bookstore; Taipei: Chinese Bookstore.

[13] See: R.Z. Qiu. Morality in Flux. *Kennedy Institute of Ethics Journal* 1991; 1: 16–27.

- The first *National Conference on Social, Ethical and Legal Issues in Human Assisted Reproductive Technologies* was held in Yueyang, Hunan Province, in November 1988.

From the above, we can see that the growth of bioethics in China has been a progressive process, initiated by the 1979 Guangzhou Conference, and, by 1988, there were the beginnings of a rich resource network of bioethics in China.

There were three events which brought scientists, decision-makers and the public together to address bioethics in an important debate:

(1) In April 1994 Professor Chen, the Minister of Health, submitted a report on a draft of the *Maternal and Infant Health Care Law* (then called '*Eugenic Law*') to the legislature (the *National People's Congress*). This report was so strongly controversial, and caused such major protest from abroad, that it seriously threatened the organisation of the *18th World Congress of Genetics* in Beijing. Many genetics colleagues outside China threatened to boycott it for the eugenic nature of the law. Bioethicists joined the efforts of Chinese geneticists to thoroughly reappraise the draft report, and to make sure that it drew a line between a healthy birth as the parents' preference, and eugenics as a state programme which would be imposed upon citizens. Subsequently, the official promise to rectify the defects in the law allowed the Congress to be successfully held.[14]

(2) When medical and public health professionals organized a group to draft a recommendation on AIDS policy, bioethicists were included, and drafted the recommendation which was submitted to the government with the appendix: *Ethical Framework for Evaluating Actions on AIDS*. The recommendation was subsequently accepted by the

[14] R.Z. Qiu. 2004. China: Views of a Bioethicist. In *Genetics and Ethics in Global Perspective*. D. Wertz & J. Fletcher, eds. Dordrecht: Kluwer: 187–207; R.Z. Qiu. 2004. Does Eugenics Exist in China? Ethical Issues in the Law on Maternal and Infant Health Care. In *Bioethics: Asian Perspectives — A Quest for Moral Diversity*. R.Z. Qiu, ed. Dordrecht: Kluwers.

government. Since then, the government's AIDS policy has been reviewed, and subsequently there have been further radical improvements in HIV/AIDS treatment in China.

(3) As early as 1998, bioethicists, together with scientists, submitted a recommendation on the *Ethical Governance on Human Assisted Reproduction*. However, the then Minister of Health and the Director of State *Commission on Family Planning* responded that the recommendation were agreeable, but that there was more urgent work to do. At the Science Conference which was held in 1999 in Kunming, participants, including scientists, bioethicists and lawyers, called for ethical governance on human assisted reproduction again. This time MOH accepted the recommendations, and this resulted in the *Regulation on Human Assisted Reproduction* in 2000.[15]

After these three events, bioethicists have been more and more confident to be players in the debates on the life sciences and biotechnology, and have taken an active role together with scientists, physicians and policy-makers. Stem cell research and development raised a range of ethical issues, such as: should we do human reproductive cloning or human therapeutic cloning? What is the moral status of human embryo? How should we get human eggs for stem cell research? Should this research be reviewed and approved by an ethical review committee? How should we dispose of the used human embryo after collecting stem cells? Should stem cell therapy be tested by clinical trials before wide application in clinics? And how should stem cell research and its clinical application be regulated? In 1999, bioethicists began to initiate action to draft a recommendation on ethical governance in stem cell research both in Beijing and Shanghai, but without agreement between them. However, before we turn to this development, there are two questions that have to be answered.

The first question is: is it necessary and desirable to regulate biomedical research and biotechnologies, including stem cell research, for the purpose of protecting patients and human subjects? The second is: if biomedical research and biotechnologies need to be regulated, why do we

[15] R.Z. Qiu *et al.* 2000. *Dilemmas Facing Bioethics in the 21st Century*. Beijing: High Education Press.

not draft our own guidelines, using Chinese cultural characteristics, and putting aside international guidelines which have been formulated based on input mainly from Western ethicists?

After years of debate, a consensus in China has eventually been reached in answering the first question: it is desirable to regulate biomedical research. The point of consensus is that, on the one hand, contemporary biomedicine and biotechnology realises promises, and proliferates advanced and effective diagnostics, therapeutics and preventive methods to save millions of patients from diseases; but on the other hand, it risks violating the patients' rights and interests in its development and application. This is because this kind of scientific progress usually involves commercialisation, leading to frequent conflicts of interests between physicians (scientists) and patients (human research participants). The purpose — and necessity — of the regulation is both to develop biomedicine and biotechnology for the purpose of helping patients, and to protect the rights and welfare of patients and human subjects involved. Some scientists advised the authority that the development of ethical norms for protecting rights and welfare of patients would impede scientific progress. They also suggested that, while there have been strict and stringent ethical norms in place for biomedical research and biotechnology in the fields of science and technology in advanced countries, China should concentrate on catching up, and indeed, surging ahead without constraints, in advancing its scientific and technological endeavours. This advice is wrong and dangerous. It is wrong because it opposes the ethical norms to the development of science and technology. It is dangerous because it will put our own science and technology at stake, since it will lose its essential integrity and public — and international — support. The scandals, for example, of Woo-Suk Hwang[16] case in Korea and the Jin Chen[17] case in China, convincingly illustrate these points.

[16] N. Wade *et al.* 2005. Korean scientist said to admit fabrication in a cloning study. *New York Times* 16 Dec. Available at: http://query.nytimes.com/gst/fullpage.html?sec=health&res=9B07E2DD1630F935A25751C1A9639C8B63&fta=y [Accessed 25 Jun 2009]; N. Wade *et al.* 2006. Researcher faked evidence of human cloning, Koreans report. *New York Times* 10 Jan. Available at: http://www.nytimes.com/2006/01/10/science/10clone.html [Accessed 25 Jun 2009].

[17] R. Fisher. 2007. Fraudbusters. *New Scientists* 10 Sep: 64–65.

The consensus on answering the second question is: although China has unique cultural traditions, it is imperative to comply with international ethical guidelines on biomedical research involving human subjects, because the international guidelines were in origin a result of communication and negotiation among experts from different countries and different cultures from all over the world, including China. The fact that we have to take the cultural context into account when implementing international guidelines and underlying basic principles, gives no reason to reject their general applicability.[18]

In 1999, the *Recommendation on Ethical Principles and Regulatory Recommendations on Human Embryonic Stem Cell Research*[19] which were drafted by bioethicists from the Program in Bioethics, Chinese Academy of Social Sciences, Centre for Bioethics, Chinese Academy of Medical Sciences/Peking Union Medical College, Health Science Centre, Peking University and the Ethics Committee of the Human Genome Project China in Beijing, were submitted to the Ethics Committee of the Ministry of Health. A few years later, in October 2001, bioethicists from the Ethics Committee of the Chinese National Human Genome Center in Shanghai drafted the *Proposed Ethical Guidelines for Human Embryonic Stem Cell Research.*[20] Neither of these drafts was officially approved at the national level; although both informed the basis of the *Ethical Guiding Principles for Research on Human Embryonic Stem Cells* jointly approved and promulgated by the Ministry of Science and Technology (MOST) and the Ministry of Health (MOH) on 24 December 2003. More recently, were the *Regulation on Scientific Misconduct* (MOST 2006), as well as the *Regulation on Ethical Review of Biomedical Research Involving Human Subjects* (MOH 2007), promulgated.

There are two sides of the Chinese policy on stem cell research and development. One side of it is the *ambition* to be a world power in life sci-

[18] X.M. Zhai *et al.* Capacity Building in Ethical Review in China under International Context: Ideas and Practices. *Chinese Medical Ethics* 2008; 2: 3–6.

[19] Research Center for Bioethics, PUMC. 2001. Ethical Principles and Regulatory Recommendations on Human Embryonic Stem Cell Research. *Newsletter* (1): 3.

[20] Ethics Committee of the National Human Genome Center (Southern). Proposed Ethical Guidelines for Human Embryonic Stem Cell Research. *Medicine and Philosophy* 2001; (6): 8–9.

ences, biomedicine and biotechnology. A huge amount of resources is invested in these three areas. Some schools of basic medicine in medical colleges became 'schools of stem cell research and development' with grants from MOST amounting to tens of millions of Chinese dollars. In 2006, there were 41 projects of stem cell research and development run by hundreds of scientists, at 41 institutes or research centres of universities and academies and approved by MOST.[21] Facilitating this ambition is to build an alliance among industry, research and education. Many biotechnological institutes are integrated with biotechnological industries with the hope that research results will be rapidly translated into industrial products and used in clinics.

The other side of Chinese policies on human embryonic stem cell research is *caution*. It was emphasised that biotechnology should be regulated and the governance should be complied with international guidelines. And articles on prohibition/permission and requirements in *Ethical Guiding Principles for Human Embryonic Stem Cell Research* (hereafter, the *Ethical Guiding Principles*, and detailed below) do comply with international guidelines.

REGULATORY GAPS AND CHALLENGES

The current policy on stem cell research, as seen in the *Ethical Guiding Principles* (2003)[22] is to try to maintain a delicate balance between scientific freedom and ethical constraints, while maximising scientific freedom and minimising ethical/regulatory constraints. There are two relevant regulations in China in respect to stem cell research:

Regulations on Human Assisted Reproductive Technologies 2003 — Procedures Prohibited:

Human gametes, zygote and embryos trading
Surrogate motherhood

[21] See: http://www.cncbd.org.cn/ [Accessed 25th June 2009].
[22] MOST & MOH. 2003. *Ethical Guiding Principles for Human Embryonic Stem Cell Research*.

Sex selection without medical indications
Hybrid creation between human species and other animals
Gene manipulation on human gametes, zygotes and embryos for reproductive purposes
Union between sperms and eggs from close relatives
Human cytoplasmic transfer and cell nuclear transfer for treating infertility
Creating chimeras for research purposes
Human reproductive cloning
Human gametes, zygotes or embryos donated to others or for research without informed and voluntary consent

Ethical Guiding Principles for hESC Research (2003) — Procedures Allowed (A) or Prohibited (P):

Human reproductive cloning	P
hESC derived from spared gamete or embryos after IVF	A
hESC from foetal cells from accidental spontaneous or voluntarily selected abortions	A
hESC from embryos obtained by somatic cell nuclear transfer technology or parthenogenetic embryos	A
hESC from germ cells voluntarily donated	A
Embryos thus obtained, it's *in vitro* culture period within 14 days	A
To hybridise human germ cells with germ cells of any other species	P
Buy or sell human gametes, fertilised eggs, embryos and foetal tissues	P
Conducting hESC research without review and approval of the protocol by an IRB	P

However, in the *Ethical Guiding Principles* there is no article which mentions licensing, scientific and ethical qualifications, registry, reporting, oversight or punishment in the case of violations. It means that the implementation of these principles is *voluntary,* and not compulsory, and without enforcement either.

As a result, these regulations may not strike a balance between scientific freedom and ethical/regulatory constraints.

Regulatory Gaps

After five years' implementation of the *Ethical Guiding Principles* we seem to go back to the beginning: is it necessary or even imperative to regulate stem cell research and development? There are several options before us: turn to *laissez-faire*, libertarian, or 'wait-and-see' policies; continue with the existing *Ethical Guiding Principles*; create general regulations and guidelines without specific reference to stem cell research and development; or create a specific and enforced stem cell regulation. Our suggestion is to follow the last option.

The assumption underlying our answer is that biomedicine and biotechnology in general, when integrated with industry/commerce in particular, have the tendency to violate patients' welfare and rights. So they need to be regulated or governed. Stem cell research and development is so unique that governance is needed because of its possible impact upon humanity. And the governance should strike a balance between facilitating scientific progress and providing ethical and practical safeguards, between research freedom and the interests of patients, subjects and society. In this respect, the *Ethical Guiding Principles* are inadequate.

The meanings of 'governance' includes forming of rules, their application, enforcement and the settling of conflicts over such rules; the process of decision-making and the processes by which decisions are implemented; paying more attention to the values and the quality of decision-making involved, as different from management. And 'good' governance implies values and standards of quality. *Good* governance is an ideal which is difficult to achieve, but actions must be taken to work towards this ideal. 'Bad' governance would be an exercise of power that does not respect the appropriate values and standards. The elements of good governance include:

- Building an infrastructure of governance;
- Developing official laws, regulations or guidelines, prescribing:

Substantial issues: obligations including informed consent, confidentiality/privacy, ethical review, benefit-sharing, conflict of interest, quality assurance, duties of researchers, permissions and prohibitions etc.; and
Procedural issues: licensing, register, reporting, stem cell products testing, clinical application, international collaboration, etc;

- Establishing ethical review committees;
- Implementation: capacity building, education/training;
- Effective oversight;
- Incentives and disincentives (including enforcement and legal sanctions); and
- Setting up a specific regulatory body with a budget.

The experiences of the implementation of the *Ethical Guiding Principles* show that the policy of maximising scientific freedom and minimising ethical constraints is not desirable and largely inadequate — it makes oversight impossible. How many institutions in China are doing human embryonic stem cell research? How many institutes among them are qualified, and how many not? Nobody knows! As the *Ethical Guiding Principles* do not specify the scientific and ethical qualifications an institute must meet when they want to do human embryonic stem cell research, and there is no legal imperative to be licensed from any regulatory bodies, thus, there is no imperative to find out. Furthermore, the *Ethical Guiding Principles* do not require the scientists and their institutes to register researchers, to submit annual reports, or to register any embryonic stem cell or cloned cell lines with regulatory bodies — it would therefore be difficult to regulate research effectively. The *Ethical Guiding Principles* specify which research conduct is permitted and which is prohibited, but how many institutes are observing these specifications? Furthermore, in view of new scientific advances and ethical debate, for example, with respect to cybrids and chimeras, the *Ethical Guiding Principles* on permission and prohibition should be updated. This will be discussed in detail in the next section.

The *Ethical Guiding Principles* requires that any protocol proposing to carry out human embryo stem cell research must be reviewed and approved by an IRB. But how effective and comprehensive is this ethical review?

What guidelines do IRBs use to review the protocol? How is the IRB established? How many IRB are qualified in their composition and functioning, and in their capacity for scientific and ethical review? How many are not? Have all members been trained? The donation of gametes or embryo used in human embryonic stem cell research should be voluntary, and valid informed consent must be obtained. Now, what is the process of informed consent in those institutes which conduct human research? And what does the written informed consent form look like? Documentation of the provenance of oocytes and stem cell lines and human embryo or human/animal embryo creation/disposition is necessary for oversight. It may include:

- Origin of the oocytes;
- The process of informed consent;
- The origin of the stem cell lines;
- The dates of, and the means used in the creation of human embryos or human/animal mixtures, and information in respect to their disposal.

New Emerging Issues and Challenges

We are not only faced with regulatory gaps, but also faced with huge ethical and governance challenges presented by rapid advancement of science and technology (and stem cell research in particular). The emerging issues we have to address include: hybrids and chimeras, parthenogenesis, genetic modification/modification of chromosomal DNA, induced Pluripotent Stem cells (iPS cells), artificial gametes from adult cells, PGD and pre-implantation tissue typing, designer babies, the translation of stem cells science from bench to bedside, medical tourism, and oocyte trading over vast Internet networks.

In August 2003, Professor Huizhen Sheng, of the Shanghai Second Medical University, published a paper in *Cell Research* in which she reported that they successfully transferred human skin cell nucleus into a rabbit denucleated egg, created about 400 human/animal embryos, and derived stem cells.[23] Before publication she had sent her paper to *Science*,

---

[23] H.Z. Sheng *et al.* Embryonic Stem Cells Generated by Nuclear Transfer of Human Somatic Nuclei into Rabbit Oocytes. *Cell Research* 2003; 13(4): 251–263.

Proceedings of the National Academy of Science and other journals, but it was rejected. Why? Was her work suspected to be a fraud, or unethical, because of the crossing of species boundaries or violation of human dignity?

Did Professor Sheng's work violate the *Regulations* on *Human Assisted Reproductive Technologies* (2003) in which the creation of hybrids between human species and other animals is prohibited, or the *Ethical Guiding Principles* (2003) in which hybridising human germ cells with germ cells of any other species is prohibited? No; because what Sheng created was not a true hybrid between human and animal, but rather a cytoplasmic hybrid or cybrid — a new entity which was not anticipated by the *Regulations* or *Ethical Guiding Principles*. But further to the question, we may pertinently ask: is the creation of cybrids ethically justifiable?

The major argument against the creation of cybrids was the possibility of crossing the species line between human animals and non-human animals. In Chinese culture and language there is a line between human and beast which may not be crossed. In the media, and when journalists report cybrid cases, they prefer to use the term 'human-beast combined embryo', which conveys a misleading message to the public.[24] However, some Chinese bioethicists argue that the line between human animal and non-human animal can be crossed under certain circumstances, and that human/animal cybrids created for research purposes should be permitted, because of certain scientific benefits and potential social benefits, and there is no noticeable harm to any stakeholder. But two constraints ought to be observed: the 14-day limit; and that the cybrid should not be implanted into a human or animal. They argue that the framework that can be used to make a decision on whether human/animal embryo research should be prohibited or permitted is not based on crossing a

[24] See the titles 'The earliest human-beast embryo made in China' (最早人兽胚胎「中国造」) Zaobao.com 4 Apr 2008. Available at: http://www.zaobao.com/special/newspapers/2008/04/hongkong080404h.shtml [Accessed 25 Jun 2009]; and 'The earliest human-beast embryo was made in China but now disconnected' (中国最早进行'人兽混合胚胎'研究现已中断(图)) Rednet.cn 27 Sep 2009. Available at: http://china.rednet.cn/c/2007/09/27/1332488.htm [Accessed 25 Jun 2009].

species line between human and non-human animal, which itself derives an objection from fuzzy concepts of 'naturalness', 'repugnance', 'slippery slope', or 'human dignity', but on the non-maleficence and beneficence principles. Hybrid/chimera research should be permitted in view of the benefits it may bring to human welfare and scientific advancement, but be prohibited only in the case where a harm greater than minimum will be brought to the hybrid/chimera itself (as a marginal person), or to other living entities involved. Based on the non-maleficence principle it was suggested that:

- Prohibiting all kinds of hybrid/chimera research cannot be ethically justified;
- Human/animal cybrid creation should be permitted;
- Animal/human chimeras should be permitted because of scientific benefits and potential social benefits (human disease model, research in stem cell motion, regulation, differentiation, and xenotransplantation research, etc.) and no noticeable harm to any stakeholder. But the research should be restricted to non-human animals which are not too close to humans in evolution; and the number of human stem cells which are to be injected into non-human animal should be as few as possible;
- True hybrid research should be still prohibited because of harm which may be caused;
- Animal/human cybrids should not be permitted when it involves the waste of human eggs and is scientifically unnecessary;
- Human/animal chimera research should not be permitted if it will entail possible harm to the human embryo.[25]

---

[25] R.Z. Qiu. 2007. *Ethical Issues in Human Embryonic Stem Cell Research, presented at the Sino-German Workshop on Stem Cell Research in Shanghai on 23 Sep*; R.Z. Qiu. 2007. *The Historical, Social and Philosophical Background of Chinese Policies Regarding Human Embryonic Stem Cell Research, presented at the BIONET Workshop on Stem Cell Research in Shanghai on 10 Oct*; R.Z. Qiu. 2007. Ethical Issues in the Frontiers of Life Sciences. *Wenhui Daily*, 14 Oct; and X.M. Zhai. 2009. *Ethical Issues in Human Embryonic Stem Cell Research, presented at the Cultural and Education Section, British Embassy in Beijing, 31 Mar.* Available at: www.ebiotrade.com [Accessed 3 Apr 2009].

CLINICAL APPLICATION OF STEM CELL PRODUCTS: THE CONCERNS OF UNDER REGULATION

A biotechnology company B 'invented' neural stem cell therapy to treat neural diseases such as Parkinson's disease or spinal injury. They work within dozens of hospitals in China to provide neural stem cell products to patients. They advertise their research, attracting a number of patients from China and abroad, whom then go to 'B approved' hospitals for 'treatment'. Each course will involve four to six injections and cost about 50,000 Chinese dollars (EURO 5000) for Chinese, and about US$25,000 for Western patients. The company B has never sought the approval of MOH, a review by any IRB, or, it would seem (based on the lack of dissemination of validated scientific research), valid informed consent.[26]

In mainland China, there may be 100–150 health institutions which offer stem cell therapies which are alleged to work. It is difficult to ascertain whether the stem cell products offered are effective, because no third party has tested them, and the methods and results have yet to be published in reputable journals. They usually recruit patients by advertisements on the Internet. In these advertisements, the stem cell therapies are described as 'magic bullets' which can cure any diseases. The patients they enroll are sometimes illiterate or semi-literate; they sometimes come from rural areas and with little awareness of the scientific controversy; and often the patients are desperate with untreatable, debilitating, and ultimately fatal illnesses. They do not know how to assess the efficiency of therapy (or that those in a position to do so have so far failed

---

[26] D. Cyranovski. Stem Cell Therapy Faces More Scrutiny in China. *Nature* 2009; 459(14): 146–147; S. Kiatpongsan & D. Sipp. 2009. Monitoring and Regulating Offshore Stem Cell Clinics. *Science* 2009; 323: 1564–1565; N. Zamiska. 2007. Stem-Cell Refugees: Seeking Hope in Chinese Stem Cells: Treatments May Not Work or Even Be Safe, but Dozens Make the Trek Each Month. *Wall Street Journal* 2 July. Available at: http://online.wsj.com/article/SB118334242884354943.html [Accessed 25 Jun 2009]; Stem-Cell Refugees: Yanks are Flocking to China for Therapy. *Business Week* 12 Feb 2007. Available at: http://www.businessweek.com/magazine/content/07_07/b4021061.htm [Accessed 25 Jun 2009]. Of course, institutions other than B company provide stem cell therapy too, see J. Qiu. 2007. To Walk Again: Can China Transform Therapy for Spinal Injury? *New Scientist* 10 Nov: 57–59.

to ascertain such evidence), or how to claim their rights when they feel they have been deceived. One reason is that in mainland China, the therapeutic misconception has tended to be common. Physicians and investigators have deliberately confused clinical trials with medical care, thereby avoiding any ethical review and the informed consent process, but with the intention to make money from uninformed patients. And no regulation on the relationship between drugs/equipment manufacturing companies and physicians and investigators or IRB members has been developed.[27]

Some stem cell therapies, like the use of bone marrow to treat leukaemia, have been available as routine treatments for some time. But most stem cell research, and human embryonic stem cell research in particular, has not reached the same stage of clinical translation. So bioethicists in China have argued that, before clinical application or clinical trials of stem cell products, there must be a strict approval process and monitoring so as to secure the scientific and ethical validity, and principally, to protect the patients' health and welfare. The translation of stem cell research to clinical application must go through clinical trials. Before proceeding with clinical trials, a favorable benefit to risk ratio must be obtained, and the examination of pre-clinical studies in animal models and with foetal tissues is also needed. The risks to human subjects of stem cell therapies have been well documented in animal studies; this may include tumour formation, inappropriate stem cell migration, immune rejection of transplanted stem cells, injuries during operation, and infection. And tumour formation and inappropriate stem cell migration must be minimised before obtaining a favourable potential benefits to risk calculus and to provide human subjects with a reasonable choice before they enroll

[27] In major regulations such as the *Regulation on Scientific Misconduct* (2006, MOST), as well as the *Regulation on Ethical Review of Biomedical Research Involving Human Subjects* (2007, MOH), no article prescribes the relationship between drugs or equipment manufacturing companies, or physicians, investigators or IRB members. See also X.M. Zhai. 2009. *Ethical Issues in Human Embryonic Stem Cell Research, presented at the Cultural and Education Section, British Embassy in Beijing, 31 Mar.* Available at: www.ebiotrade.com [Accessed 3 April 2009].

in clinical studies.[28] It is imperative that the media be used to convey this message to the public.[29]

CONCLUSION: HOPE FOR FUTURE REGULATION

In March 2009, the *Regulation on Clinical Application of Medical Technologies*[30] was promulgated by MOH. In this regulation, medical technologies are classified into three categories: (1) those in which clinical application is safe and efficacious with minimum risks and which may be administrated by the institution (hospital); (2) those in which clinical application is safe and efficacious but with high risks; and they must be administrated by the provincial bureau for health care; and (3) those in which safety and efficacy are uncertain, have high risks, may entail major ethical issues and use scarce resources; and so they must be administrated by the MOH. 'Being administrated' means the institution's capacity of clinical application of a given medical technology and the results of clinical trials must be reviewed and examined by a specific team appointed by the provincial bureau for health care (for medical technologies in the second category) or MOH (for medical technologies in the third category). Cloning therapy, autogenic stem cell therapy, gene therapy, heterogenic stem cell transplantation, detoxification and mental illness treatment with brain surgery are under the third category of medical technologies. According to this regulation, xeno-stem cell therapy, xero-gene therapy, and human somatic cloning technology are prohibited from clinical application.[31]

The regulation will be helpful to validate the scientific basis of stem cell therapy and increase protection of the patients' interests and welfare,

---

[28] R.Z. Qiu. 2008. *Common Grounds and Differences in Ethics and Governance of Reproductive Technologies and Stem Cell Research in China and Europe, presented at the BIONET Conference on Reproductive Medicine and Stem Cell Research in Changsha on 1 Apr*; and X.M. Zhai. 2009. *Ethical Issues in Human Embryonic Stem Cell Research, presented at the Cultural and Education Section, British Embassy in Beijing, 31 Mar.* Available at: www.ebiotrade.com [Accessed 3 Apr 2009].

[29] 'Expert is calling for the governance of stem cell therapy'; www.ebiotrade.com/newsf/2009-4/20094291502.htm [Accessed 3 April 2009].

[30] http://www.moh.gov.cn.

[31] http://www.moh.gov.cn.

but it is still inadequate. At the meeting of *Ethics Committee of Ministry of Health* in March 2009, the Committee gave approval for a team headed by Dr./Professor Ching-Li Hu, the former Associate Director of WHO to draft a specific regulation on stem cell research and its clinical application. It is expected that the team will submit their draft to the Committee at the end of this year, and after approval it will be submitted to the MOH. We hope that this will then confer sufficient protection for patients enrolled in stem cell therapy.

LIST OF CHINESE LAWS AND REGULATIONS:

Minister of Health (MOH): Regulations on Human Assisted Reproductive Technologies, 2000, 2003

MOH: Regulation on Clinical Application of Organ Transplantation Technology, 2005

MOH: Regulation on Ethical Review of Biomedical Research Involving Human Subjects, 2007

MOH: Regulation on Clinical Application of Medical Technologies, 2009.

Ministry of Science and Technology (MOST)/MOH: Protecting Human Genetic Resources, 1998

MOST/MOH: Ethical Guiding Principles for Human Embryonic Stem Cell Research, 2003

National People's Congress (NPC): Civil Law: General Principles, 1986.

NPC: Law of Succession, 1985.

NPC: Criminal Law, 1979.

NPC: Maternal and Infant Health Care Law, 1994

NPC: Family Planning and Population Law, 2001

State Council: Regulation on Medical Institutions, 1994

State Council: Regulation on Marriage Registry, 2003

State Council: Regulation on AIDS Prevention and Control, 2006

State Council: Regulation on Organ Transplantation, 2007

State Food and Drug Administration (SFDA): GCP for Clinical Trials, 1999, 2003

14

NEITHER A 'PERSON' NOR A 'THING': THE CONTROVERSY CONCERNING THE MORAL AND LEGAL STATUS OF HUMAN EMBRYOS IN JAPAN

Satoshi Kodama and Akira Akabayashi

INTRODUCTION: NEITHER A 'PERSON' NOR A 'THING'

Until now, there have been only very cursory explanations (based on English language newspaper articles and the like) of Japanese policies and regulations regarding cloning and stem cell research, and the process through which they were formed.[1] One reason for this is that records of

---

[1] See for example: L. Walters. Human Embryonic Stem Cell Research: An Intercultural Perspective. *Kennedy Institute of Ethics Journal* 2004; 14: 3–38. L.P. Knowles. A Regulatory Patchwork — Human ES Cell Research Oversight. *Nature Biotechnology* 2004; 22: 157–163. The following article by a Japanese philosopher is an exception: M. Morioka. 2006. The Ethics of Human Cloning and the Sprout of Human Life. In *Cross-Cultural Issues in Bioethics: The Example of Human Cloning*. H. Roetz, ed. Amsterdam, The Netherlands: Rodopi: 1–16. In this article, Morioka explains (1) details of one of the main reports by the *Bioethics Committee* as well as the *Law Concerning Regulations Relating to Human Cloning Techniques and Other Similar Techniques*, (2) results of the government's public opinion survey on cloning in 1998, and (3) some opinions of prominent scholars and journalists in Japan following establishment of the law. He lastly considers the meaning of and ideas behind the phrase 'sprout of human life', which our present chapter will also touch upon. However, our present chapter differs from his in that it looks at discussions of the *Bioethics Committee* leading up to the establishment of the *Law Concerning Regulations Relating to Human Cloning Techniques and Other Similar Techniques*, based primarily on records of proceedings.

administrative proceedings in Japan are released in Japanese only. Therefore, this chapter will analyse the discussions of the *Bioethics Committee* leading up to the establishment of the *Law Concerning Regulations Relating to Human Cloning Techniques and Other Similar Techniques*, based primarily on records of proceedings, and also examine the background of Japan's eclectic solution, which established human embryos as the 'sprout of human life'. The first section provides background information about the structure and activity of the *Bioethics Committee* in Japan. The second section examines discussions surrounding the regulation of human cloning. The third section examines the discussions of human embryonic research. The final section considers the conflict between the advocates and sceptics of human embryo research.

THE BIOETHICS COMMITTEE OF THE COUNCIL FOR SCIENCE AND TECHNOLOGY

The birth of Dolly, the cloned sheep, was reported worldwide in February 1997. The communiqué issued by the Denver Summit of the G8 held in June of the same year acknowledged concerns about the creation of cloned humans, and noted the necessity of both domestic and international efforts to regulate cloning. In September, the *Bioethics Committee* was established as a division of the *Council for Science and Technology* within the former Japanese Prime Minister's Office. The *Council for Science and Technology* itself had been established to act in an advisory capacity to the Prime Minister, aimed at the overall promotion of the government's science and technology policy.[2]

In January 2001, with the major restructuring of the central government, the *Bioethics Committee* was reborn under the *Cabinet Office's Council for Science and Technology*, and was later renamed the *Expert Panel of Bioethics*. Up to that point, the *Bioethics Committee* met a total of ten times, with each meeting lasting approximately two hours. The first meeting was held on October 30, 1997, and the last was held on June 14, 2000.

---

[2] The *Council for Science and Technology.* Available at: http://www.mext.go.jp/b_menu/shingi/kagaku/index.htm [In Japanese; accessed on 29 Apr 2009].

The committee initially had 17 members, including the chair. In addition to life science specialists, medical researchers, and clinicians, it included a writer and researchers in the fields of law, philosophy, religion, and economics. Most of the committee members held positions at the level of Professor or Professor Emeritus. The committee's first chair was Wataru Mori (former president of the University of Tokyo and a pathologist), but he completed his term as a member of the *Council for Science and Technology* midway through. Hirō Imura (former president of Kyoto University and an internal medicine specialist) replaced him in time for the Committee's fourth meeting. Due to requests from committee members hesitant to make discussions public, the committee initially did not allow outsiders to observe the proceedings, and only made a summary of the proceedings available, with the names of individual speakers kept anonymous. However, the committee gradually shifted toward public disclosure of information. Beginning with the eighth meeting, the committee was completely open, even allowing observers to attend.

The *Bioethics Committee* was a standing committee. While there had previously been a number of government bioethics committees convened, such as the *Provisional Commission on Brain Death and Organ Transplantation* (1990–1992), the committee established in 1997 was the first standing bioethics committee at the level of the Prime Minister's Office. Furthermore, compared to the bioethics committees existing at the ministry level (at the former *Ministry of Education, Science and Culture* or the former *Ministry of Health and Welfare*, for example), this committee was designed to discuss bioethics from a broader perspective and formulate Japan's fundamental principles and policies on bioethical issues.[3] Although this standing committee was created to discuss bioethical issues

---

[3] Chair Wataru Mori made the following remark concerning the *Bioethics Committee's* role at the beginning of the first meeting: 'As I understand, there are at the moment several committees dealing with bioethical issues within the ministries and agencies, such as the Ministry of Education, Science and Culture and the Ministry of Health and Welfare. While these committees work out the details of research or clinical regulations, we, the *Bioethics Committee*, are here to discuss bioethical issues from a broader perspective. For instance, we need to decide whether or not there should be legislation on a certain issue, and what stance Japan should take on certain bioethical issues'. Authors' translation of http://www.mext.go.jp/b_menu/shingi/kagaku/80821.htm [In Japanese; accessed on 29 Apr 2009].

in general, its main purpose at first was to discuss the ethical implications of cloning.

The committee established subcommittees when necessary, resulting in the formation of three. The *Cloning Subcommittee* convened 12 times from February 17, 1998 to November 17, 1999, and produced a report titled 'Fundamental Policy on the Production of Human Individuals Using Cloning Techniques' (11.17.1999). The *Subcommittee on Human Embryo Research* was formed following the creation of human embryonic stem cells in the United States (US) in November 1998, and again in the following month in Korea, where it was reported that a human embryo was successfully cloned. This subcommittee met 14 times from February 9, 1999 to March 6, 2000, and produced a report titled 'Fundamental Policy on Human Embryo Research Focused Primarily on Human Embryonic Stem Cells' (3.6.2000). The chair of these two committees was Yoshio Okada (Professor Emeritus, Osaka University), an authority on cellular biology. In addition, and in light of advances in human genome research, the *Human Genome Research Subcommittee* was formed and chaired by an internal medicine specialist, Fumimaro Takaku (Professor Emeritus, University of Tokyo). This committee convened six times from January 28, 2000 to June 7, 2000, and released a report titled 'Fundamental Principles of Research on the Human Genome' (6.14.2000). Public comment was sought on each of these reports, and these comments were taken into consideration during revisions made by the subcommittees and parent committee (i.e. *Bioethics Committee*).[4]

A description of the debates and discussions is given below, based primarily on records of the proceedings of the *Bioethics Committee*.[5]

---

[4] For instance, in February 2000, the draft report 'Fundamental Policy on Human Embryo Research Focused Primarily on Human Embryonic Stem Cells' was sent to about 400 organisations, including academic societies, civil society organisations and local governments to elicit opinions. The draft report was also obtainable via the Internet for anyone who was interested. All in all, there were 88 comments. The *Subcommittee on Human Embryo Research* prepared responses to each comment and changed the wording of the draft report when necessary. These changes, as well as comments to the draft report, were considered in the eighth *Bioethics Committee* meeting (3.13.2000) prior to finalising the draft.

[5] The proceedings are available from the following webpage (only in Japanese). http://www.mext.go.jp/b_menu/shingi/kagaku/rinri.htm [Accessed on 29 Apr 2009].

COMMITTEE DISCUSSIONS REGARDING THE REGULATION OF HUMAN CLONING

The two main points that were debated with respect to regulations on human cloning were: (1) whether 'human dignity' could be used as the basis for such regulations and (2) whether regulations should be in the form of laws or administrative guidelines.

The main points of the discussions regarding the regulation of human cloning that took place within the *Cloning Subcommittee* are summarised as follows. First, the committee discussed the issue of human cloning separately from the issue of animal cloning. They considered animal cloning to be highly useful and beneficial, and determined that regulation was not urgently needed. In the case of human cloning, on the other hand, although there are individuals with identical genetic characteristics (i.e. identical twins), the subcommittee concluded that the intentional creation of clones for *reproductive purposes* violates human dignity. The subcommittee's reasoning was that nuclear transplantation cloning is a form of asexual reproduction, and thus lacks the element of 'chance at the genetic level' that accompanies normal sexual reproduction. The subcommittee also concluded that the production of cloned organs for transplants should be prohibited, because this also involves the creation of human clones (implanting cloned embryos in the uterus). However, the subcommittee decided that cloning for the purposes of investigating cellular structure should be permitted, because such research is of great value, and, lacking any reproductive ends, does not violate human dignity.

The draft of the report produced by the *Cloning Subcommittee*, 'Fundamental Policy on the Production of Human Individuals Using Cloning Techniques', concluded the following regarding the regulation of human cloning:

> 'The production of human clones, due to what accompanies this production, could lead to the breeding of humans, could turn humans into a means to an end, and/or into tools. This can also result in a deviation from the ways of thinking about reproduction, i.e. asexual reproduction. This will bring about disruption of the family order and cause problems related to the safety of those born. Furthermore, the serious issue unique

> to human cloning is the intentional production of people with duplicate genetic characteristics. This may lead to the violation of the resulting cloned child's human rights, and clearly violates the constitutional principle of respect for individuals. Therefore, the intentional production of cloned human individuals should be completely prohibited due to the magnitude of the negative effects, and it would be appropriate to regulate cloning using the binding force of law'.[6]

On the other hand, the committee concluded that research that did not involve the creation of individual clones should be regulated using administrative guidelines and not prohibited by law, because it was very likely that such research would prove to be highly useful in the future.

Human Dignity

Upon receiving the report from the *Cloning Subcommittee*, the *Bioethics Committee*'s discussion focused primarily on the meaning of 'dignity' and the significance of making distinctions between human beings and animals.

First, there were questions about whether 'dignity' could serve as the legal basis for regulation. In particular, as the following comment demonstrates, the issue was whether or not the German principle of 'human dignity' can be derived from the Japanese constitution.

> 'The very question of whether the German principle of "human dignity" exists in the Japanese constitution has been controversial, although the constitution does contain the principle of respect for the individual. I think it is a bit difficult to go straight from the idea of human dignity to specific legal regulation. On the other hand, I think it would be easier to set up legal regulations based on the idea of harm to

[6] Authors' translation of http://www.mext.go.jp/b_menu/shingi/kagaku/rinri/cl912271.htm [In Japanese; accessed on 29/Apr/2009]. The draft report did admit that reproductive cloning of human individuals, if ever successful, would be useful for assisted reproduction and organ transplantation. However, the subcommittee argued that the negative effects associated with reproductive cloning far outweighed its usefulness.

> others, or disruption of public order, although there are also strong counter arguments against that as well'.[7]

Related to this first problem, a second issue emerged when it was pointed out that a clear rationale should be given for permitting the creation of animal clones while forbidding those of human. The next comment, for example, was typical:

> 'The report says it is wrong to produce offspring without the involvement of both sexes, and to intentionally produce individuals that are genetically identical. In fact, we are already doing this with animals. By this logic, we are violating the dignity of animals, so I think we need to clearly explain why it is wrong only in the case of humans'.[8]

Other comments also demonstrate scepticism toward drawing a well-defined line between humans and animals, and as the following quote shows, some argued that this way of thinking was Western rather than Asian:

> 'There can be no doubt that the idea that humans possess a special mission different from animals is emphasised within the Christian tradition. I think it is also true that it was on this basis that the modern concept of human dignity was established. So I think it's natural that this idea should seem out of place when considered from an Asian, or Japanese, perspective'.[9]

Through these discussions, the *Bioethics Committee* came to define human cloning as both a violation of human dignity, and a violation of human rights (*vis-à-vis* the children born through cloning). The connection

---

[7] Authors' translation of a quote by an anonymous member of the Bioethics Committee at the third meeting [21 Apr 1998]. http://www.mext.go.jp/b_menu/shingi/kagaku/808212.htm [In Japanese; accessed on 29 Apr 2009].

[8] Authors' translation. Ibid.

[9] Authors' translation. Ibid.

between human dignity and human rights was pointed out by Kyoto University Law Professor Ryuichi Ida (a specialist in constitutional and international law), who was a member of both the *Cloning Subcommittee* and the *Human Embryo Subcommittee*. Professor Ida explained that human rights were at the core of the principle of human dignity.[10] Sophia University Law Professor Saku Machino (an expert in criminal law), echoing Professor Ida's opinion, commented as follows:

> 'Basically, there are two steps, I think... First, we have human dignity, which is a very abstract value — the value of our civilisation. And then, we have a *violation* of human dignity, which takes a concrete shape when individual rights are violated, as Professor Ida has just mentioned. That's how we conceive the relationship between human dignity and human rights'.[11]

Legal Regulation or Administrative Guidelines?

Both the *Cloning Subcommittee* and the *Human Embryo Subcommittee* ultimately supported legal regulation over administrative guidelines. The reasoning behind this was explained by Professor Machino. His argument can be summarised as follows:

> Although administrative guidelines have an advantage in that they can be applied more flexibly than laws, they lack binding power insofar as they have no legal basis. Thus it is not possible to penalise violators through the use of sanctions. In the case of legal regulation on the other hand, those orders can be imbued with binding force. Laws enacted by the National Diet [i.e. the Japanese Parliamentary Assembly] also have an advantage over administrative guidelines because they are established through democratic procedures. In the case of cloning regulation in particular, it is really best if these things are debated in the Diet, as it

[10] At the sixth meeting of the Bioethics Committee [21 Nov 1999]. http://www.mext.go.jp/b_menu/shingi/kagaku/rinri/gijiro6.htm [In Japanese; accessed on 29 Apr 2009].

[11] Authors' translation. Ibid.

> may limit constitutional rights such as freedom of scholarship or reproductive rights.
>
> On the other hand, as a general rule the fact that something is immoral does not alone justify the use of legal coercion. To justify such a step, there must be a violation of interests protected by law. But the creation of human clones violates the principle of 'respect for individuals', in the sense that 'all people must be respected as unique entities with unique personalities' because it is an activity that involves creating humans with genetic characteristics copied from people already existing. And thus it violates Article 13 of the Constitution, which states that, 'All people shall be respected as individuals'. The creation of chimera embryos or hybrid embryos by fusing human and animal embryos also damages the integrity of the human species, and the production of incomplete individuals is an act that violates the dignity of those produced. Therefore this could be said to violate the respect for individuals stipulated in Article 13.
>
> Nonetheless, the drawback of legal regulation is that it may have a chilling effect on research. Thus it is best to legally prohibit only the creation of human clones, and regulate research using human embryos with administrative guidelines.[12]

Following this discussion, the *Bioethics Committee* ultimately released a short document entitled, 'Regarding the Production of Human Individuals through Cloning', dated December 21, 1999.[13] Its main points were as follows: (1) cloning by transplantation of somatic cell nuclei will be prohibited, but clones made using nuclear transplantation from early embryos and the creation of multiple individuals through the division of

---

[12] Summarised and translated by the authors, based on the transcripts of Machino at the fifth meeting of the Bioethics Committee [29 Sep 1999]. http://www.mext.go.jp/b_menu/shingi/kagaku/rinri/gijiro5.htm [In Japanese; accessed on 29 Apr 2009]. Concerning the nature and significance of Japan's administrative guidelines on biomedical research, see: B.T. Slingsby *et al.* Administrative Legislation in Japan: Guidelines on Scientific and Ethical Standards. *Cambridge Quarterly of Healthcare Ethics* 2004; 13: 245–253.

[13] http://www.mext.go.jp/b_menu/shingi/kagaku/rinri/cl00215.htm [In Japanese; accessed on 29 Apr 2009].

early embryos will be regulated by means other than law, (2) creation of individual organisms using chimera or hybrid embryos will be prohibited, (3) guidelines will be drawn up by the *Human Embryo Subcommittee* in order to regulate the production of human embryos for research purposes, and (4) these points will be reviewed in three to five years given the need for international harmony and release of information to the public.

HUMAN EMBRYO RESEARCH

The draft of the report, 'Fundamental Policy on Human Embryo Research Focused Primarily on Human Embryonic Stem Cells', released in March 6, 2000 by the *Subcommittee on Human Embryo Research*, states that human embryos (including cloned embryos) are the 'sprout of human life' and would require considerate, rather than frivolous, treatment. Therefore research should be permitted within an appropriate regulatory framework.[14] The expression 'sprout of human life' (*seimei no houga)* was first used in the draft of the law on cloning technology within the *Cloning Subcommittee* that met on May 12 of the previous year. Within the subcommittee it was explained that the concept of 'sprout of life' is different from 'life' itself, and research using human embryos should be permitted in certain situations because 'the harm in violation of embryos that are no more than a sprout of life is minute relative to that of foetuses or humans'.[15]

The subcommittee's report stated the following:

> 'This subcommittee holds that human embryos existing outside of the uterus are the sprout of human life and require careful handling, but they are still at a different stage than foetuses or post-natal humans. Therefore, embryos which have been set to be disposed of can be used

---

[14] http://www.mext.go.jp/b_menu/shingi/kagaku/rinri/ki00306.htm [In Japanese; accessed on 29 Apr 2009].

[15] Authors' translation of an early draft of the above report [dated 28 Jul 1999]. Available at: http://www.mext.go.jp/b_menu/shingi/kagaku/909011.htm [In Japanese; accessed on 29 Apr 2009].

> in research deemed scientifically and morally appropriate... Particularly in light of the establishment of embryonic stem cell research, which requires a swift response in Japan and is the source of high hopes for regenerative medicine, we judge after considerable consideration that the use of human embryos should be permitted'.[16]

The subcommittee suggested that specific regulations on research using human embryos include the following: (1) only frozen surplus embryos would be used, (2) consent from the couple would be required, (3) no compensation would be provided for the embryos, (4) research would be limited to basic research initially, and no clinical research would be performed, and (5) research would require review by an ethics committee. Furthermore, as embryonic stem cells do not result in creation of an individual human, the committee deemed that legal regulation was not necessary and opted for more flexible guidelines. In addition, the subcommittee proposed a moratorium on the use of cloned embryos for the following reasons: (1) it might lead to the creation of human clones,[17] (2) the creation and subsequent destruction of a cloned embryo for research purposes is, morally speaking, on par with doing the same thing to a human embryo and hence undesirable, (3) stem cell research using surplus embryos, which is less problematic than use of cloned embryos, should proceed first, and (4) based on the results of research using surplus embryos, the propriety of using cloned embryos should be re-examined.

'Sprout of Human Life'

A fascinating exchange occurred regarding the expression 'sprout of human life', between committee member Norio Fujisawa, a prominent researcher of Greek philosophy, and legal scholar Ryuichi Ida.

---

[16] Authors' translation of http://www.mext.go.jp/b_menu/shingi/kagaku/rinri/ki00306.htm [In Japanese; accessed on 29 Apr 2009].

[17] The authors are unaware of any discussions on the 'slippery slope' argument against therapeutic cloning in the proceedings of the committees, although there may well have been such discussions in academia and elsewhere in Japan.

Fujisawa noted:

> 'Consider the issue in really commonsensical terms: from the standpoint of science you can rationalise it in all sorts of ways and argue that an embryo is the sprout of life, but not life. Yet, I think that maybe to the ethical sensibility of a normal person, they might be inclined to think that the sprout of life is the same as life'.[18]

To which Ida responded as follows:

> 'Well, of course, if born, this becomes a "person". And legally it is possible a foetus would be treated as a person as well. However, a human embryo itself has not yet become a foetus..., so I think it is extremely difficult to judge whether this should be thought of as being the same as a person... Because it is at the embryo stage, a stage at which it has not yet fully developed into a foetus, isn't it rather difficult to call it human life? Having said that, an embryo is not just a "thing" either; if it divides, it will naturally become a person. This is why we used the expression "sprout of human life", and thus in a sense it describes an intermediate stage on the way to becoming a person... In embryonic stem cell research, embryos are created, and the created embryos are destroyed. If the embryo was deemed to be human life, then to take it to an extreme, these researchers would be committing murder. The Embryo Protection Law in Germany, for instance, reflects such a position, and thus human embryo research is not possible there. But to hold the position of wanting to conduct human embryo research if possible, or even to a certain extent, you essentially draw a line to signify that it is acceptable to do certain types of research but not others. In this case, I think that a rationale — that embryos are not human life — is necessary to some degree. And that is why I say that human embryos are the sprout of human life'.[19]

---

[18] At the seventh meeting of the Bioethics Committee [22 Feb 2000]. http://www.mext.go.jp/b_menu/shingi/kagaku/rinri/gijiro7.htm [In Japanese; accessed on 29 Apr 2009].
[19] Authors' translation. Ibid.

In response, Fujisawa asked:

> 'So then, in terms of ancient philosophical concepts, there's potentiality and actuality. Are you saying that embryos basically constitute the potentiality of life, but not the actuality?'[20]

Both Ida and the Chair, Imura, responded that Fujisawa was correct. It's not clear whether the two of them fully understood Fujisawa's question, which was based on the thinking of Aristotle. However, the exchange suggests that the expression 'sprout of human life' is close to the discussion of 'potentiality', which has been the centre of contention in debates over the artificial termination of pregnancy in English-speaking countries. Thus, a human embryo is potentially a person, but it is not yet a person. Therefore, its destruction is not the same as murder.[21]

In the end, this report was accepted by the *Bioethics Committee*, and the committee's views were compiled in a final report, 'Regarding Human Embryo Research Focusing Primarily on Human Embryonic Stem Cells'.[22] At the same time, the *Regulation of Human Cloning Techniques* bill drafted by the government in accordance with the reports by the *Cloning Subcommittee* and *Human Embryo Subcommittee* was presented and explained, and the committee was adjourned. The bill was

---

[20] Authors' translation. Ibid.

[21] The *Bioethics Committee* thus introduced a new category for the moral status of the embryo. A similar idea had been expressed in the West by the phrase 'pre-embryo', i.e. the embryo before the primitive streak appears. (See for example: R.A. McCormick. 1991. Who or What is the Preembryo? *Kennedy Institute of Ethics Journal* 1991; 1: 1–15. C.A. Tauer. 2004. II. Embryo Research. In *Encyclopedia of Bioethics 3rd edition*. S.G. Post, ed. New York, NY: Macmillan Library Reference: 712–722.) Both ideas were used to justify research using early embryos. The differences are that the idea of a 'pre-embryo' presupposes that the embryo *is* a person (the *pre*-embryo is not a person yet), whereas the concept of 'sprout of human life' does not assume that the embryo is a person, but rather is something which will *become* a person in the future. The primitive streak was brought up on numerous occasions by the *Bioethics Committee* and subcommittees, but no explicit comparison of the two ideas was made.

[22] http://www.mext.go.jp/b_menu/shingi/kagaku/rinri/ken00313.htm [In Japanese; accessed on 29 Apr 2009].

submitted to the National Diet on April 14, 2000. The *Law Concerning Regulations Relating to Human Cloning Techniques and Other Similar Techniques* was passed on November 30, 2000, and went into effect on June 6, 2001.[23]

LIFE SCIENCES AND BIOETHICS: CHECKS *OR* BALANCES?

The conflict between champions of human embryo research and sceptics began to clearly emerge as a series of objections were raised by some committee members with respect to the report from the *Subcommittee on Human Embryo Research*. The primary objections of the sceptics can be summarised as follows: (1) that the *Bioethics Committee* had not adequately discussed the issue, (2) that they should wait for national public opinion on the matter to develop, (3) that the discussion had focused only on short-term usefulness, without discussing the long-term outlook, and (4) that mere lip service was being paid to ethical considerations.

For example, scholar of religious studies Susumu Shimazono (University of Tokyo) made the following comments:

> 'How much was the matter discussed in this parent committee?...I certainly don't think that sufficient time was allotted for deliberations...This is a very serious issue. How are we to define a human embryo as the sprout of human life? Will it be permitted to create them and destroy them? If it will be allowed, what will the conditions be? I think we're dealing with a very fundamental issue, and it should be considered carefully...What is life? What does it mean if human life is newly born? What does the 'sprout of life' mean? What does it mean for these to be used scientifically? Concerning even the single issue of embryonic stem cells, shouldn't this be properly considered through a national discussion? I think opinions need time to develop and mature'.[24]

---

[23] http://www.cas.go.jp/jp/seisaku/hourei/data/htc.pdf [In English and Japanese; accessed on 29 Apr 2009].

[24] Authors' translation of a quote from the eighth meeting of the Bioethics Committee [13 Mar 2000]. http://www.mext.go.jp/b_menu/shingi/kagaku/rinri/gijiro8.htm [In Japanese; accessed on 29 Apr 2009].

In addition, committee member Fujisawa used an analogy to nuclear physics as follows:

> 'Do we really have the right to tamper with the most basic core unit of life, in which case the core unit for matter is the atomic nucleus, and that for life is the cell nucleus...? Humanity tampered with the atomic nucleus of substances, and paid a high price for that. Who can guarantee that the same sort of thing won't occur as a result of tampering with and manipulating the cell's nucleus? And, I think it's possible that the consequences will place an extremely heavy burden on future generations'.[25]

In response, the advocates stressed that they certainly did not begin from the conclusion that the research should be promoted, and stated that the subcommittee adequately discussed the status of the human embryo. Some advocates pointed out the fact that human embryo research is already being conducted in the field of reproductive medicine, and thus it would be difficult to enact a comprehensive ban, while others stressed that regenerative medicine could possibly save the lives of 'patients standing right in front of their eyes'. The chair, Imura, supported making a decision quickly, emphasising as a clinician that there was a need to advance regenerative medicine.

The conflict between the advocates and sceptics was also apparent in the discussions of the introduction to the report written by the *Human Genome Research Subcommittee*, 'Fundamental Principles of Research on the Human Genome'.[26] The conflict concerned the *raison d'être* of the *Bioethics Committee*.

Committee member Fujisawa, who was sceptical of the ethical acceptability of this kind of research, made the following remark, from the

---

[25] Authors' translation. Ibid.

[26] Discussions on human genome research are beyond the scope of this chapter. The draft of the fundamental principles was revised based on public comment and published officially on June 14, 2000. The only section that has been officially translated in English can be found at: http://www.mext.go.jp/b_menu/shingi/kagaku/rinri/pri00614.htm [In English and Japanese; accessed on 29 Apr 2009].

perspective that ethics was supposed to serve as a 'check' on science, and apply the brakes in order to prevent science from running amok:

> 'Simply put, I think that bioethics committees were formed to serve as a check on the runaway development of science. There are all these new forms of science and technology, and if left alone, who knows how far they'll be taken? So on the other hand, the idea of human dignity is made to function as a check of that... As I've said at times before, when ethics battles with science and technology, ethics often loses and science continues on ahead. So amidst these circumstances, scientific research isn't free, really. Human dignity, or human value, is the most important thing, and now science must remain within that framework. So in a sense, science is not free'.[27]

Both Shimazono and Fujisawa, likewise sceptical, argued that researchers must come to realise that they have the power to 'play God'.

In response, embryo research advocate, Chair Imura, expressed his understanding that bioethics, rather than serving as check on the life sciences, was meant to weigh the benefits and harms derived from the life sciences, and strike the proper balance.

> 'I think that bioethics is supposed to evaluate the benefits and harms...incurred in the real world application of the myriad technologies found in the truly advanced field of life sciences, and make the most appropriate judgment possible. So I don't think it is meant to be a unilateral check on science, but rather that it should carefully consider both the harms and benefits and make an adequate judgment. Many new technologies have a tendency to come with various negative effects. But where the benefits are great, I think we must think of a way to minimise the harm as much as possible. And that is why we develop various guidelines and regulate science in all sorts of ways'.[28]

---

[27] Authors' translation of a quote from the tenth meeting of the Bioethics Committee [June 14, 2000]. http://www.mext.go.jp/b_menu/shingi/kagaku/rinri/gijiro10.htm [In Japanese; accessed on 29 Apr 2009].

[28] Authors' translation; Ibid.

Despite the conflict, the report on fundamental principles of human genome research passed the committee with only minor revisions in its introductory remarks. The conflict between the advocates and sceptics continued into the new *Expert Panel of Bioethics*, and became even more pronounced.

CONCLUSION

The *Bioethics Committee* that convened over three years beginning in 1997 discussed regulations on cloning technology and research using human embryos, as well as the proper form of human genome research. Products of their efforts included three reports based on deliberations of the three subcommittees. Furthermore, the committee's discussions prompted the drafting of the *Law Concerning Regulations Relating to Human Cloning Techniques and Other Similar Techniques*. The creation of human clones became prohibited by law, while administrative guidelines were to be drafted for research using human embryos. Drafting of these guidelines was postponed, however, and discussions continued in the *Expert Panel of Bioethics*.[29,30]

---

[29] As of June 2009, embryo research is permitted under conditions stipulated by administrative guidelines as mentioned below. (1) The Ministry of Education, Culture, Sports and Science and Technology (MEXT) published *Guidelines Concerning the Establishment and Use of Human ES Cells* in September 25, 2001, which required all research using human ES cells to be approved by both the ethics committee at the institution and that of the government. The requirement, however, has been relaxed recently, and now only approval from the ethics committee at the institutional level is necessary (according to the revised guidelines effective as of May 20, 2009). (2) The *Expert Panel of Bioethics* report, *Fundamental Policy on Handling of Human Embryos* (July 2004), banned the creation of human embryos for research purposes except for research on infertility. Based on that report, the MEXT and Ministry of Health, Labour and Welfare (MHLW) published a joint report in January 2009. Guidelines that regulate infertility research involving the creation of human embryos is expected to follow soon. (3) In March 2009, the *Expert Panel of Bioethics* approved MEXT's draft guidelines allowing the creation of cloned embryos for therapeutic research, ending the moratorium on creation of cloned embryos.

[30] In line with its domestic policy, Japan urged to put an international ban on reproductive cloning of humans at the *UN Ad Hoc Committee on the Convention Against Reproductive*

Several issues surfaced during discussions of the committee and subcommittees. First, the relationship between the subcommittees and parent committee was not clearly defined. The parent committee was originally expected to be a body that would discuss issues from a macroscopic point of view. Yet, in the end, the committee made only relatively minor revisions to the reports produced by the subcommittees, and it is likely that the definitions of 'human dignity' and 'sprout of human life' were not fully discussed. This was partially attributed to the time intervals between sessions.

Although the *Bioethics Committee* was established as a standing committee, at times eight or ten months passed between meetings. This problem was pointed out during one of the later meetings, and it was therefore decided that the committee would convene at least once every three months. Even so, when one considers that the *Expert Panel of Bioethics* later met once a month, the intervals between meetings of the *Bioethics Committee* were too long and the time devoted to the issues too short, making it difficult to adequately discuss the topics.

Still another issue, one exacerbated by the lack of time and discussion, was that the conflict between embryo research advocates and sceptics did not wither away. While the sceptics' perspective was that the *Bioethics Committee* existed as a 'check' on scientific recklessness, the advocates' position was that the committee was there to strike a 'balance' between benefit and harm. This conflict was never resolved and continued within

---

Cloning of Human Beings in February 2002 (see http://www8.cao.go.jp/cstp/tyousakai/life/haihu15/siryou3.pdf, accessed on 01 Jun 2009). However, Japan voted *against* the General Assembly's *UN Declaration on Human Cloning* on March 8, 2005, along with countries such as the United Kingdom, the Republic of Korea and China. The *Declaration*, by which 'Member States were called on to adopt all measures necessary to prohibit all forms of human cloning inasmuch as they are incompatible with human dignity and the protection of human life', was adopted by a vote of 84 in favour to 34 against, with 37 abstentions (see http://www.un.org/News/Press/docs/2005/ga10333.doc.htm, accessed on 01 Jun 2009). Japan did so because the *Declaration* was difficult to interpret as to whether it allowed the creation and use of human cloned embryos for research and therapeutic purposes, which was in principle permitted by the *Expert Panel of Bioethics* in July 2004 (see http://www.mext.go.jp/b_menu/shingi/gijyutu/gijyutu1/006/gijiroku/05061001/002_7.htm, only in Japanese, accessed on 01 Jun 2009).

the *Expert Panel of Bioethics*, reaching its climax when the Panel decided to enforce a unilateral decision without consensus in favour of research using human embryos.

Had the *Bioethics Committee* more time for discussion, would the situation have been any better? The authors' speculation is that things might not have been that different, for the compromise it struck between advocates and sceptics of embryo research was, like it or not, very Japanese in a distinct way. The *Committee* introduced the Western idea of human dignity, which leans toward absolutist ethics and suggests a total ban on the use of human embryos as well as the creation of cloned embryos. However, by coining the symbolic phrase 'sprout of human life', the *Committee* found an eclectic solution. Although this term may not be a commonsensical one, it nevertheless allowed the *Bioethics Committee* to approve research using human embryos while demanding that researchers exercise due respect in handling them. Accepting the Western idea of human dignity and at the same time making ambiguous the Western dichotomy of things and persons, the *Committee* made it possible for ethics and science to reconcile with each other, at least for the time being.

ACKNOWLEDGEMENTS

The authors would like to express their thanks to Dr. B. T. Slingsby for his insightful suggestions.

15

A TALE OF TWO COUNTRIES: CZECH AND SLOVAK STEM CELL BIOPOLICIES

Peter Sýkora

INTRODUCTION

Only ten years since the breakup of a common state, the Czech and Slovak biopolicies regarding research on human embryos and human embryonic stem cells (hESC) found themselves completely at opposite poles. While in Slovakia such research is banned, it is permitted in the Czech Republic. What are the reasons for such opposite biopolicies in two countries, which, until recently, shared seven decades of a common state and legislation, and which are culturally as well as linguistically very close? Is the answer hidden in the development of those first ten years after the separation of Czechoslovakia; or should we search for the reasons in a more distant history?

Immediately after the dissolution of Czechoslovakia in 1993, the same laws of the common state remained valid in both successional states. However, in the course of the following years, two antagonistic processes started to influence legislation in both countries: first, the natural diversification which was caused by the accumulation of different amendatory acts to the same laws as well as by the process of creating completely new and different acts; second, at the same time, the convergence of national legislations started due to the accession procedure of both countries to the European Union, which involved also accommodation and implementation of the European legislation. Slovakia and Czech Republic joined the EU in 2004.

The legislative situation in the field of health care in both countries has been affected mainly by its transformation from an ineffective and highly indebted post-communistic health care system to the Western European standard. Furthermore, in recent years, the Slovak and Czech Republics, along with other post-communistic countries, have been facing unprecedented challenges to the health care legislations caused by new developments in biomedicine.

It is becoming obvious that these countries have chosen different strategies to cope with the 'bioethical deficit' in their health care legislation, and the issue of hESC research provides a good example of this. In the years 2004 and 2005, Slovakia passed two legislative acts which banned research on human embryos in a very general way, and classified this research as a serious criminal offence. On the other hand, the Czech Republic opted for a different strategy to fight the existing deficit in bioethical legislation, and adopted a new and specific act on hESC research in 2006. The new act allowed research on hESC under exact specified conditions, and defined the competences of a newly created *Bioethics Committee*, whose roles would include competence in franchising the issuance of licenses for hESC research.

The explanation of the differences between the Slovak and Czech hESC biopolicies may seem to be, at first glance, trivial — the difference being explained as a result of religious differences between these two countries: on the one hand, there is a modern and atheistic Czech Republic with no ideological objections to human embryo research, while on the other hand, there is a traditionalistic and Catholic Slovakia for which embryo research is inevitably objected to on religious grounds.

The aim of this paper is to demonstrate that the differences in biopolicies between the Slovak and Czech nations may be the result of a much more complex situation than that suggested by the mere differences in religion and secular regulation. This case study presents a comparison of the key political and historical developments in the Czech Republic and Slovakian regulatory policies; and concludes that a probable key factor responsible for the opposite biopolicies in these countries is the impact national research lobbies had on the preparation of each country's legislation.

HISTORICAL AND CULTURAL CONTEXT

Czechoslovakia — the common state of Czechs and Slovaks in the centre of Europe — was, on 1 January 1993, after seven decades of its existence, divided into two independent states: the Czech Republic consisting of the western part of the state inhabited by Czechs and Moravians (ca. 10.3 million inhabitants) and Slovakia in the east, inhabited by Slovaks and a Hungarian minority (ca. 5.3 million inhabitants). Both republics are modern Western-type parliamentary democracies, and are full members of the European Union, Council of Europe, NATO, OECD and other important regional and international organisations.

The Czech and Slovak nations are very linguistically and culturally similar West European nations. However, their destinies unwound differently over the centuries. Slovakia was an integral part of the Kingdom of Hungary under the ascendancy of Hungarians for 900 years starting from the end of the ninth century. Meanwhile, in the tenth century, Czechia (Bohemia) and Moravia together created the Czech Kingdom, which was an important part of the Holy Roman Empire. By the last half of the 17th century, the Habsburgs took both the Czech and the Hungarian thrones, and due to this, Czechia and Slovakia became part of one Empire — the Habsburg Monarchy. In 1867 under pressure from the Hungarians, this Monarchy was transformed into the Austro-Hungarian Empire. Czechoslovakia as a common state of Czechs and Slovaks was created in 1918 as the result of a new post-WWI organisation of Europe, which included the dissolution of the Austro-Hungarian Empire.

It is important to note that the status of Czechs and Slovaks was not equal in Czechoslovakia. From the inception of the common state, Czechs, who were in majority and better established politically, economically and culturally, predominated Slovaks in all these aspects in the state. Furthermore, the political endeavour to create, out of Czechs and Slovaks, one common Czechoslovak nation encountered resistance from the Slovaks, who, following the cultural and economical progress within Czechoslovakia, started to develop higher political ambitions. These separate ambitions were in the end exploited by the National Socialist German Government, which in spring 1939, split Czechoslovakia: Czechia and Moravia became part of the Third Reich, and Slovakia was proclaimed as a new 'independent' state, but in fact just one of Germany's puppet states.

Czechs and Slovaks re-established their common state directly after the World War II. In 1947, two years after the re-establishment of Czechoslovakia, communists seized power and established a totalitarian communist regime which lasted for following 42 years. The efforts of Alexander Dubček to liberalise communism in Czechoslovakia were violently repressed by the invasion of the Soviet and other armed forces of the Warsaw Pact nations on 21 August 1968. Democratisation and liberalisation ultimately arrived 21 years later, after the fall of the Berlin Wall in December 1989. At this time, the communist regime in Czechoslovakia was rejected by the people, and the political dissident, Václav Havel, became the new president. However, the disagreements between Czechs and Slovaks regarding the political and economic organisation of a common state grew steadily, and finally led to the split of Czechoslovakia in 1993, in the so-called 'Velvet Divorce'.[1]

LEGISLATION

Situation in Slovakia

Characteristics

Research on hESC in Slovakia is banned and criminally prosecutable; although there is no explicit legislation concerning hESC. In the post-communist countries of Central and Eastern Europe, there is a general lack of modern bioethical legislation that properly addresses the fast paced progress in the field of biomedicine; and Slovakia is no exception to this group. Slovakia implemented six new health care laws during 2003–2004, including the new *Health Care Act*. The strategy of the then Minister of Health, who authored the health care reform, was to focus on the organisational and economic aspects of the health care. His intention was to put aside all bioethically controversial topics (e.g. induced abortion, assisted reproductive technologies, pre-implantation genetic

[1] For more details on recent Slovak history and Czech and Slovak relations see: K. Henderson. 2002. *Slovakia. The Escape from Invisibility*. London-New York: Routledge.

diagnosis), about which he could expect a strong resistance among the Christian-Democrats (a coalition partner in the government at that time). Such a situation could have endangered the entirety of the health care reform.

The strategy proved to be a success, and all six laws passed in the parliament without any complications. Following this the Ministry of Health began to prepare a single expansive law on bioethics, which was to include all modern and often ethically controversial issues of health care that had yet to be addressed. However, this act encountered resistance in its preparatory stage and never reached the final format needed to be submitted to Parliament. One of the consequences of this is the fact that Slovakia still does not have a law addressing assisted reproduction, despite the fact that it has been routinely carried out for years there.

The Ban on Embryonic Stem Cell Research

The ban on embryo research was introduced to Slovak legislation in a somewhat non-systematic way, *via* 'small' amendments hidden in the shadow of other major legislative changes. In this way, a specific formulation was 'smuggled' into the new *Health Care Law*[2] No. 576 from the 2003–2004 health care reform. In the text referring to the protection of certain persons from possible abuse in biomedical research, a very general formulation about the protection of embryos was added, which in fact, banned research on embryos and on hESC. A section of this law referring to biomedical research says, in §26 Article 10, that researchers are not permitted to perform biomedical research on: 'a) *a living foetus or an embryo*; b) an arrested or imprisoned person; c) a soldier performing compulsory military service, alternative or preparatory service or a person performing civilian service; d) mentally ill person; and e) a foreigner'.[3] In this simple manner, human embryos and foetuses were added to the text of the law to the same category together with other 'persons' without any sort of explanation or comment.

[2] Zákon o zdravotnej starostlivosti č.576/2004 Z.z (*The Heath Care Law No. 576/2004 Coll.)* from 21 Oct 2004, effective from 1 Jun 2006 .

[3] Ibid. Unofficial translation, italics added.

The 2004 health care law only 'slightly' changed the §42 Article 3 of the previous Health Care Law No. 277 from 1994. In the 1994 law, human embryos and foetuses were listed among persons protected against medical tests without therapeutic purposes.[4] Those persons included pregnant women, minors and persons deprived of full legal competence, persons detained or imprisoned, persons in military service (regular or substitute) or civil service, and foreigners. In the new 2004 Law, the term 'medical tests' was replaced by the term 'research'. The term research is explicitly defined in the same paragraph:

> 'Bio-medical research includes every research activity in the field of biology, medicine, pharmacy, nursing care, midwifery and psychology which can influence physical or mental health of a person taking part in this research (hereinafter 'research participant')'.[5]

The shift in meaning is obvious: from medical tests on human persons to biomedical research covering also embryos and foetuses.

From the context, one could assume that this paragraph refers to embryos *in utero* — in the womb of a pregnant woman — and not to embryos *in vitro*, which are used in biomedical research. But the law does not define the term embryo. Moreover, in Slovak legislation there is no distinction between embryo *in vivo* and *in vitro.* Therefore, it is generally understood, that the term embryo in this paragraph is used in its generic meaning, which covers both types of embryos — *in vivo* and *in vitro.* Based on this presumptive interpretation, the concern prevails that courts, inexperienced in such term-differentiation, could interpret the term embryo in its generic way. This is even more likely to happen since human embryos and foetuses are listed in the legislation together with other human persons.

Although to date no case has arisen in which the Slovak courts would have to make a decision in such an issue, the Slovak government in its official statement already accepted such an interpretation. Based on the

---

[4] Zákon o zdravotnej starostlivosti č.277/1994 Z.z. z 24. augusta 1994 *(The Health Care Law No. 277/1994 Coll.)*.

[5] Ibid: §42: Requirements for the medical tests without therapeutical purposes.

initiative of the Christian-Democratic Minister of Education the government was presented in November 2003, with a proposal for the official statement of the Slovak Republic for the negotiations in the Council of the European Union for Competitiveness.[6] The goal was to prepare an official Slovak position on the question of whether the European Union should financially support research on hESC within its Sixth Framework programme (FP6). During its session on 19 November 2003, the Slovak government approved the proposal stating that the Slovak Republic disagrees with the EU proposal to fund research on hESC, including the procurement of stem cells from human embryos and from the so-called surplus embryos, because this research contravenes the current Slovak legislation.

In the substantiation, it was stated that, despite to the fact that the Slovak Republic 'does not have in its judicial system any specific provisions, which would explicitly regulate the matter of biomedical research, including the procurement and use of stem cells from human embryos created as a result of medically assisted *in vitro* fertilisation (so called surplus embryos)', there is a suggestion that Slovak Regulation can 'adequately apply at least the provisions of the *Convention of the Council of Europe on Human Rights and Biomedicine* (Oviedo 1997) respectively the provision of §42 Article 3 let. c) Of the Act No. 277/1994 Coll. on health care'.[7]

The substantiation is very obscure. First, the *Convention on Human Rights and Biomedicine* does not ban research on hESC procured from surplus IVF embryos: it bans the *creation* of embryos for research purposes only. Second, the Health Care Law No. 277/1994, which was in

---

[6] *Stanovisko Slovenskej republiky k riešeniu bioetických problémov výskumu na kmeňových bunkách získavaných z ľudských embryí, Úrad vlády SR č. UV-10470/2003 (The Official Statement of the Goverment of Slovak Republic on funding research involving procurement hESC. Government Office of The Slovak Republic).* Documents in Slovak available at: http://www.rokovania.sk/appl/material.nsf/0/7E65C05F68BD595BC1256DE20041BD59?OpenDocument [Accessed 11 Jun 2009].

[7] *Stanovisko Slovenskej republiky a Zdôvodnenie návrhu stanoviska (The Official Statement of the Goverment of Slovak Republic and Substantiation of the Statement proposal).* Document in Slovak available at: http://www.rokovania.sk/appl/material.nsf/0/21EA251E3EBB89E1C1256DE2004204F2/$FILE/Zdroj.html [Accessed 11 Jun 2009].

force at that time, did not formulate a prohibition of research on surplus embryos either.

The restrictive positions of the Slovak Republic within the international organisations, like the UN and the EU, were thereafter based on this official statement of the Slovak government. The Slovak Republic requested a universal ban on European funding of research on hESC within the Sixth and the Seventh Framework Programme (FP6 and FP7), and together with Austria, Lithuania, Malta and Poland, voted against hESC research during the European Council decision.[8] Slovakia also signed the 'Declaration of Ethics' prepared by Italian Prime Minister Berlusconi, together with Austria, Germany, Malta, Poland and Italy, in November 2005, which called on the European institutions to exclude hESC research from financing under FP7.[9]

Biomedical research on embryos is explicitly banned also by the new Slovak *Penal Code* No. 300/2005 effective since 1 January 2006.[10] In accordance with the code's section dealing with unauthorised experimentation on humans and cloning of human beings, anyone who performs an experiment with the aim of 'obtaining new medical knowledge, elaboration of new methods or confirmation of a previously formulated hypothesis', for clinical investigation of drugs without authorisation, 'or performs such experiments on a human foetus or embryo' will be punished with imprisonment for one to five years. The sentence can increase up to 12 years, if the perpetrator has made a 'benefit', although the term benefit has not been defined in detail.[11]

In fact, the law says nothing explicitly about hESC research, or about specific aspects of the hESC research. It seems that the main aim of the

---

[8] European Communities. 2007. *European Group on Ethics in Science and New Technologies to the European Commission. Opinion No. 22: Recommendations on the ethical review on hESC FP7 research projects*: 32.

[9] European Communities. CORDIS. 2006. Italy Withdraws from Ethical Declaration on Embryonic Stem Cell Research. *Cordis News* 2 Jun. Available at: http://cordis.europa.eu/fetch?CALLER=EN_NEWS&ACTION=D&SESSION=&RCN=25751 [Accessed 15 Jun 2009].

[10] *Slovak Penal Code, Law No. 300/2005* from 20 May 2005 in Zbierka zákonov č.300/2005, čiastka 129.

[11] Ibid: 3031, §161, Par. 1–3.

law submitter was to protect human embryos from the moment of conception. Therefore the ban on procurement of hESC would follow from the law, as far as obtaining hESC would lead to the destruction of human embryos. However, the law obviously does not cover the hESC research on hESC lines created before the law, or on hESC lines imported to Slovakia from abroad. Since at the present there is general concern about the possible free interpretation of these legislatively undefined biomedical terms by Slovak courts, Slovak scientists are afraid they might break the law, and therefore refrain from performing any hESC research.

Ban on Therapeutic Cloning

One of the research programmes within the hESC field is creation of new blastocysts using somatic cell nuclear transfer (SCNT), often referred to in press as 'therapeutic cloning'. Human cloning is prohibited in Slovakia by the *Penal Code* in a similar way as embryo research: by the use of generic terms. The *Penal Code* makes no distinction between reproductive and therapeutic cloning; it basically prohibits the cloning of human beings in whichever stage of their ontogeny:

> '[A]ny intervention aiming to create a human being *at any stage of its formation*, which is genetically identical to another human being whether living or dead'.[12]

Punishment for the violation of this law would include imprisonment for three to eight years; but since the destruction of a blastocyst can be considered the infliction of an actual grievous bodily harm or induction of death, the punishment can be increased to imprisonment for eight to 15 years.

The wording of the ban is ostensibly very similar to the text of the *Additional Protocol on the Prohibition of Cloning of Human Beings* (Paris, 1998) to the *Convention on Human Rights and Biomedicine*, which Slovakia signed and ratified, except that words 'at any stage of its

[12] Ibid: 3031, §161, Par. 2 (italics added).

formation' have been inserted into the Slovak Penal Code text. This fact is often used as an argument for prohibition of cloning — namely that the Slovak *Penal Code* only confirms what Slovakia already committed itself to on an international level. Once again we need to look at the way the Slovak bioethical legislation is created — via 'slight' modifications of already accepted texts, which remain unnoticed by parliament.

In the substantiation of the Penal Code, it is stated that:

> '[A] state has the duty to protect apart from the security of its citizens and its own national security also the security of the civilisation which it is part of. To the fundamental elements of our civilisation belong also the protection of human dignity and protection of the family'.[13]

According to the proponent, which was at that time a Christian-Democratic minister of justice, 'cloning of humans is experimentation with human life, which does not have an own father nor mother and is as such in contrary to the principles of our civilisation'.[14] And therefore it has to be classified as a penal offence.

The law does not make a distinction between reproductive and therapeutic cloning, but in the substantiation to the law, it is explicitly stated that the term cloning includes both reproductive and therapeutic cloning. Interestingly enough, during the legal review process, only the *Ministry for Regional Development and Construction* was against the inclusion of therapeutic cloning into the ban, but it later withdrew its objections. During the debate about this law, there was not a single voice pointing to possible criminalisation of scientific research in Slovakia.

In the same period of time as the final preparations of this new Penal Code were taking place, Slovakia supported Costa Rica´s proposal on the universal ban on human cloning at the UN. It is of note that this proposal

---

[13] *Dôvodová správa k Vládnemu návrhu zákona, ktorým sa mení a dopľňa zákon č. 140/1961 Zb. Parlamentná tlač č.151, 7 JAN 2003 (The Substantiation Report to the new Penal Code Proposal*). Available at: http://www.nrsr.sk/appbin/NRCPT.ASP?WCI=NRCPT_Workitem&WCE=Master=551&WCU=VO=3|HPO_List=-1 [Accessed 11 June 2009].

[14] Ibid.

did not distinguish between reproductive and therapeutic cloning. In contrast, the Czech Republic supported the alternative Belgian proposal, which banned reproductive cloning, but proposed to leave the decision about therapeutic cloning to domestic legislation.[15]

Extraterritorial Application of Penalty Code

Of special concern is that the new Penal Code also bans international scientific cooperation on human embryo research. The law introduced a new principle to the Slovak legal system, one with which the Slovak legislation was until then unfamiliar — the element of exterritorial application of a criminal law. This means that each Slovak citizen or each foreigner with permanent residence within the territory of Slovakia can be prosecuted for the violation of the above described paragraphs, even on the territory of another state, where such actions are not considered illegal.

According to a legislative analysis requested by the *Cancer Research Institute* of the *Slovak Academy of Sciences*, based on this principle, the Penal Code bans the international collaboration of Slovak scientists in the research field of embryonic and hESC research.[16] If, for example, a Slovak scientist moves within the scope of international collaboration to perform research leading to procurement of hESC from surplus embryos to the neighbouring Czech Republic, with which the Slovak scientific community has traditional and long lasting close connections and where such research is legal, when the scientist returns to Slovakia, he or she could be prosecuted for it.

---

[15] S. Mayor. United Nations Fails to Agree on Human Cloning. *British Medical Journal* 2004; 329 (7473): 996; Fifty-Ninth General Assembly Plenary, 82nd Meeting (AM). 2005. *Press Release GA/10333: General Assembly Adopts United Nations Declaration on Human Cloning by Vote of 84-34-37*. 8 Mar. Available at: http://www.un.org/News/Press/docs/2005/ga10333.doc.htm [Accessed 11 Jun 2009]; Peter Sýkora. Dilema terapeutického klonovania v OSN (Dilema of a Therapeutical Cloning in the UN). *Domino fórum* 2004; 13: 15 (In Slovak).

[16] V. Jancura. 2007. Slovenským vedcom hrozí za výskum trest (Slovak Scientists Face a Sentence for Doing Research). *Pravda* 22 May: 3 (In Slovak).

A particularly troublesome fact is that there was virtually no discussion about this new legislation which introduced the ban on hESC research in Slovakia. Both bioethically relevant sections of the new laws remain completely overshadowed by other, seemingly more important, topics brought by these laws. In the case of the *Health Care Law*, the debate was dominated by health care service privatisation; and in the case of the Penal Code, the discussion focused on the new principle of 'Three Strikes And You're Out' in criminal proceedings in the Slovak legal system.[17]

Situation in the Czech Republic

Characteristics

Research on hESC is explicitly allowed in the Czech Republic as is stipulated by a special law passed in 2006. According to this law, hESC can be procured from surplus embryos derived from assisted reproduction clinics, but it is illegal to create new embryos for this purpose. It is permitted to import and export hESC lines, but it is prohibited to do so with embryos.

The particular law regarding hESC was passed in April 2006 and it entered into force on 1 June 2006.[18] The passage of this bill was also used by the Czech Republic as a chance to update bioethical legislation related to embryo research. With this law, the Czech Republic concurrently amended numerous other legislative acts which complemented the new

---

[17] After three convictions, a manditory life sentence is handed down. Among more then 100 articles on new Penal Code proposal there is no a single one on bioethical aspects. Cf. K. Boďová. *Rekodifikácia tresného práva (k tlač 656, 720), Výberová rešerš z knižničného systému Tinlib, Kancelária Národnej rady Slovenskej Republiky, Parlamentná knižnica, Bratislava, október 2004 a máj 2005 (Recodification of the Penalty Code. Bibliographic search from Tinlib database. Library of the Slovak Parliament*, Oct 2004 and May 2005).

[18] *Zákon o výzkumu na lidských embryonálních kmenových buňkách a souvisejících činnostech a o změně některých souvisejících zákonů, Datum přijetí: 26. dubna 2006, Datum účinnosti od: 1. června 2006 (Act Nr. 227/2006 Coll. on Research on Human Embryonic Stem Cells and Related Activities and on Amendment to Some Related Acts from 26 April 2006, effective from 1 Jun 2006*) Částka: 75/2006 Sb., pp. 2850–2861.

law on hESC research. For example, assisted reproduction was also addressed in a law.

The goal of the new Act was to set up the conditions for research on hESC (the law does not refer to embryo research *per se*). In its first sections, the Act introduces important definitions of the basic terms, explaining, for example, what are embryonic stem cells and their lines, what their research is, what is a human embryo and a surplus embryo. The definitions make a distinction between human embryos *in vitro* and *in vivo*. While the human embryo is defined in general as a 'totipotential cell or their groupings that is able to develop into a human individual' (§2, d), hESCs are defined as pluripotential cells descended from human pre-implantation embryos created *in vitro*: 'all the pluripotential stem cells that are descended from human pre-implantation embryos created outside a human body'(§2, b).

The conditions for research on hESC are specified as follows (§3):

(1) Research on hESC may be conducted only on the basis of a permission issued by the *Ministry of Education, Youth and Sport*. This research may be conducted only at workplaces with the permission for hESC research.
(2) Research on hESC may be conducted only:
    a) on imported hESC lines, that were imported based on a permission from the Ministry and only for research purposes under this Law; or
    b) on hESC lines derived from surplus human embryos from the Czech medical institutions that perform assisted reproduction in their accredited centres.
(3) Manipulations with hESC must not lead to creation of a new human individual (reproductive cloning).
(4) Both hESC lines and human embryos intended for the procurement of hESC must be protected against theft or unauthorised use.

The law also defines specific conditions under which the procurement of hESC for research purposes is permitted (§8). The surplus embryos to be used must not be older than seven days, they must be provided by centres of assisted reproduction, and the woman and man, from whom the surplus embryos are obtained, must give their informed and written consent for research use. The conditions for such written consent are defined in this law in §9. There will be no reward paid to the donors of the surplus embryo (§9, 5), but all 'costs associated with acquiring the consent to use surplus embryos for obtaining hESC' shall be reimbursed to the centre for assisted reproduction by the legal entity authorised to conduct research (§9, 6).

The law underlines, that hESC for research purposes may only be imported into the Czech Republic in the form of cell lines and that such import of lines shall be subject to the approval by the *Ministry of Education, Youth and Sport* (§10). Export from the Czech Republic may be performed only with a valid permission, and only lines registered in the territory of the Czech Republic may be exported purely for the purpose of additional research (§11). The export of embryos is explicitly prohibited (§11,7).

The law defines the conditions for the acquisition of a licence for research (e.g. scientific level of research has to be guaranteed, impossibility to achieve the scientific results by a different method, scientific project is ethically admissible), export and import of hESC lines, registration of hESC lines and their competence (§13), and control over the compliance with this law (§14).

Non-compliance with this law is classified as an administrative offence. A fine up to CZK 20.000 (cca 750 EUR) may be imposed for an offence in the case of an individual, while in the case of an institution, the fine may be anywhere from 500.000 up to two million Kč (19.000–75.000 EUR). The *Ministry of Education, Youth and Sport* is authorised to issue the permissions, to carry out inspections, and to control or impose fines in accordance with this law.

The new law on hESC research demanded important additional changes in other Czech laws — new amendments to the *Penal Code*, the *Law on Public Health*, and the *Law on Research and Development Support from Public Funds* and to the *Family Law*. Above all, the Czech *Penal Code* from 1961 (the *Czech Penal Code* No. 140/1961 Coll.) was revised by inserting paragraph §209b, which prohibits the manipulation of human embryos leading to reproductive cloning as well as modification of the human genome. There is also a ban on the creation of hybrid human-animal embryos. The violation of this law is punishable by imprisonment of one to three years, or by a ban on professional activity, or by a financial penalty. The punishment is increased in the case of repeated violation or if the offence is committed in the setting of organised crime or for financial profit. In the case that the perpetrator has made a major financial gain or if the offence has international interconnection, the punishment can be imprisonment for up to eight years or the forfeiture of property or both.

Important to notice is that the new amendment of the *Health Law* from 1966 (*Health Law* Nr. 20/1966 Coll.) added a new extensive text of the paragraph §27 d–h, which regulates the conditions for assisted reproduction, and that were not covered by existing law. According to this law, centres of assisted reproduction, which can provide surplus embryos, need to have the accreditation from the *Ministry of Health* of the Czech Republic. Another change in law was the amendment of the 2002 *Law on Research Support* (Nr. 130/2002 Coll. about Research and Development Support from Public Funds) which created a new specialised body — the *Bioethics Committee* — to advise the *Research and Development Council* of the government by examining ethical dimension of licence applications for hESC research (in §35 new Articles 7 and 8.). As of today, the *Bioethics Committee* has granted permission to perform research on hESC to two Czech institutions: the *Institute of Experimental Medicine* in Prague and the *Department of Biology* at the Faculty of Medicine of the Masaryk University and has declined one application.[19]

The debate during 2005–2006 in the Czech parliament[20] regarding the hESC research law proposal, which was submitted by the Social-Democratic *Minister of Education,* focussed on the fact that the Czech Republic ranks as a world leader in hESC research, and that without the

---

[19] *Records from Sessions of the Bioethics Committee of the Council for Research and Development* from 22 Feb 2007 and 12 Jun 2007 (in Czech). Available at: http://www.vyzkum.cz/FrontClanek.aspx?idsekce=31893 [Accessed 11 Jun 2009].

[20] See the history of *Act Nr. 227/2006 Coll. on Research on Human Embryonic Stem Cells Proposal in the Czech Parliament*. Available at: http://www.psp.cz/sqw/historie.sqw?T=1071&O=4 [Accessed 24 Jun 2009].

approval of such legislation, the continuation of their excelling reputation in this research field would end. A major argument used by the proponents was the fact that the *Academy of Sciences of the Czech Republic* (ASCR), which enjoys significant prestige in the country, officially declared support for hESC research.

On the other hand, Christian-Democratic MPs expressed disapproval of this law in Parliament. The Vice-Chairman of the lower House of Parliament criticised the efforts of scientists to use human embryos as research material. He was alluding to the warning voices of European philosophers, and who did not share the optimism of the scientific public regarding such research. Another Christian-Democratic MP criticised the fact that this confirmed that utilitarian ethics prevails in Czech society to the detriment and continued disregard, of the fundamental status of the embryo. Other critics referred to a petition organised by the Pro-Life organisation 'Hnutí pro život České republiky'[21] (Pro-Life movement of the Czech Republic), and to a letter of some Czech scientists, who requested to impose a moratorium on hESC research.[22]

In reaction to objections from Christian-Democrats, the *Minister of Education* argued that surplus embryos intended to be used in hESC research would be destroyed anyway, so why not use them in a meaningful and positive way? But it is obvious that Czech Christian-Democrats interpreted the discussion on hESC research as an extension of the debate about abortions. They criticised the uncontrolled (unlimited) freedom of research and utilitarian ethics in society, which focuses mostly on benefits. The act was finally passed at the end of April 2006 with 115 legislators voting for its adoption and 30 representatives voting against it.[23]

---

[21] http://www.prolife.cz/?a=24&id=24 [Accessed 19 June 2009].

[22] The letter is mentioned by Tomáš Kvapil MP during a parliamentary debate on hESC research act proposal. See Stenoprotokol, 48. schůze, čtvrtek 27. října 2005, Digitální parlamentní knihovna (The Shorthand record from the 48th session of the Czech Parliament, 27 Oct 2005). Available in Czech at: http://www.snemovna.cz/eknih/2002ps/stenprot/048schuz/s048359.htm [Accessed 19 June 2009].

[23] 55. schůze, 218. hlasování, 26. 4. 2006, 10:57 Vl.n.z. o výzkumu na lidských embryon. kmen.buňk (55th Session of the Czech Parliament, voting No. 218, 26 Apr 2006). Available at: http://www.psp.cz/sqw/hlasy.sqw?G=43620 [Accessed 24 Jun 2009].

SEARCHING FOR REASONS

Catholic Slovakia versus an Atheistic Czech Republic?

Where should one look for reasons to explain the diametrically different positions on hESC research found in the Czech Republic and Slovakia? The first answer that comes to mind is the different status of religion to be found in these two countries. The Czech Republic is one of the most atheistic states in Europe. In the 2001 population census as much as 59% of the Czech population claimed to be atheist. In the same year in a census carried out in Slovakia, only 13% of the Slovak citizens considered themselves to be atheists, and almost 70% of the population claimed to be Roman Catholic.[24] Does this indicate that the hESC research ban in Slovakia is a consequence of the size of the Roman Catholic denomination in the country, as is the case in Ireland or in neighbouring Poland? Slovakia is often considered to address bioethical issues in a very similar manner to these two countries — both are countries with dominant Roman Catholic Church influences — because Slovakia voted with them against the funding of hESC research in the EU. On the other hand, it may be easy to explain a pro-research hESC biopolicy in the Czech Republic simply as a consequence of the country's dominant atheism.

The Eurobarometer survey on biotechnology in 2005 (approximately 1000 respondents in each EU Member State) included a number of questions that directly examined the opinions of EU citizens on stem cell research.[25] This survey revealed that in terms of their familiarity with hESC research, the citizens of Slovakia and the Czech Republic are equally proportionate to EU countries with the lowest degree of public awareness (together with the new Baltic Member States and Greece).

There is a difference, however, in the level of public support for embryonic stem cell research between the Slovak and Czech populations. Having 65% of its questioned population approving of hESC research, the

---

[24] A. Kvasničková. 2005. *Náboženstvo ako kolektívna pamäť: prípad Slovenska a Čiech (Religion as a Collective Memory: The Case of Slovakia and Czechia).* Bratislava: Comenius University: 23 (in Slovak).

[25] G. Gaskell *et al.* 2006. *Europeans and Biotechnology in 2005: Patterns and Trends. Final Report on Eurobarometer 64.3.*

Czech Republic thus ranks amongst those EU countries with the highest level of research support, and which comprises of one third of all member states, and is close to Italy with 66%. Belgium and Sweden rate highest with 73% and 72%, respectively, whereas Estonia and Slovenia are at the bottom with 32% and 31%, respectively. Slovakia on the other hand, with 54%, ranks somewhere in the middle. Together with Germany and Cyprus, Slovakia ranks below the UK with 62%, but above both Poland with 47% and Austria with 45%.[26]

Do these differences reflect people's view on the ontological and ethical status of early human embryo? As many as 60% of all Slovakian participants agreed with the statement that 'Immediately after fertilisation the embryo can already be considered to be a human being'. This level is the same as that of Belgium. In the Czech Republic, 11% less of those surveyed agreed with the above statement (see Table1). Furthermore, 17% more Czechs than Slovaks did not consider the early human embryo to be a human being. These results correlate well with the 11% higher support for hESC research among Czechs than Slovaks and with the 14% higher disapproval rate of hESC research among Slovaks (see Table1).[27] Surprisingly though, there is only a 5% difference between those who agreed with the statement in the Czech Republic and in Poland, although according to the Polish Constitutional Court, the Polish Constitution protects the human being from conception and consequently abortion is illegal in Poland. Therefore it is important to take a country's position on abortion into consideration.

The differences between the views of Czechs and Slovaks on abortion seem to be similar to the differences in the Eurobarometer polls on embryonic stem cells. Results of public opinion polls on abortion in both countries have been quite similar for many years, regardless of important differences of religion.

There were very small differences in public opinion on abortion between Czechs and Slovaks in the common state. Based on surveys conducted in Czechoslovakia in 1991, 61% of the country's population was

[26] Ibid: 32 (Figure 14).

[27] Ibid: 32–34 (calculation based on Figures 14 and 15).

Table 1: Opinions on Stem Cell Research, Ontological Status of Human Embryo and Abortion in Czech Republik, Slovakia and Poland

Country	Approve hESC Research with Usual Government Regulation or if More Tightly Regulated (%)	Do Not Approve hESC Research Under Any Circumstances or Except Under Very Special Circumstances (%)	Totally Agree or Tend to Agree with the Statement that Immediately after Fertilisation the Embryo can Already be Considered to be a Human Being (%)	Totally Disagree or Tend to Disagree with the Statement that Immediately after Fertilisation the Embryo can Already be Considered to be a Human Being (%)	In Support of a Liberal, Pro-choice Abortion Law in 2007 (%)
Czech Rep.	65	22	49	43	72
Slovakia	54	36	60	26	58
Poland	47	26	54	25	23

Source: Adapted data from Eurobarometer 64.3 and the country opinion polls.[28]

[28] See notes 25–33.

in the favour of unrestricted abortion and only 4% of the citizens were requesting its complete ban. Results from 1991 also showed that differences between Czechs and Slovaks were minimal: 63% of Czechs and 56% of Slovaks were in favour of abortions (7% difference). And as subsequent polls demonstrated this percentage has not changed significantly in following years.[29]

We can compare this opinion poll data with those from Poland, where only 22% of Polish citizens were in support of unrestricted access to abortion.[30] Polls conducted in separate states after splitting of Czechoslovakia confirmed that close similarities in public opinion on abortion remained between the Czech and Slovak Republics.

The recent results of opinion polls from 2007 and 2008 have shown that a higher percentage of respondents, 72% and 75% respectively, in the Czech Republic are in the favour of an unrestricted access to abortion, as compared to 63% in 1995.[31] In similar respects, 58% of respondents in the Slovak Republic considered the existing liberal abortion law (which is same as in the Czech Republic) to be either adequate or even too authoritarian, and only 16% of respondents answered that it is 'too lenient' in the

---

[29] S.L. Wolchik. 2000. Reproductive Policies in the Czech and Slovak Republics. In *Reproducing Gender*. S. Gal and G. Kligman, eds. Princeton, NJ: Princeton University Press: 58–91.

[30] In Poland 15%–26% for free access to abortions and 9%–17% for absolute ban of abortions in 1991–1998 according to the CBOS Polling Center Surveys, Warsaw. E. Zielinska. 2000. Between Ideology, Politics, and Common Sense: The Discourse of Reproductive Rights in Poland. In *Reproducing Gender*. S. Gal and G. Kligman, eds. Princeton, NJ: Princeton University Press: 40; see also: D. Duch. 2000. *Ustawa antyaborcyjna w Polsce, Funkcjonowanie, skutki spoleczne, postawy i zachowania Raport — Wrzesien 2000.* Available at: http://www.federa.org.pl/publikacje/raporty/aborcja2000/aborcja2000_6.htm#top [Accessed 28 Feb 2009].

[31] M. Škodová. 2009. Public Opinion about Foeticide and Euthanasia. Press Release. *Public Opinion Research Centre of the Institute of Sociology of the Academy of Sciences of the Czech Republic.* 1 Jun. http://www.cvvm.cas.cz/index.php?disp=zpravy&lang=1&r=1&s=&offset=&shw=100924 [Accessed 16 Jun 2009] Full text with graphs is available in Czech only at: http://www.cvvm.cas.cz/upl/zpravy/100924s_ov90601.pdf [Accessed 16 Jun 2009]; Poll: Czechs more tolerant of abortion than euthanasia. *Prague Monitor Daily* 2 Jun 2009. Available at: http://praguemonitor.com/2009/06/02/poll-czechs-more-tolerant-abortion-euthanasia [Accessed 16 Jun 2009].

opinion poll carried out by the Institute for Public Affairs of Bratislava in 2007. It is noticeable how these figures resemble those from the 2003 opinion poll.[32] Again for comparison, only 23% Poles were for unrestricted, pro-choice, access to abortion in the 2007 opinion poll.[33]

In contrast to the Czech Republic, the passing of restrictive hESC research legislation in Slovakia took place in the shadow of the final stage of the six-year-long decision-making process at the Constitutional Court concerning the compliance of the Abortion Law with the Slovak Constitution. In spite of the fact that the Czech Republic inherited the same Abortion Law as Slovakia from Czechoslovakia, and the Czech Constitution also adopted the same text about protection of life from the Czechoslovak Constitution, Christian-Democrats in the Czech Republic, as well as Pro-Life activists, have not referred the abortion issue to the Constitutional Court as they did it in Slovakia.

Both Slovakia and the Czech Republic belong to a group of countries with liberal abortion legislation. Slovak, as well as Czech law, inherited from Czechoslovakia a law that allows abortions to be performed upon a woman's demand up to the 12th week of her pregnancy. Abortions in Czechoslovakia started to be regulated by the Abortion Law from 1957 (Act Nr. 68/1957 Coll.) and later by a more liberal Abortion law from 1986.

After the formation of an independent Slovakia, Christian-Democratic representatives tried to use the revision of the Slovak Constitution in 2001 as an opportunity to change the Slovak Constitution in a way that it would prohibit abortions explicitly. They intended to replace the original text of the Constitution (a whole section about human rights originally inherited from the 1991 post-Communist amendments to Czechoslovak

---

[32] In 2003 only for 11% of respondents the Slovak liberal abortion law was 'too lenient', for 49% was 'just fine' and for 23% was even 'too strict'. For the 2003 and 2007 survey data see: Z. Bútorová. 2008. *She and He in Slovakia. Gender and Age in the Period of Transition*. Bratislava: Institute for Public Affairs: 62–63.

[33] For more data on the opinions about abortion in Poland during the years 1999, 2002, 2005, 2006 and 2007, see: Public Opinion Research Center (CBOS). 2007. Opinions About Abortions. *Polish Public Opinion*, Oct: 2–3. Available at: http://www.cbos.pl/EN/publications/public_opinion_2007.php [Accessed 16 Jun 2009].

constitution) according to which human life is 'worthy of protection already before birth' (Section 15, Article 1, second clause)[34] with a new formulation, according to which 'human life has the right to be protected since [sic.] conception'. This would virtually mean a ban on induced abortions. However, a great majority of Slovak MPs rejected this proposal.

Then Christian Democrats turned their strategy upside down — they claimed that a change of constitution is not necessary because even according to existing constitution abortion is not allowed. In 2001, The Constitutional Court accepted the proposal of 31 members of Slovak Parliament led by a Christian Democrat MP (who later became a Minister of Justice and a proposer of the new Penalty Code analysed above) that the abortion law is not in accordance with the Slovak Constitution.

The Christian Pro-Life movements in Slovakia grew more active and strong following the six years it took the Constitutional Court to make a decision, and abortion became a topic of heated debates in media. An umbrella-organisation *Forum of Life* (Fórum života) was created by 14 non-governmental organisations in 2001. It was based on a previous pro-life initiative: the so called 'Declaration of the Rights of the Conceived Child'. The Declaration is founded on the statement that each human being has the right for legal protection from the moment of its conception. The Declaration was supported by the influential Bioethics Committee of the Slovak Roman Catholic Bishops as well as by numerous politicians.

As far as hESC research is concerned, the position of the *Forum of Life* is in accordance with the general Pro-Life philosophy:

> '[T]hese experiments downgrade the conceived human being to material for different trials and procedures. Such manipulation is in conflict with the value of the human life, with the personal dignity of the human being, with its integrity and identity, and therefore we disapprove it'.

It is interesting, that not all advanced interventions are rejected. Genetic interventions, which would, for example, repair defective genes with the

---

[34] 'Everyone has the right to life. Human life is worth protection even before birth'. *Constitution of the Slovak Republic*, Art. 15, par. 1. English version available at: http://www.concourt.sk/en.do [Accessed 16 Jun 2009].

aim to treat handicapped individuals, are acceptable. It is not clear whether this covers only somatic genetic changes or if it includes also germ line modifications.[35] However, interventions that lead to the destruction of an existing human individual, in their view, an embryo from the moment of its conception, as it is the case of the hESC procurement, are of course unacceptable.

The next, mostly symbolic political event was the adoption of the *Declaration on Sovereignty of EU Member States in Cultural and Ethnical Issues* by the Slovak Parliament in 2002. The Declaration was once again an initiative of the Christian-Democratic MPs.[36] It demanded that decisions in the EU about cultural and ethical questions concerning:

> 'the protection of life and the dignity of the human being from the conception to the death, protection of the family and the institution of the marriage as the basic stone of the society, as well as decisions about matters related to these in the field of health care, upbringing and education'.

And therefore, such decisions would remain within the competency and sovereignty of the Member States. The document reflects concerns that some politicians had about the EU membership of Slovakia. These concerns were, firstly, the result of poor knowledge of European legislation which already respects national legislation and tradition in cultural and ethical issues. Secondly, they were a result of disproportionate fears about the Western liberalism arriving from Brussels to Slovakia and destroying traditional conservative values.[37] In spite of the fact that *the Declaration* was addressed to the European Parliament, its message was meant to reach a domestic audience. *The Declaration* has no legally binding

---

[35] *Genetická manipulácia, klonovanie a kmeňové bunky (Genetic Manipulations, Cloning and Stem Cells).* Available at: http://www.forumzivota.sk/geneticka-manipulacia [Accessed 16 Jun 2009].

[36] http://www.kdh.sk/article.php?dokumenty::zvrchovanost [Accessed 16 Jun 2009]; http://www.kdh.sk/article.php?dokumenty::zvrchovanost-dovodova-sprava [Accessed 16 Jun 2009].

[37] P. Sýkora. 2002. Vykročenie k teokratickému štátu 1. a 2. časť' (Towards a theocratic state, part 1 and 2). *SME* 6 and 7 Feb.

implications, has been mostly ignored by the public, and did not have any direct impact on a later discourse on bioethical issues.

An anti-abortion campaign culminated in 2007, just before the decision of the Constitutional Court on abortions was expected to come. Until that moment, an unknown pro-life organisation *European Centre for Bioethical Reform* started a provocative billboard campaign with the title 'Right for Life'. The organisation posted 500 large and colourful billboards around Slovakia showing a photograph of the torn apart body of a human embryo after an abortion. A large majority of Slovak society deplored the campaign as aggressive and unethical; and many Christians refused it as contra-productive in pro-life issues. Finally, the statutory body responsible for the supervision of ethics in advertising decided to cancel it. The campaign continued with a second, more moderate version in 2008 with the title 'Stop Genocide' (the Slovak version of the originally American *Genocide Awareness Project*), where the billboards compared abortions with mass graves from Nazi concentration camps, and from Cambodia, Rwanda, and Yugoslavia.

By the end of 2007, after six years of decision-making, the Constitutional Court finally decided that the effective Abortion Law was not in contradiction with the Slovak Constitution (nine judges were in favour of this decision, five judges voted against and added differing statements of disapproval). The Constitutional Court underlined in its substantiation, that the Slovak constitution distinguishes between everyone's right to life (the Slovak Constitution, Art. 15, first clause) and the protection of unborn life (the Slovak Constitution, Art. 15, second clause), and it rejected the creation of a new subject of law: i.e. the embryo and foetus, in addition to the already existing legal entities — the natural person and legal person. It also underlined that:

> '[F]rom the constitutional imperative, which establishes the legislator's duty to protect human life before birth, does not arise the conclusion that the legal protection of the foetus to mother should be the same in each stage of its prenatal development'.[38]

---

[38] *Constitutional Court of the Slovak Republic. PL. ÚS 12/01 from 4 December, odst.21.* Available at: http://www.concourt.sk [Accessed 16 Jun 2009] .

Different Status of Science in the Czech and Slovak Republic

A more detailed analysis of the Czech and Slovak situation exposes three important differences that can be considered closely, and which are related to the differing roles played by the scientific communities in the process of hESC research legislation approval: the existence of a scientific group lobbying to promote the research and use of hESC, overall national support for science and research; and the status of science within society in general. It would appear that the divergence in hESC biopolicies was, in fact, not determined by the different religiosity of the Czech and Slovak populations, but, more likely, due to the role that the scientific community played within the legislative process concerning hESC. While the scientific community in Slovakia remained passive and left the formulation of the bioethical legislation to the politicians, Czech scientists actively participated in the legislative process from its beginning, while being at the same time involved in the promotion of the scientific view on hESC research among politicians and the public.

The Supporting Statement of the Czech Republic Academy of Sciences of the Czech Republic

The Academy of Sciences of the Czech Republic (ASCR) was established in 1992 as the Czech successor of the former Czechoslovak Academy of Sciences. Today, the ASCR is a complex of 54 public research institutions, and employs over 3500 researchers.[39] The ASCR enjoys immense prestige within Czech society as the cutting-edge national scientific institution. As such, the release of an official supporting statement concerning hESC research by this highly respected institution in February 2005 played an important role in the legislative process.

According to the official ASCR statement, the support of research on all cell types including the ‘hESC derived from human blastocysts’ is essential. Furthermore, the statement underlines the equally important

---

[39] http://www.cas.cz/en/information.php [Accessed 11 Jun 2009].

necessity to create a legislative framework for hESC research. Two restrictions on research were proposed:

(1) The procurement of hESC must be performed exclusively on surplus human blastocysts which will not be further used for fertility treatment and with the informed consent of the donors.
(2) Research regulations must be a result of the consensus between scientists, physicians, ethicists and lawyers.[40]

In contrast to the specifications outlined above, the Slovak Academy of Sciences (SAS,)[41] which is a national research institution similar to the ASCR, completely ignored the issue of hESC research. Not only did the SAS not release any official statement, the whole problem of hESC research and ethics was not discussed in the Slovak scientific community. The process that culminated in the restrictive legislation in Slovakia took place without input from the scientific community, and without public discourse.

The Impact of Pro-Research Lobbying on hESC Biopolitics

The Czech Republic had an influential group of scientists supporting hESC research connected to non-governmental organisations and supporting medical research. No such group existed in Slovakia. In 2000, a Czech civic association *Macropulos* was created, with the goal to support brain research.[42] However, this association reacted on the potential that regenerative medicine could offer in the future and redirected its focus to the support of hESC research and its transfer into the clinical practice in 2003. This association collaborates with physically handicapped persons within the framework of the project 'Wheelchair invalids for themselves'

[40] *Stanovisko Akademie věd České republiky k výzkumu na embryonálních kmenových buňkách získaných z lidských embryí. Přijato na 57. zasedání akademické rady Akademie věd České republiky dne 22. února 2005 (The Official Statement of the Academy of Sciences of the Czech Republic on hESCR from 22 February 2005).*

[41] http://www.sav.sk/index.php? [Accessed 11 Jun 2009].

[42] www.makropulos.cz [Accessed 11 Jun 2009].

(Vozíčkari sobě), who could actively participate in clinical trials which test experimental treatments of spinal cord injuries.

Another non-governmental organisation, 'Cell therapy' (Bunečná terapie) has actively supported hESC research since the end of 2003. The statute of this association says:

> 'The association is a voluntary, independent, non-political organisation uniting specialists and persons concerned, who are active in the promotion of hESC research and its applications in treatments of patients with the help of cell therapy and tissue replacements'.[43]

Members of this association are scientists from numerous research institutes — *the Institute of Experimental Medicine* in Prague, *Motol University Hospital* in Prague, and *the Department of Tissue Engineering at the Medical Faculty of Charles University*. The association is also linked to the commercial sphere through the *Agropol Group company*. The administrative board of the association is chaired by Prof. E. Syková from the Institute of Experimental Medicine of the ASCR in Prague.

The Institute of Experimental Medicine of the ASCR plays a key role in hESC research in the Czech Republic. It is led by Professor Eva Syková, a prominent Czech neuroscientist. The Institute is an internationally recognised cutting-edge research centre, one of the EU's Centres of Excellence. The Institute's Department of Molecular Embryology was the first laboratory in the Czech Republic to create new hESC lines from human blastocysts in 2003.[44] The research at the Institute is also dedicated to the potential use of hESC in the treatment of neurodegenerative diseases. In 2004 the Institute, together with other academic and medical workplaces, created the common institution — 'The National Research Centre for Cell Therapy and Tissue Repair' to support the practical application of basic biomedical research in potential regenerative medicine, and by the end of 2008, had opened the first business incubator in the field

[43] *Stanovy občanského sdružení 'Bunečná terapie'*. Čl.IV, Odst.1. Available at: http://www.bunecnaterapie.cz/stanovy [Accessed 11 Jun 2009].

[44] http://www.iem.cas.cz/article.asp?nArticleID=407&nLanguageID=2 [Accessed 16 Jun 2009].

of biomedicine in the Czech Republic. Guests at the official opening included the Czech Prime Minister and the chairman of ASCR. The institute communicates its research goals and achievements via the Internet to the public.[45]

In contrast, there is no equivalent research institution specialised in hESC research in Slovakia, nor are there non-governmental organisations linked with scientists' groups supporting this research. Furthermore, there is no comparable support for hESC research from government, and in fact, there is very low support for any scientific research in Slovakia in general.

Funding of Science and Research in the Slovak and Czech Republics

The extent to which science and research are funded and supported is much greater in the Czech Republic than in Slovakia. Slovakia ranks among the EU countries with the lowest support for research. In terms of the GERD indicator (percentage of GDP per capita allocated to science and research) Slovakia gives almost four times less financial resources than the Czech Republic. For example, in the year 2006, US$340 per capita was spent in the Czech Republic as compared with US$87 in Slovakia, the average of 27 EU member countries (EU27) was US$492 per capita. The situation is similar regarding the growth dynamics of science and research funding: for the years 2000–2006, the growth rate in the Czech Republic was more than three times higher than that in Slovakia (average yearly growth in the Czech Republic 11.1%, in Slovakia 3.4%, EU27 average 4.4%).[46]

In terms of GDP, Slovakia funded its scientific and research activities in 2005 with a total amount of 0.51% of its GDP, and in the following year

[45] Open science (in Czech) is the title of the web page which brings information about the Institute of Experimental Medicine to a public, see http://www.otevrena-veda.cz/ov/index.php?site=uem [Accessed 16 Jun 2009].

[46] *Mezinárodní srovnání výdajů na VaV. Český statistický úřad. (International Comparison of Gross Domestic Expenditure on Research and Development. Czech Statistical Office).* Available at: http://www.czso.cz/csu/redakce.nsf/i/mezinarodni_srovnani_vydaju_na_vav; http://www.czso.cz/eng/edicniplan.nsf/aktual/ep-9?opendocument#96 [Accessed 16 Jun 2009].

with only 0.49 % of the GDP. It ranked at the bottom of 27 EU countries, together with Bulgaria (0.45% of GDP) and Romania (0.45% of GDP). In the same year, the Czech Republic allocated three times more with respect to percentage of GDP, that is 1.54% of GDP. The Czech Republic is clearly attempting to reach the level in the R&D funding comparable with the average of the most developed countries of the EU. In the years 2000–2006, the Czech Republic's expenses for science research increased 0.33 percent points, while during the same period of time in Slovakia, they decreased funding 0.16 percent points, which represents the highest decrease amongst all the countries of the EU.

One could assume that the extraordinarily low investment in science and research in Slovakia reflects the poor economic development of the country, but the truth is just the opposite. Slovakia experienced its most successful economic growth in its history during the 2000–2006 years: starting from 1.4% GDP growth in 2000 to 8.5% in 2006. It is true that at the same time the Czech economy was generally more productive than that of Slovakia (it should be noted that the Czech part in Czechoslovakia was already economically stronger than the Slovak part). The comparison of the relative GDP values per capita in PPS compared with the average in the EU (EU27 average is 100%) shows that the GDP per capita in the Czech Republic was 13.9 percent points higher than in Slovakia (77.4% versus 63.5% in 2006). However, during this same period, the dynamics of the growth of the Slovak economy was higher: GDP per capita increased by 8.9% in the Czech Republic between 2000 and 2006, while it increased by 13.4% in Slovakia.[47] These numbers clearly reflect the long-term pro-research strategy of the Czech government.[48]

---

[47] European Communities, EUROSTAT. *Real GDP Growth Rate, Growth Rate of GDP Volume, Percentage Change on Previous Year*. Available at: http://epp.eurostat.ec.europa.eu/tgm/table.do?tab=table&init=1&plugin=1&language=en&pcode=tsieb020 [Accessed 16 Jun 2009].

[48] However, notice a recent crisis meeting of Czech scientists led by the Academy of Science to stop a government plan for drastic budget cuts in science funding for next years due to the global financial and economic crisis. See: Q. Schiermeier. 2009. Czech Researchers Angry Over Government Changes. *Nature* 460, 9 Jul: 157. There are no similar crisis meetings of Slovak scientists which would react to a long-term government underfinancing the science and universities.

Overall Perception of Science in Society

Unfortunately, there is no specific sociological research available that compares the general status of science in the Czech and Slovak societies. One can only form conjectures based on indirect factors, for example on the extent to which science is popularised in a society.

Within the Czech Republic several domestic magazines focusing on popular science are published, and most of them are of outstanding quality, having both high circulation and a significant readership. These journals are part of a long tradition of science popularisation which dates back to the second half of the 19th century, when the emancipation of Czech science was seen as an important part of the emancipation of the Czech nation itself. In 1853 the influential Czech biologist J.E. Purkyne established a journal popularising biology called *Živa (*Life*),* which is still published today. Another example is the journal *Vesmír* (Universe), which popularises all scientific fields and is also published up to the present day. Slovakia, on the other hand, does not have such tradition.

After World War II, new popular science magazines for younger generations began to be published in Czechoslovakia mostly in the Czech language, for example, the journals *VTM* (Science and Technology for Youth) and *ABC for Young Naturalists and Technicians*, both of which remain in print. Similar Slovak magazines (e.g. *Elektrón*) slowly disappeared from the market. The Czech popular science magazines survived because of their better quality, and they were read amongst the Slovak youth. In general, after the breakup of Czechoslovakia the Slovak interest in Czech magazines endured, while the Czech interest in Slovak magazines, which had always been very low, disappeared completely. The same is true for popular science magazines.

Several new popular science magazines have appeared in the Czech Republic (none in Slovakia) in recent years. For example, the new monthly '21st century' (*21.století*), which has a similar layout as the British monthly magazine *Focus* soon became the most popular science magazine.[49] In

[49] The popular science monthly '*21. století*', with its circulation about 80,000 copies, has the highest readership (about 380,000 readers) from all popular science magazines in the country. According to the Audit Bureau Circulation CZ and the survey of Mediaproject. See *Magazine 21. století* 2009: 3.

comparison to this, at present in Slovakia only one scientific magazine exists — *Quark,* and one journal specialising in the popularisation of astronomy — *Kozmos* (existing for 40 years). However, Czech magazines, including popular science magazines, are distributed widely in Slovakia and read by many Slovak readers.

What is also important is the presentation of science in national newspapers. Once a week all major Czech newspapers include a periodic specialised section focusing on science. The science supplement inserted into daily *Lidové noviny* (*LN*) may be considered to be an analogy with the well-known science section in the *New York Times*. This newspaper supplement, as well as the previously mentioned journal *21st Century*, often contains articles that promote the significant successes achieved recently by Czech scientists (e.g. article headlines like: 'Czech scientists will improve carp meat' — *LN* 22.12.2008, 'Czech found shark teeth in Antarctica' — *LN* 13.1.2009, 'Czechs discovered how cancer emerges' — *LN* 15.4.2009 and similar) and such information slowly builds up in the public an image of successful Czech science. Slovak newspapers also have science sections in their editions (e.g. daily *SME*), but these sections are usually put together from brief press news. Science related topics regularly appear also in a very popular semi-tabloid weekly *Plus Sedem dní* (Plus Seven Days).

A similar situation exists for the popularisation of science in electronic media. While Czech public service broadcasters — both television and radio — have been broadcasting for years regular programmes popularising science (e.g. the weekly programme *Meteor* on the Czech Radio 2, and the programmes *Popularis*, *Planeta věda*, *Prizma*, and *Čaj pro třetího* on Czech Public television),[50] the equivalent Slovak public radio and TV stations do not broadcast any similar programmes.

Since the year 2002, a competition called *Česká hlava* (Czech Head) exists in the Czech Republic. Its aim is to create a sort of national Nobel prize awards. Each year awards are given to the best Czech scientists and technicians in a big TV show broadcast at primetime. This project is

---

[50] V. Kratochvílová. 2006. Véda v České televizi (Science in Czech television). *Akademický bulletin*, 4/2006. Available in Czech at: http://abicko.avcr.cz/cs/2006/4/11/veda-v-ceske-televizi.html [12 Jun 2009].

overseen by a *Česká hlava* foundation with a board of distinguished Czech scientists led by the Professor Eva Syková, above mentioned director of the Institute of Experimental Medicine. In addition there is also a regular TV programme that has the same title *Česká hlava and* which focuses on the promotion of excellent Czech scientists.[51]

Similar difference can also be found between Czech and Slovak Internet portals devoted to the popularisation of science. Whether one considers the websites of the print-media with science sections mentioned above, or web portals specialised to popularise science, one will find higher quantity, as well as quality, among Czech websites as compared with Slovak ones.[52]

The Key Role of a Pro-Research Lobby

A common sense explanation of the opposite hESC biopolicies in Czech and Slovak Republics looks for the reasons in the contrasting traditionalist Catholic character of Slovakia, on the one hand, and the modernistic, liberal and atheistic character of the Czech Republic, on the other. However, the very similar liberal position of the population in both countries on abortion, as expressed in abortion legislation and opinion polls, make this explanation doubtful. Based on an atheistic-catholic scheme, one would expect Christian-Democratic politicians to be better represented in the Slovak rather than in the Czech parliament. Surprisingly, in both national parliaments Christian Democrats have been represented for a long time by almost the same proportion: around 10%.

Therefore, I suggest that we have to look somewhere else for the explanation of the differences in these two biopolicies. As is described above, there is a striking difference in the roles which science and scientists play in the society of each country. Could this difference explain the

---

[51] http://www.ceskahlava.cz/index.php?mainpager=who&csum=13550aaa [Accessed 12 May 2009]; http://www.ceskatelevize.cz/ivysilani/1185979869-ceske-hlavy/ [Accessed 12 May 2009].

[52] In Czech Republic e.g.: http://www.lidovky.cz/ln_veda.asp, http://www.osel.cz/, http://scienceworld.cz/, in Slovakia: http://www.equark.sk/index.php?cl=mainclass&iid=1.

permissive Czech hESC law compared to the very restrictive legislation in Slovakia?

It has already been demonstrated by Michael Mulkay, in his brilliant study *The Embryo Research Debate*[53] that the most important factor for the creation of the well-known liberal *Human Fertilisation and Embryology Act* (1990) in the UK was the active role played by a pro-research lobby during the human embryo legislation process in the 1980s. This is rather surprising, since science enjoys significant public support in Britain and the government is traditionally pro-research oriented. Furthermore, ethics does not seem to be a principal obstacle to the progress of science in the UK. In the words of Roger Brownsword: 'ethics tends to be a loose package of pragmatic-utilitarianism set alongside respect for privacy, consent, confidentiality and non-discrimination'.[54] Despite all of this, hESC research would have very likely been banned in Britain in the 1980s if a lobby of scientists advocating embryo research had not been formed.

In short, the British Parliament rejected the proposals of the Warnock Committee in 1984, which recommended the continuation, but formal regulation, of embryo research.[55] The majority of British MPs preferred a total prohibition of such research. This was the consequence of the activities of a well organised *anti-abortion lobby*, which was connected to many members of the Thatcher's conservative party and which had a large majority in the Parliament at that time.[56] The anti-abortion lobby introduced a proposal for the *Bill for Protection of Unborn Children*. This proposal received the support of 238 MPs of the House of Commons in its second reading, while only 66 representatives were against. The scientific and medical community was shocked by this vote and it immediately realised that it was crucial to mobilise itself, if the possibility to perform

---

[53] M. Mulkay. 1997. *The Embryo Research Debate*. Cambridge: Cambridge University Press: 17–41.

[54] R. Brownsword. 2005. Regulating Stem Cell Research in the United Kingdom: Filling in the Cultural Background. In *Crossing Borders. Cultural, Religious and Political Differences Concerning Stem Cell Research — A Global Approach*. W. Bender, Ch. Hauskeller & A. Manzei, eds. Münster: Agenda Verlag: 418.

[55] For more details, see Mulkay, *op. cit.* note 54, pp. 20–42.

[56] Ibid: 17–18, 22–24.

research on embryos were to be saved in Britain. In November 1985 a non-governmental association of scientists, physicians and representatives named *Progress* was created. The association immediately started a campaign in the House of Commons that aimed to raise support for embryo research among the representatives and the public via a media campaign. At the same time *the Medical Research Council* (MRC) together with *the Royal Society of Obstetricians and Gynecologists* created the *Voluntary Licensing Authority* (VLA), which started to issue the first licences for the research using IVF embryos, to make the public aware of the fact that this research was no longer without control. The scientific community also changed its attitude towards the Warnock Report and decided to support its main recommendations. Finally, scientists succeeded in convincing MPs to vote in favour of a permissive embryo research policy. In 1990 *Human Fertilisation and Embryology Act (*HFEA) passed in both Houses of the British Parliament with a large majority.[57]

The situation repeated itself on a smaller scale more recently when the first significant revision of the 1990 Act began in 2003.[58] After a number of high-profile court cases, it was becoming increasingly clear that the 1990 Act was becoming progressively more disconnected with scientific discoveries.[59] And moreover, the urgency for an outcome of this revision was further provoked by the requests of British scientists who demanded that the HFE Authority issue licences on the use of hybrid animal-human embryos for research in 2007.[60] This request triggered an extensive discussion in British media about whether this does not divert from the original scope and competency of the Human Fertilisation and Embryology Authority. The tabloid press started to publish pictures of human-animal monsters similar to those described in the horror movie,

---

[57] Ibid: 37–41.

[58] See Holm & Natasha Hammond-Browning, this volume.

[59] See: R. Brownsword. 2008. *Rights, Regulation, and the Technological Revolution.* Oxford: Oxford University Press: Chap. 6.

[60] 'The Christian Legal Centre Claims that the HFE Authority Acted Beyond Its Powers' in: *BBC News*. 2008. Legal Challenge to Hybrid Embryos. 9 Apr. Available at: http://news.bbc.co.uk/go/pr/fr/-/2/hi/uk_news/7337910.stm. [Accessed 12 May 2009].

The Island of Dr. Moreau, based on a story by H.G. Wells. As a reaction to the growing concerns of the public about such research the government started to prepare an amendment to the Act, which would ban the creation of hybrid embryos.

Again, the scientific community managed to mobilise itself quickly and efficiently. In a letter addressed to the newspaper *The Times* a group of 45 scientists, academics and politicians, led by three Nobel prize winners (Paul Nurse, John Sulston and Tim Hunt) opposed the government's intentions to ban research on hybrid embryos. Moreover an unprecedented letter to the government was written by *The Association of Medical Research Charities* and signed by 223 medical charities and patient organisations. The British Medical Association pronounced itself in a similar manner opposed to the ban. Under this pressure, 336 to 176 MPs voted against a proposed ban on animal-human embryo research in May 2008.[61]

Once again it was shown, at least in case of the UK, that the systematic activity of a pro-research lobby is able to reverse the attempts of the government and parliament to ban promising, although ethically controversial, scientific research. Based on this it is reasonable to suggest that in the Czech Republic the key factor in the passing of permissive hESC research legislation was the active role played by the Czech pro-research lobby in society. In contrast, no such lobby existed in Slovakia and therefore there is a restrictive hESC biopolicy in place.

CONCLUSION

After the dissolution of Czechoslovakia in 1993, and from the outset of both the Slovak and Czech Republics, each shared almost identical legislation, including health care laws. However, after ten years of independent development in the field of hESC research, their biopolicies were to find themselves diametrically opposed. It seems that the key factor responsible for the contemporary permissive hESC research legislation in the Czech

[61] UK Lawmakers back Hybrid Embryo Research. *Associated Press*. 19 May 2008. Available at: http://www.msnbc.msn.com/id/24715997 [Accessed 12 May 2009].

Republic was not the modernistic, liberal and atheistic character of this particular country, but was in fact the active role played by the pro-research lobby, together with high status of science in Czech society. Also authors of the 2005 Eurobarometer study on hESC research concluded that 'the main religious denomination of the country (which we might expect to be related to the climate of public opinion of the country) does not appear to be a decisive factor in shaping attitudes towards embryonic stem cell research'.[62]

One can only speculate about the outcome had the Czech researchers not been proactive and if the Czech Christian-Democratic politicians, supported by country's pro-life organisations, had demanded a ban on hESC research. Could the Czech Republic have ended up with a restrictive biopolicy similar to that of Slovakia?

And vice versa, it seems that the key factor responsible for the restrictive hESC biopolicy in Slovakia was not the country's traditional Catholicism, as one might expect considering Slovakia's dominant Roman Catholic denomination. Evidently the passive role of its research community, the lack of public debate on hESC research, as well as the low status of science in society and the corresponding low level of governmental support for research were all more instrumental in the prohibitive outcome. Had all these factors been more corroborative, and had the Slovak scientific community and the Slovak Academy of Sciences continually raised their voices from the very inception of the legislative process, would Slovak hESC biopolicy have been permissive?

In other words, does all this mean that in general, in the absence of a respected and influential pro-research lobby, there is no ideological opponent supportive of the pro-scientific position who could thus succeed in surmounting nascent public opposition at a national level to bioethically controversial scientific research? This situation seems to be prevalent, at least in modern European countries with Christian traditions, regardless of whether or not the society is so-called conservative or liberal unless there is no ideologically blind government (cf. hESC biopolicy in the US during Bush administration). Even in a liberal society a few conservative

---

[62] G. Gaskell *et al.* 2006 *op. cit.* note 25, p. 32.

activists or politicians can open a national debate on ethically controversial research with contentions over human dignity and the protection of human life, which, in their opinion, should ultimately result in the absolute ban of such research. Where there is no well organised national pro-research lobby in existence, presenting counter-arguments and highlighting the prospective benefits of the research to both the lay public and to the political representatives of a country, there is a danger that even a so-called liberal country with a pragmatic non-ideological government might accept restrictive biopolicy.

ACKNOWLEDGEMENTS

This work was supported by the Slovak Research and Development Agency (APVV) under the contract number LPP-0017-06. I am very grateful to Veronika Šablicová, Ash Coupland, Benjamin Capps and Alastair Campbell for their very helpful comments on earlier drafts. The final stage of the work was done during my stay as a Visiting Professor at the Centre for Biomedical Ethics, National University of Singapore, Singapore in January–March 2009.

INDEX

3Rs animal welfare; replacement, reduction and refinement 241, 250–252

abortion, 444, 456, 458–462, 464, 472, 473
Academy of Sciences of the Czech Republic (ASCR), 456, 465–468
accountability, 4, 7, 12, 39
Additional Protocol to the Convention for the Protection of Human Rights and, Dignity of the Human Beings with Regard to the Application of Biology and, Medicine, 1998, 147
Ad Hoc Committee of the Sixth (Legal) Committee (UN), 124, 125
Advanced Therapy Medicinal Products (ATMP), 60
Alder Hey, 217, 222
animal rights, 14
animal welfare, 20, 21, 23
Animal Welfare Act 2006, 252–254, 256, 266, 274
animalisation, 304, 305, 318
Animals (Scientific Procedures) Act 1986, 249, 250, 253, 255, 256, 266
anti-theory, 15
Artificial Reproductive Technology (ART), 69, 72, 73, 77–82
Audi, Robert, 321, 324, 325, 327–331, 333–336, 338, 339, 341, 342, 344, 346–348, 356
Australia, 17, 125, 128, 144, 189, 190, 192, 202
Austria, 105, 448, 458
authority, 192, 196, 198–202

Belgium, 106, 128–130, 149, 458
Bioethics Advisory Committee (BAC, Singapore), 12, 123, 132–134, 145
bioreactor, 57, 58
blastocyst, 449, 465–467
Brownsword, Roger, 4, 38, 43
Buddhism, 396
Bush, George W., 34–36, 130–132

California Institute for Regenerative Medicine (CIRM), 34, 37, 131, 364, 365, 367–369

California Stem Cell Research and Cures Initiative, 361, 366
Capps, Benjamin, 1, 19, 20, 30
Cattaneo, Elena, 102
Cell Nuclear Replacement (CNR), 63, 65, 67–69, 71–75, 79, 80
centralised (federal), 368, 369, 371
Chalmers, Donald, 7, 8
character, 340, 341, 356
chimera, 7, 23, 29, 33, 43, 44, 51, 52, 72, 74, 279–282, 284, 285, 288–300, 303, 304, 308, 310, 317–319, 379, 383, 410, 412, 413, 415
  animal model, 284
  animal-human, 287, 288, 290, 298, 306
  embryonic, 279, 283, 287, 291, 298, 303, 304, 310, 314, 317–319
  human-non-human embryonic, 279, 298, 303, 304
  inter-species, 284–286
  intra-species 284, 285
  mythology, 279, 281, 282, 317
  spontaneous, 285, 304
China, 44–48, 53, 128, 133
Christian Democrat, 445, 447, 450, 456, 461–463, 472, 476
civic
  engagement, 339
  responsibility, 344
  voice, 325, 334, 335, 339, 352
clinical translation, 417
Clonaid, 128
Comment on Reproductive Ethics (CORE), 139, 381, 384
commodification, 2, 14, 26, 30, 33
Confucian, 45, 47, 396, 399–402
consent, 73, 80, 84, 86, 87, 89, 91, 93, 207–210, 212–221, 223, 224, 226–235, 237–239
Constitutional Court, 458 (Poland); 461, 464 (Slovakia)
Convention for the protection of Human Rights and dignity of the human being with regard to the application of biology and medicine, Convention on Human Rights and Biomedicine, 99, 101, 113, 118, 447, 449
cord blood, 29, 31–33
  banking, 33
Costa Rica, 129, 130
Council of Europe, 13, 49, 249
Cutas, Daniela, 8, 9, 13, 48
cybrid, 412, 414, 415
Cyprus, 458
cytoplasmic hybrid research, 379
Czech Republic, 50, 51, 53, 441–443, 451, 452, 454–458, 460, 461, 465–472, 475, 476
Czechoslovakia, 441, 443, 444, 458, 460, 461, 469, 470, 475

decentralised (USA), 368, 369
Declaration of Helsinki, 229, 237
deliberative democracy, 341
democratic governance, 360, 362
Denver Summit of the G8, 422
Department of Health, UK, 60, 390
developmental biology, 279, 287
dialogue, 341
disembodiment, 14
Dolly, 422
Donaldson Report (UK), 382
Donum Vitae, 345, 347, 349–352

Dublin Well Woman (European Court of Human Rights), 112

E112, 111
embryo question, 7, 13, 23, 33, 35, 36, 45, 49, 53
empirical ethics, 14–17
engineered tracheal tissue, 57–59, 62
epigenetic, 312, 314, 318
Estonia, 458
ESTOOLS, 102
ethical
  being, 340, 341
  citizenship, 324, 325, 329, 331, 333–335, 339, 344, 352, 356
  deliberation, 322–325, 338, 339, 341, 354, 356
  discourse, 339, 341
  framework, 187
  inquiry, 341
  rationality, 321, 339, 340, 344, 348, 356
  vacuum, 6
Ethics Discussion Group, 185
ethics of citizenship, 324, 333
Eurobarometer survey, 457
European Convention on Human Rights, 113
European Directive 86/609/EEC, 249
European Group on Ethics and New Technologies (EGE, European Union), 10
European Medicines Agency (EMEA), 60
European Union (EU), 9, 13, 20, 35, 49, 51, 60, 61, 147, 150, 151, 441, 443, 447
EuroStemCell, 102
evidence based, 363
experimental neuroscience, 172, 180, 181, 184
expert, 196, 198, 202
exploratory openness, 339, 341, 342, 344, 354
extraterritorial jurisdiction, 8, 9

fallibility, 332, 336, 339, 340, 348, 349, 351, 352
federalism, 34, 359, 360, 368, 370, 373, 375
  rejuvenated, 34, 359, 360, 370, 375
foetal stem cell, 29, 30
Framework Programme 6 (FP6), 447, 448
Framework Programme 7 (FP7), 448
France, 124, 126, 147, 149
Fukuyama, Francis, 133

GDP, 468, 469
Gene Therapy Advisory Committee, (GTAC, UK), 60
generic rights, 237
genetic essentialism, 196
GERD, 468
German Stem Cell Act, 105
Germany, 100–102, 104, 124, 126, 129, 147, 149, 444, 448, 458
Gewirth, Alan, 237
Good Manufacturing Practice (GMP), 60

Hammond-Browning, Natasha, 43
Hashmi, 137–140, 142
Heath Care Law No. 576/2004 Coll. (Slovakia), 445
HeLa cell, 210, 215
Hinxton Group, 95, 98

HIV, AIDS, 405, 406, 419
Ho, Calvin, 11–13
Hollander, Anthony, 5, 6, 15
Holm, Søren, 43
Holy See, 125, 126
Homo sapiens, 289, 305
Honduras, 132
human admixed embryo, 23, 43, 378, 386
human being, 282, 300, 302, 303, 306, 313, 315, 316, 318
human cloning, 7, 11, 46, 51, 63, 65, 77, 78, 81, 448–451, 453
human dignity, 11, 26, 47, 121–123, 127, 146, 147, 149, 305, 308, 318, 425–428, 436, 438, 439, 450, 477
human embryo, 70, 73, 74, 77, 81, 121, 123, 138, 142, 143, 145, 288, 290, 291, 298–302, 304, 307, 310–319, 400–403, 406, 412, 413, 415
human Embryonic Stem Cell (hESC), 63, 69, 70, 72, 76, 77, 80, 83, 84, 92, 164, 166, 174, 175, 441, 442, 444, 445, 447–449, 451–459, 461–463, 465–468, 472, 473, 475, 476
Human Fertilisation and Embryology Act (UK), 42, 52
 the 1990 Act, 136, 138, 140, 144, 381–383, 385
 the 2008 Act, 382, 386, 388, 393
Human Fertilisation and Embryology Authority (HFEA, UK), 12, 123, 136–140, 379, 474
human flourishing, 324
Human Tissue (Quality and Safety for Human Application) Regulations, 2007, 391
Human Tissue Authority (HTA, UK), 60, 388, 390
humanisation, 304, 305, 318
Humanzee, 289, 307
Hwang, Woo Suk, 18, 19
hybrid, 7, 23, 25, 26, 43, 44, 51, 52, 279, 292, 293, 295–303, 310, 410, 413–415
 embryo, 172, 174, 177, 178, 377–384, 386, 387, 389–393

immortal cell line, 19
immutable mobile, 11, 12, 123
India, 128
induced Pluripotent Stem Cell (iPS Cell), 2, 19, 30, 44, 68, 71, 72, 92, 207, 223, 231, 240, 377, 378, 380, 387, 388, 390, 392, 393
innovative research, 5
institutional, 200
institutional ethics of citizenship, 333
Institutional Review Board (IRB), 410, 412, 413, 416, 417
instrumental, 242, 245, 256
interdisciplinary bioethics, 188
International Society for Stem Cell Research (ISSCR), 8, 64, 84–86, 88–90, 93, 103, 393
 Guidelines for the Clinical Translation of Stem Cells (2008), 85, 86, 88–90, 93
Interstate Alliance on Stem Cell Research (IASCR), 367, 373
intrinsic, 242, 277
Ireland, 100, 112–116
Islamic, 129, 130
Israel, 128
Italy, 102, 104, 108, 448, 458

Japan, 46–48, 53
John Hopkins Berman Institute of Bioethics, 95
Judeo-Christian, 130
justice, 288
Justice as Fairness, 258, 262–265, 267–269, 271–273, 276

Kerridge, Ian, 17
Kure, Joseph, 23

Lacks, Henrietta, 210, 212, 214, 216, 220, 232
Latin America, 105
Law Concerning Regulations Relating to Human Cloning Techniques and Other Similar Techniques (Japan), 422, 434, 437
legitimacy, 2, 3 ,8, 14, 15, 18, 28, 34, 38, 40, 53, 140, 149, 189, 192, 195, 196, 200–202
- administrative, 360, 362
- legal, 322
- moral, 341, 356
- political, 323, 336

legitimation, 199, 202
legitimisation, 12
Lethal-Dose 50 test, 251
licence (embryo research), 73, 77, 79, 80
Life Not Worth Living (LNWL), 242, 243, 258, 268, 269, 271, 274–278
Life Worth Living (LWL), 242, 258, 274–277
Lithuania, 105
Lockhart Report (Australia), 191
Lomax, Geoffrey, 34–37
Lysaght, Tamra, 17

Mackenney, Jonathan, 19, 20, 30
Malaysia, 125, 128
Medical Research Council (MRC, UK), 380
Medicine and Healthcare Products Regulatory Agency (MHRA, UK), 60
Mertes, Heidi, 96–98, 103–106, 116
mesenchymal stem cell, 58
Mexico, 125
Mo cell line, 211
Moore, John, 210–216, 220, 221, 223, 232, 234
moral
- argumentation, 322–324, 336, 352, 356
- awareness, 342, 344
- consciousness, 342–344
- identity, 342
- imagination, 342
- intuition, 343
- perception, 342, 354
- reasoning, 322, 341
- status, 97, 280, 281, 288, 306, 314, 345
- traits of character, 340

multidisciplinary research, 172, 181, 184
Munthe, Christian, 8, 9, 13, 48
Muslim, 129

narratives, 17
National Academies Guidelines for Stem Cell Research (USA), 366
National Institutes of Health (NIH, USA), 64, 81, 83, 84, 366, 373–375
non-human animal, 20, 27, 241–246, 256, 261–264, 267, 269–272, 275, 277

normative discourse standards, 339
novelty, 294
Nuffield Council on Bioethics (UK), 235

Obama, Barack, 36
ontology, 279–281, 295, 297, 298, 304–306, 308, 309, 311, 312, 314–319
Open Door, 112
organ transplantation, 285
original position, 259–265, 267, 268, 271, 272, 276

Pennings, Guido, 96–98, 103–106, 116
personalised tissue, 58
personhood, 400, 401
pluripotent stem cell, 64, 68, 72, 86
Poland, 100, 105, 150, 151, 448, 457–460
policy oriented (loop) learning, 363
political neutrality, 333, 334
Polkinghorne Report (UK), 30
power, 189, 195, 196, 199, 201, 202
pre-embryo, 433
preformistic position, 312, 318
preimplantation genetic diagnosis (PGD), 136, 138–145, 152, 153
principle of secular motivation, 325, 330, 331, 336
principle of theo-ethical equilibrium, 325, 331, 333, 337, 338
privacy, 19, 209, 211, 222, 227, 233, 234, 236–239
procedural, 6, 28, 29, 34, 36–38, 40, 42
    ethics, 321–325, 334, 338–341, 344, 345, 348, 352, 354–356
    integrity, 362
procedure, 208, 209, 211, 212, 214, 216, 217, 220, 228, 229, 232–235, 239
process transparency, 363, 364
'pro-choice', 47
'pro-life', 47
property, 19, 209, 211–214, 218–220, 228, 234–236, 238, 239
proprietary rights, 220, 234
pro-research lobby, 466, 472, 473, 475–477
Protection of Animals Act 1911, 252
public
    agency, 360, 362, 364, 365
    debate, 189, 192, 195, 197, 202, 205, 321, 324, 325, 328, 334–338, 342, 343
    discourse, 189, 192, 193, 195, 197, 199, 201, 204
    ethics, 29, 40
    good, 399
    interest, 17, 38, 41
    policy, 193, 197, 199, 321, 323–326, 328, 330, 331, 335, 337, 339, 351, 356
    speech, 335, 344, 352
    understanding, 18

qi (vital force), 400, 401
Qiu, Renzong, 44, 45, 48
qun (capacity for social relationships), 401

R (on the application of Quintavalle) v. Secretary of State for Health, 142
Radin, Margret, 219–221, 228, 234, 236
Rawls, John, 20, 21, 258–270, 272, 323, 329

Rawlsian, 243, 272
reflective equilibrium, 337, 338, 340, 348, 356
regenerative medicine, 63, 65, 70, 283, 286
regulatory
challenge, 7
haven, 3, 6, 16
religion, 321, 324, 326–328, 330, 331, 333, 338, 341–344, 353, 355, 356
reproductive cloning, 2, 11–14, 45, 46, 51, 66, 81, 121, 122, 124–127, 129, 132, 133, 145–148, 150
Retained Organs Commission (UK), 217
rhetoric, 189, 195–199, 202
rights, 324, 325, 332, 334, 335, 338, 344, 346, 350
Roman Catholic, 457, 462, 476
Royal College of Veterinary Surgeons (UK), 252
Rust vs. Sullivan (USA, Supreme Court), 114

scientific enquiry, 199
secular rationale, 321, 325–332, 334–337, 342, 344, 346–349, 351, 356
shen (psyche), 400, 401
Singapore, 12, 49, 52, 104, 122, 123, 126–128, 130, 132–135, 145, 148, 150, 152
slippery slope, 127
Slovak Academy of Sciences (SAS), 451, 465, 466, 476
Slovakia, 50, 51, 105, 441–445, 447–452, 457–466, 468–473, 475, 476
Slovenia, 100, 458
sociology in bioethics, 157, 158
'soft law', 73, 81
somatic cell nuclear replacement (SCNR), 100, 107
somatic cell nuclear transfer (SCNT), 189–191, 196, 202–204
somatic stem cell, 2, 29
South Africa, 128
South Korea, 18, 125, 128, 133
Spain, 125–127
species, 279–282, 284–286, 288, 289, 292, 294, 296–298, 302, 303, 306–308, 310, 311, 314, 317, 318
boundary, 306
integrity, 14
speciesism, 27
specified embryo, 301
Sprout of human life, 422, 430–434, 438, 439
state-based research programme, 359, 361, 366
stem cell, 283, 312
therapy, 68, 82, 84, 85
Stem Cell Policy and Ethics Program (SCOPE, USA), 95
suffering, 241–243, 246, 247, 249–255, 257, 258, 261–264, 267–272, 274–278
Sweden, 100, 106, 128, 458
Switzerland, 128
Sykora, Peter, 50–52

tao, 401
Taoism, 396
technocratic, 4
technological determinism, 337, 353
Teoh, Chin Leong, 28, 29
Testa, Giuseppe, 102

The Netherlands, 100, 125
therapeutic cloning, 11, 12, 24, 29, 45, 46, 66, 80, 121–128, 130, 131, 133, 135, 145–147
ti (the physical body), 400, 401
tissue engineering, 58, 59
Tissues Directive (EU), 9, 10, 35, 76, 231, 388, 390, 391
transgenic creature, 294
translational
  ethics, 167, 172, 181, 184
  research, 6, 13, 14, 157–160, 162, 163, 167, 168, 172, 173, 180, 181, 184, 186
transplant, 6
trust, 195, 197, 198, 202
Tunisia, 105

UK Biobank, 231, 232, 234–236, 239
UK Regulatory Route Map for Stem Cell Research and Manufacture, 61, 391
UK Stem Cell Bank, 387–390
UN Declaration on Human Cloning, 11, 121, 122, 146–150, 395, 438
United Kingdom (UK), 5, 12, 14, 20, 23, 26, 30, 42, 43, 106, 112, 113, 115, 123, 128, 132, 134, 135, 137, 138, 140, 144, 146, 148, 152, 243, 248, 249, 252, 254, 255, 263, 269, 278, 377–379, 381, 382, 387–393
United Nations (UN), 4, 10–12, 49, 121–124, 132, 146, 148, 150, 395, 398
United Nations Educational, Scientific and Cultural Organisation (UNESCO), 147, 152
  International Bioethics Committee 152
United Nations General Assembly (UNGA), 124, 126, 130–133, 151
United States of America (USA), 33–36, 102, 105, 108, 110, 114, 115, 119, 125–132, 134, 359, 361, 362, 366, 368, 370, 371, 373–375
Universal Declaration on the Human Genome and Human Rights, 1997, 147
US Food and Drug Administration (FDA), 374
utilitarian, 200, 205, 209, 213–215, 219, 226, 229, 233, 234, 237, 238, 245, 248, 255, 258

values, 197–202
'Velvet Divorce', 444
Veterinary Surgeons Act 1966 (UK), 252–254
virtue, 321, 324–327, 329–331, 333–342, 344, 345, 348, 349, 352–356

Wainwright, Stephen, 14, 15, 18
Warnock, Mary, 12
Warnock Report, Committee of Inquiry into Human Fertilisation and Embryology (UK), 140, 141, 145
welfare, 241, 242, 250, 252, 266, 267
Williams, Clare, 14, 15, 18

Xun Zi, 401

yang, 400
Yeates, James, 20–22
yin, 400
"yuck" factor, 24

Zhai, Xiaomei, 44, 45, 48